Antiviral Agents, Vaccines, and Immunotherapies

Antiviral Agents, Vaccines, and Immunotherapies

Stephen K. Tyring

University of Texas Health Science Center, Houston, Texas
Center for Clinical Studies, Houston, Texas

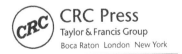

CRC Press
Taylor & Francis Group
Boca Raton London New York

CRC Press is an imprint of the
Taylor & Francis Group, an **informa** business

CRC Press
Taylor & Francis Group
6000 Broken Sound Parkway NW, Suite 300
Boca Raton, FL 33487-2742

First issued in paperback 2019

© 2005 by Taylor & Francis Group, LLC
CRC Press is an imprint of Taylor & Francis Group, an Informa business

No claim to original U.S. Government works

ISBN-13: 978-0-8247-5408-2 (hbk)
ISBN-13: 978-0-367-39374-8 (pbk)

Visit the Taylor & Francis Web site at
http://www.taylorandfrancis.com

and the CRC Press Web site at
http://www.crcpress.com

Preface

The development of antiviral drugs is still in its infancy with rapid changes and progressive milestones encountered almost daily. By the time this book is distributed, new drugs may have already been added. This is particularly true for the antiretroviral drugs, which seem to be growing in number exponentially to the casual observer trying to keep abreast of recent advances in this field. As this book is going to press, the United States Food and Drug Administration granted accelerated approval of Epzicom and Truvada. Epzicom is a fixed-dose combination of the antiretroviral drugs Ziagen (abacavir sulfate) and Epivir (lamivudine). Truvada is a fixed-dose combination of Emtriva (embricitabine) and Viread (tenofovir disoproxil fumarate). In keeping pace with these advances, the book will survey the latest in antiretroviral drugs, general antiviral therapies, the antiviral vaccines, and immunotherapies used for treatment, and prophylaxis of viral infections.

The book begins with a review of the current state of antiviral management (therapy and prophylaxis) and discussion of the challenges for the future. The second chapter discusses the major categories as well as the indications, adverse reactions, and drug interactions of each specific medication of the antiretroviral drugs. Chapter Three delves into the treatments available for other viral infections, such as herpes simplex virus, varicella zoster virus, cytomegalovirus, human papilloma virus, chronic viral hepatitis, and others. The book then concludes with a discussion of the vaccines that are currently available and being developed and gives an overview of the use of immunoglobulins and monoclonal antibodies for antiviral therapy.

The last two decades have been the most dynamic in the history of viral infections and their management. During this time the eradication of the epidemic form of the most deadly viral infection known to medicine, smallpox, was announced. Ironically, this landmark achievement was followed almost immediately by the observation of a new viral pandemic that currently infects 46 million people, i.e., HIV/AIDS. Within the past decade several new emerging viral diseases, e.g., West Nile virus, SARS, avian influenza, etc., have challenged our ability to recognize and manage these infections. Unfortunately, antiviral drugs have been effective for only a few groups of viruses up until now. Most antiviral drugs do not produce a cure, but rather allow control of the infection. An exception to this observation has recently been seen with the combined use of pegylated interferon alpha and ribavirin, which allows virologic cures for the majority of hepatitis C patients who successfully complete therapy. However, the limitations of antiviral therapy, including the high costs of drugs, make the need for prevention even more urgent. The most cost effective means of prevention are public health measures, such as proper sanitation/clean drinking water, mosquito control, testing blood/blood products, not sharing needles, and safer sex/condom use. In addition, vaccines provide the most effective and cost-efficient means of preventing infectious diseases. The greatest success story in medical history was the eradication of epidemic smallpox, which was due to a combined effort of public health measures and an effective vaccine. For such combined efforts to eradicate other viral diseases, such as measles and polio, the challenges are not only to reach the susceptible populations but also to overcome unfounded prejudice against vaccines. At the same time, new technologies will lead to the development of new prophylactic vaccines, particularly for infections such as HIV, human papillomaviruses, and herpes simplex viruses, ushering in a whole new set of arsenals in the fight against viral infections. It is my hope that *Antiviral Agents, Vaccines, and Immunotherapies* will serve as a valuable tool for the clinician and the basic scientist in better understanding the current management protocols of viral diseases as well as greater possibilities for the future.

Stephen K. Tyring, MD, PhD, MBA

Acknowledgements

The efforts of Nancy Bell, PhD, for all aspects of the editing and production process are deeply appreciated. I wish to thank my wife, Patricia Lee, MD, for her support, encouragement, and dedication throughout the writing and publication of this book. In addition, I wish to thank my mentor (and a pioneer in antiviral research), Samuel Baron, MD, Professor (and Chairman Emeritus) of Microbiology/Immunology and Internal Medicine at The University of Texas Medical Branch, Galveston, Texas, for his guidance, suggestions, and wisdom over the past 25 years. Without such outstanding people, the publication of *Antiviral Agents, Vaccines, and Immunotherapies* would not have been possible.

Contents

Antiviral Agents, Vaccines, and Immunotherapies

Chapter 1

Introduction

Public health measures should always be the first line of defense against viral infections and should include clean drinking water, proper sewage disposal, vector control, testing of blood and blood products, nonsharing of needles, hand washing and use of disposable gloves, and safer sex/condom usage/abstinence (Fig. 1.1). Global travel has made the rapid implementation of these measures paramount. The rapid spread of the SARS (severe acute respiratory syndrome) corornavirus and avian influenza are recent examples of the problem of viral globalization. In a similar manner, the West Nile virus and monkeypox virus made their appearance in North America. In addition, new viruses are being described for previously recognized diseases, such as the role of human metapneumovirus as the second most common cause of infant respiratory infections. For viral diseases for which they are available, vaccines can be added to the list of measures to prevent viral diseases and should be used in combination with the other interventions. Antiviral drugs, however, can be considered a

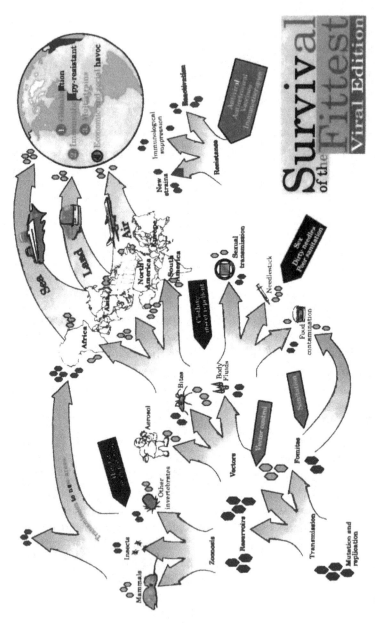

Fig. 1.1 Transmission of viral diseases.

second line of defense against viral infections because they are generally not viracidal, because they are much more expensive than other forms of intervention, and because they are usually most beneficial when used acutely (which limits the time in which the patient can obtain them).

A prototype successful vaccine was the use of vaccinia to eliminate epidemic smallpox from the world. Starting with Jenner's use of cowpox to prevent smallpox in 1797 through the last epidemic case of smallpox, treated in 1977, this accomplishment could easily be considered the single greatest achievement in medical history. Even in the 20th century, hundreds of millions of persons died from smallpox and hundreds of millions more suffered marked morbidity, such as blindness. Thus, by extrapolation into the 21st century and beyond, an infinite number of lives and dollars will have been saved by this landmark event. It is important to remember that no antiviral drug was approved for smallpox and that the elimination of this deadly disease was accomplished via public health measures plus an effective vaccine.

For the 150 years after Jenner, only one other viral vaccine was developed—the rabies vaccine by Pasteur in 1885. In the 50 years between 1945 and 1995, however, 11 more vaccines were approved (Fig. 1.2). Although the rotavirus vaccine

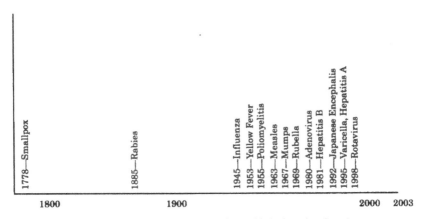

Dates for smallpox and rabies vaccines are for the first published results of vaccine usage. Remaining dates are for FDA approval of vaccine.

Fig. 1.2 Timeline of virus vaccine development.

was approved by the U.S. Food and Drug Administration
(FDA) in 1998, it was taken off the market after a few months
due to a relatively small but statistically significant increase
in the number of infants developing intussusception. Therefore, the medical-legal environment in the United States
forced the removal of a vaccine from the market that could
have saved millions of infants around the world from dying of
diarrhea. Hopefully, potentially safer versions of the rotavirus
vaccine, currently being tested, will be available in a few
years. It may be asked whether the smallpox vaccine, i.e., vaccinia, would have reached the market and saved hundreds of
millions of lives and billions of dollars if it had been required
to pass the extremely rigorous standards of the 21th century.

Although vaccinia has not been routinely administered
(and not available) to the public for more than 20 years, it is
now being offered to certain populations considered to be at
high risk in the event that the smallpox virus is used for bioterrorism. In contrast to other available vaccines, there is the
potential for morbidity, and even mortality, with vaccinia. This
potential, however, is very low if the vaccinated population
does not include immunosuppressed individuals or persons
with certain skin conditions, such as atopic dermatitis, that
compromise the epidermal barrier. Potentially safer alterna-
tives to live vaccinia for smallpox vaccination, however, are
being studied in clinical trials.

Other marked success stories with vaccines include those
to prevent poliomyelitis and to prevent measles. Polio vaccines
(plus public health measures) have eliminated polio from
North America and from most of the remainder of the world.
Unfortunately, the goal of global elimination of polio by the
beginning of the 21st century has not been met, primarily due
to the difficulty of reaching susceptible individuals in a few
war-torn parts of the world. Although the distinct advantage
exists of polio having an effective oral vaccine, polio has
proven more difficult to eradicate than smallpox because of
the numerous subclinical infections (1). The measles vaccine
has been almost as successful as the polio vaccine in the
United States, considering that fewer than 100 cases have
been reported annually in this country for the past few years.

In many parts of the world, however, measles is a major source of mortality as well as morbidity. Approximately 36 million cases of measles occurred globally in 2003. More than one million children die of measles annually, mostly in Third World countries where there is marked malnutrition and lack of vaccines.

Biological criteria that are essential for a disease to be considered a reasonable candidate for global elimination are as follows:

- The disease is specifically human, with no animal reservoir.
- The disease is acute, self-limiting, and infectious for other persons for about only a week (two exceptions exist: inclusion body encephalitis and subacute sclerosing panencephalitis).
- An effective method of intervention exists, e.g., a vaccine (2).

Measles, like smallpox, meets these criteria, but measles appears more difficult to eradicate, partly because it is more infectious than smallpox. Also, there is a period of vulnerability between passive immunity due to maternal antibodies (and concomitant resistance to measles vaccination) and the age of 12 months, the youngest age at which the vaccine is known to be effective.

Because measles vaccine is usually given along with the rubella and mumps vaccines, these viral diseases should be candidates for eradication as well. This possibility is especially important because of the severity of congenital rubella. The difficulty in diagnosis of rubella (and mumps) makes the surveillance of the eradication of these viruses more difficult. Because measles is the most infectious of the three diseases and the clinical manifestations are most easily recognized, a good surveillance system for measles potentially can serve as an effective marker for surveillance of rubella and mumps in judging the efficacy of vaccination campaigns.

Hepatitis B is also a specifically human pathogen and the vaccine is safe and effective. Indeed, hepatitis B produces extensive morbidity and mortality worldwide. Unlike other viruses that are reasonable candidates for global eradication, hepatitis B is a disease in which many persons become chronically infected early in life and become persistent or recurrent excretors of the virus. Therefore, surveillance becomes much more difficult and would involve large numbers of people who are infected but are not ill.

Some viral diseases that have effective vaccines are less likely to be eradicated because of animal reserves. Therefore, control is more reasonable than eradication. In the case of yellow fever, mosquito control is extremely important and proved very effective even before the vaccine became available. Another important factor in the control of yellow fever is the fact that monkeys constitute a jungle reservoir of this virus. Likewise, intervention in the spread of rabies involves control and containment of animal reservoirs.

In general, the risk/benefit ratio of approved vaccines is extremely favorable. In fact, the chance of major morbidity (or mortality) from these vaccines is on the order of a millionfold less than that of the diseases they are designed to protect against. Many persons in industrialized countries have reached adulthood in recent decades without knowing anyone who has suffered from measles, rubella, hepatitis B or polio. Thus, they sometimes do not believe there is sufficient justification to have their children vaccinated. Moreover, unfounded claims have surfaced linking the measles/mumps/rubella (MMR) vaccine to autism as well as the hepatitis B vaccine to certain autoimmune diseases. Extensive investigations by such independent agencies as the FDA and the Centers for Disease Control and Prevention (CDC), however, have demonstrated that there is no cause-and-effect relationship between these vaccines and the alleged diseases. Likewise, in some Third World countries, some persons refuse government-sponsored vaccination programs because they fear that politicians do not have their interests in mind. For example, some groups believe that vaccine is a form of population control and that it might make them sterile.

While many persons do not become vaccinated because they do not feel they are at risk, this false sense of security becomes even more complicated when vaccines to prevent sexually transmitted diseases (STDs) and parental consent are involved. Currently, only one vaccine to prevent an STD is available—the hepatitis B vaccine. Because hepatitis B can also be transmitted by nonsexual routes, however, it is not perceived by the public as an STD vaccine. The safety and efficacy of vaccines to prevent herpes simplex virus (HSV)-2 and human papillomavirus (HPV)-16 indicate that these vaccines could be marketed by the end of the decade (3,4). If these vaccines are not given before a girl becomes sexually active, the chance that they would benefit her is markedly decreased. On the other hand, convincing the parents that their daughter will need a vaccine against an STD is often difficult. The medical need for vaccination against HPV-16—prevention of cervical cancer—is obvious to the medical community.

The added difficulty that advocates of this vaccine face is that this relationship between HPV and cervical cancer is unknown to most of the lay public.

Although the benefits of vaccination over therapy are numerous, many persons do not become vaccinated for one reason or another and there are vaccines against only 13 viral diseases. Sometimes the cost of the vaccine is cited as a reason not to vaccinate. The cost of not vaccinating, however, is almost always greater than the cost of vaccinating.

In the past three years there have been eight major shortages of vaccines. In the 2003–2004 "flu" season, the shortage of influenza vaccine resulted from the early start of the influenza outbreak as well as the severity of the infections. In fact, influenza vaccines have been in short supply for three of the past four years. Since the beginning of 2000, there have also been shortages of vaccines for varicella and measles as well as for such bacterial diseases as diphtheria and tetanus. A report by the Institute of Medicine (IOM), a branch of the National Academy of Sciences, noted that there has been a steady erosion in the number of vaccine producers over the past three decades. In the 1970s, there were 25 vaccine makers, but in 2004 there are only five manufacturers. Most of the decline is due to slim profit margins and legislative and liability issues. Due to such small number of producers, shortages can develop quickly as a result of manufacturing problems or underestimating the expected demand.

Approximately 150 million people are considered at high risk for influenza in the United States, especially children, persons over 50 years of age and those suffering from chronic diseases. One of the big uncertainties in forecasting demand for vaccines is that only 70 million to 80 million people are vaccinated annually, leaving a large number who might panic and seek vaccination once a severe outbreak begins, as occurred during the 2003–2004 season.

Although vaccines have been available for influenza viruses for a number of years, these viruses also mutate rapidly or undergo antigenic drift. Therefore, development of an effective vaccine each year usually has limited benefit for subsequent years. Because time is needed for development and manufacture of the appropriate influenza vaccine at the beginning of each "flu" season and approximately two weeks are needed for optimal immunity after receiving the vaccine, each year vaccine manufacturers must make an educated "guess" regarding the appropriate strain of virus for which the vaccine must be made. Even more difficult is the task of determining the quantity of vaccine to manufacture.

Distribution is often a problem with influenza vaccines, because some states are usually hit worse than others. Transferring vaccines between states is a moderate problem, but during the 2003–2004 influenza season, there was a nationwide shortage which necessitated the United States to buy influenza vaccine from other countries.

Four anti-influenza medications are available for those persons who do not receive the vaccine or if the vaccine strain is significantly different than the infecting strain. These agents include amantadine, ramantadine, oseltamivir, and zanamivir. Whereas some studies suggest that such agents may help protect a person from the symptoms of influenza if started before or soon after exposure to the virus, most clinical investigators have confirmed that these drugs can shorten the duration of symptoms of influenza if they are initiated within the first one to two days of the first symptom.

Many vaccines, such as those for tetanus and varicella, have only a single supplier in the U.S. market. The influenza vaccine, including the recently available nasal spray, has only three manufacturers. At least for some vaccines, stockpiling is one solution to reducing shortages, but the CDC notes that only three vaccines (of the 10 vaccines targeted for stockpiling) were stockpiled in 2002. The vaccines that were stockpiled were for measles, mumps, and rubella, but a small amount of polio vaccine is also in storage.

Stockpiling, however, is expensive and the CDC has been conservative about developing stockpiles to minimize the financial risk. Because of seasonal strain variations, the influenza vaccine cannot be stockpiled.

One reason for manufacturers' decreased interest in vaccines is the fact that the U.S. government buys slightly more than 50% of the vaccines in the United States and keeps prices low, primarily through the Vaccines for Children program run by the CDC. Because the influenza vaccines are given to many more adults than children, the government buys a lower percentage of these vaccines. The CDC negotiates a discounted price with the manufacturer under the Vaccines for Children program. Then it allocates to each state a credit balance, which states can use to buy vaccines from the manufacturer at the discounted price. The program offers free vaccines to uninsured children under 18 years of age or to those eligible for Medicaid or care from federally funded qualified health centers.

The IOM reports that health-care providers such as physicians and clinics face unusual difficulties in carrying out vaccination programs and notes that "reimbursements for vaccines and administrative fees barely cover the costs of vaccine purchase. In many cases, providers lose money on immunization." In addition, the cost of immunizing children and vulnerable adults is escalating rapidly, as new, expensive recommended vaccines are FDA-approved. The cost of immunizing children (adjusted for inflation) has risen to $385 per child in 2001 from $10 per child in 1975, and may triple to more than $1000 per child by 2020.

The IOM concluded that the price squeeze, coupled with a heavy regulatory burden, has discouraged investment and driven drug companies out of the vaccine business. In addition, the manufacture of most vaccines involves the complex transformation of live organisms into pure, active, safe, and stable vaccines. Many vaccines must remain in a narrow temperature range during storage and delivery, called the cold chain. In addition, each lot must be tested and approved before release.

One possible attractive and potentially inexpensive alternative to vaccination by injection is the ingestion of transgenic plants expressing recombinant vaccine immunogens. Such edible plants can be grown locally and easily distributed without special training or equipment. For example, the full-length HPV-L1 protein has been expressed and localized to the nuclei of potatoes. The plant-expressed L1 self-assembles into VLPs (Virus-Like Particles) with immunological properties comparable to those of native HPV virions. In mice, ingestion of the transgenic potatoes induced a humoral response similar to that induced by parenteral administration of HPV-L1 VLPs (5). Thus, the potential exists for such vaccines to become available for use in resource-poor areas of the world, where most cervical cancer is found.

There is also the problem of legal liability. Supposedly, manufacturers are protected from lawsuits regarding pediatric vaccines, but plaintiffs' attorneys have found ways around that insulation.

All available vaccines are prophylactic; there are no approved viral vaccines that are therapeutic once symptoms develop. Some vaccines, however, can be effective if given shortly after exposure to the virus, although it is always preferable to administer the vaccine before exposure to assure that sufficient immunity develops. Vaccination after symptoms of a disease are manifested is rarely effective. This strategy, however, has been studied for the therapy of human immunodeficiency virus (HIV), herpes simplex virus (HSV) and human papillomavirus (HPV) diseases, but with limited success. A possible exception is the varicella zoster virus (VZV) vaccine, which is normally given to prevent primary varicella (i.e., chickenpox). This vaccine is currently being studied to determine whether it can be given to older individuals to prevent the reemergence of this virus in the form of shingles. Preliminary evidence is encouraging thus far.

Although therapeutic viral vaccines are not yet available, certain antiviral drugs can help prevent infection (Fig. 1.2). The first routine use of an antiviral drug to help prevent infection was the administration of antiretroviral agents to pregnant HIV-seropositive women to help reduce transmission of HIV to their infants before delivery. It is logical to consider that similar use of antiretroviral agents should reduce sexual transmission of HIV as well. In fact, investigators have reported a 60% per partnership reduction in risk of HIV infection following the widespread use of highly active antiretroviral therapy (HAART) by HIV-seropositive persons in San Francisco. Unfortunately, however, study participants doubled their rate of unprotected receptive anal intercourse, which offset the beneficial effects of HAART (6). Another potential means of preventing infection following occupational exposure to HIV is postexposure prophylaxis (PEP). After occupational exposure to blood, empirical treatment with two or more antiretroviral drugs not part of the source patient's current regimen (i.e., PEP) should be provided unless information such as HIV test results in the source patient or a detailed description of the exposure indicate that PEP is not necessary. A third drug, such as a protease inhibitor, is a recommended addition to the regimen if other factors such as deep puncture, high viral load, etc., suggest an increased risk of HIV. The source patient should be evaluated to determine the probability of HIV infection (in accordance with state and local laws and policies). The use of a quick HIV test can reduce the time needed to rule out HIV infection to a few hours or less. A useful resource for discussing treatment options and obtaining advice regarding the management of adverse effects of drugs is the U.S. National Clinicians' Post-Exposure Prophylaxis Hotline (PEPline, 888-448-4911).

The guidelines for nonoccupational HIV postexposure prophylaxis (NPEP) are less well defined, but a registry exists at http://www.hivpepregistry.org. The NPEP should never be given as a substitute for primary prevention, i.e., reduction of risky behavior. When prevention efforts have failed (e.g., condom breakage) or were not possible (e.g., sexual assault), NPEP can be an important second line of defense. Ideally, PEP or NPEP should be started within one hour, but at least within 72 hours, of exposure.

An early limitation in knowing who should receive postexposure prophylaxis was the fact that traditional laboratory tests for HIV took days or weeks to produce results. In November, 2002, the OraQuick Rapid HIV-1 test was approved. Although the test only took 20 minutes, it required whole blood. In December, 2003, the Uni-Gold test was FDA-approved as the first rapid-test product for testing blood serum, plasma and whole blood. This test, which takes only 10 minutes, had already been approved by the World Health Organization (WHO) for HIV testing in Africa. Preapproval testing demonstrated that the Uni-Gold test was 100% accurate in detecting known HIV-positive specimens and 99.7% accurate for confirming negative specimens. On March 25, 2004, the FDA approved the first rapid test for HIV in oral fluids. Therefore, these tests will guide physicians in the use of postexposure prophylaxis as well as in the use of antiretroviral agents in HIV-seropositive pregnant women to prevent transmission of the virus.

The first FDA-approved use of an antiviral agent to reduce sexual transmission of a virus came in 2003 when valacyclovir was approved to reduce the risk of transmission of genital herpes. This reduction was suspected based on the marked decline in asymptomatic viral shedding of HSV-2 in persons taking nucleoside analogs (acyclovir, famciclovir or valacyclovir) (7). In the study that led to FDA approval, 1484 immunocompetent, heterosexual, monogamous couples were enrolled: one person with clinically symptomatic genital HSV-2 and one HSV-2 seronegative partner. The partners with HSV-2 infection were randomly assigned to receive either 500 mg of valacyclovir once daily or placebo for eight months. Both partners were counseled on safer sex and were offered condoms at each visit. The susceptible partners were closely monitored for signs or symptoms of genital herpes as well as for seroconversion. The study demonstrated that daily use of valacyclovir by the source partner resulted in a 77% reduction in clinical genital herpes and a 48% reduction in HSV-2 seroconversion in the susceptible partner (8). Thus, valacyclovir was capable of reducing transmission of genital herpes with safer sex counseling and condom use.

There is little data to support the use of antiherpes medication as a "morning after pill." Although nucleoside analogs used for herpes treatment are generally very safe, they all require activation by viral thymidine kinase. Therefore, if a person is not already infected with a herpes virus, it is unlikely that the nucleoside analog would be active and thus able to prevent infection.

Although there is only one vaccine to prevent a herpesvirus infection—the varicella vaccine—numerous agents are available to treat HSV-1, HSV-2, VZV, and cytomegalovirus (CMV). Interferon-alpha (IFN-α) was approved to treat Kaposi's sarcoma before the etiology was found to be HHV-8. Therefore, IFN-α alpha is not technically approved to treat HHV-8, but it is clear that part of its mechanism of action is antiviral. Systemic use of such nucleoside analogs as acyclovir, famciclovir, and valacyclovir can be safe and effective for acute therapy of herpes labialis, herpes genitalis, primary varicella, or herpes zoster. Suppressive daily use of these agents is also safe and effective for preventing most outbreaks of herpes labialis or herpes genitalis. Topical acyclovir and penciclovir are approved for therapy of herpes labialis and are very safe, but they are minimally effective. Trifluridine is available for optical use only. Although originally proposed to have antiviral properties, n-docosanol was approved as a nonprescription drug to treat herpes labialis. A number of agents are now available to treat cytomegalovirus (CMV) infections, primarily in immunocompromised patients. These drugs include ganciclovir, valganciclovir, foscarnet, cidofovir, and fomivirsen. In general, agents used to treat herpes simplex viruses and varicella virus are safe and effective, but usually only benefit the patient while the drug is being taken. Antiviral drugs used for therapy of CMV infections, on the other hand, can have dose-limiting toxicities, primarily renal, and should be reserved for those patients for whom there is a documented indication.

Acyclovir-resistant HSV-1, HSV-2, or VZV is usually the result of a mutation or a deficiency of viral thymidine kinase (TK), the enzyme necessary to phosphorylate acyclovir. Because famciclovir, penciclovir, and valacyclovir also must be activated by TK, acyclovir resistance usually translates into resistance to all members of this class of nucleoside analogs. Foscarnet is FDA-approved for therapy of acyclovir-resistant HSV and is frequently used for acyclovir-resistant VZV infections. Although not FDA-approved for this indication, cidofovir is also recommended by the CDC for acyclovir-resistant HSV and VZV infections.

Over 100 types of HPV have been described. These infections cause either benign or malignant lesions of the skin or mucous membranes. Benign lesions can be treated with cytodestructive measures or with surgery, but often recur due to latent or subclinical HPV in clinically normal-appearing tissues. Oncogenic HPV can result in neoplasia such as squamous cell carcinoma, especially in the cervix and other anogenital tissues. Cervical cancer is the second most common cause of cancer death of women worldwide. Regular Pap smears have reduced cervical cancer in most industrialized countries by the detection of abnormal cytology and subsequent cytodestructive/surgical intervention. The sensitivity and specificity of Pap smears have increased in recent years due to the concomitant use of HPV typing. Therapy of benign and dysplastic lesions due to HPV has improved during the past decade due to the use of immune response modifiers (IRMs), such as imiquimod. Our understanding of the mechanism of action of imiquimod is partly based on the activities of IFN-α, the first antiviral agent approved for therapy of HPV infections. Interferon-alpha has antiviral action, modulates the immune system, is antiproliferative, causes phenotypic reversion, downregulates oncogenes, and upregulates antioncogenes. Exogenous interferon was effective but had many negative features, such as the necessity of administration via injection, as well as systemic side effects. Imiquimod stimulates the production of many TH1 cytokines in addition to IFN-α. Thus it has potential to be more effective than exogenous IFN. In addition, imiquimod is applied topically and has no systemic side effects. Use of IRMs as monotherapy, or in combination with traditional treatment, has led to marked clearances and has significantly reduced the recurrence rate of these lesions. The clinical effect of IRMs originates from cytokine-induced activation of the immune system. This is the initial event in an immunological cascade resulting in the stimulation of the innate immune response and the cell-medicated pathway of acquired immunity. This immune modification mediates the indirect antiviral, antiproliferative, and antitumor activity of imiquimod *in vivo*.

Whereas VLP vaccines against oncogenic HPV will probably be available before the end of this decade (4), much remains to be learned about how HPV causes cancer. The oncogenic HPV is considered necessary but not sufficient to result in a carcinoma. The role of cofactors such as helper viruses, immunity, cigarette smoking, diet, and genetics are under active investigation. A better understanding of these factors should lead to better prevention and management of HPV infections (9).

Respiratory syncytial virus (RSV) is a common childhood infection, but no vaccine is yet available. Ribavirin, however, is an approved therapy and is administered to the affected patient via an aerosol. In addition, a monoclonal antibody, palivizumab, is widely used to prevent RSV infections in high-risk infants.

Approximately 46 million HIV-seropositive persons are estimated by the WHO to be living in the world at the beginning of 2004. Another 16,000 people acquire the virus every day, and millions of orphans have lost one or both parents to the virus. Over one-third of the adult populations of some sub-Saharan countries are infected and unable to work, resulting in collapsed economies. Therefore, the need for a safe and effective vaccine to prevent HIV infection is paramount. The results of the first phase-III vaccine trial to prevent HIV, however, failed to show efficacy. The reasons for the failure of this recombinant gp120 vaccine are not completely understood, but possible explanations include its inability to induce cellular immunity to the virus, although it did induce antibodies to gp120. General problems with developing an effective vaccine against HIV are the ability for the virus to mutate rapidly and the existence of many clades of HIV throughout the world. A number of more antigenic vaccines are being developed that involve recombinant HIV proteins being associated with attenuated carrier viruses such as adenovirus, vaccinia, or canarypox.

Antiretroviral agents are now available to block replication of HIV at three different steps: 1) fusion of the virus and target cell; 2) reverse transcription; and 3) assembly of viral proteins. There are three types of reverse transcriptase inhibitors: 1) nucleoside inhibitors (e.g., zidovudine, lamivudine, zalcitabine, didanosine, stavudine, abacavir, and emtricitabine); 2) nucleotide inhibitors (e.g., tenofovir); and 3) nonnucleoside inhibitors (e.g., nevirapine, efavirenz, and delavirdine). Protease inhibitors interfere with viral assembly and include saquinavir, ritonavir, indinavir, lopinavir, nelfinavir, amprenavir, fosamprenavir, and atazanavir. The newest class of medication to be approved is the fusions inhibitors (e.g., enfuvirtide). When used in certain combinations, these agents compose highly active antiretroviral therapy (HAART). Although HAART has resulted in marked reductions in morbidity and mortality in those industrialized areas of the world where patients or third-party payers can afford the cost of approximately $20,000 per year to treat one patient, most HIV-seropositive persons live in Third World countries. Therefore, approximately 99% of the world's AIDS patients cannot afford HAART. Although some of these persons have received medication through donations from pharmaceutical companies, WHO activities, and inexpensive generic substitutes, distribution remains a problem. Most of the antiretroviral drugs have toxicities (e.g., gastrointestinal, hepatic, neurologic, pancreatic, etc.) in some individuals, while other persons have developed mutant HIV stains that do not respond to these agents. Pharmacogenetic laboratory tests, such as with single-nucleotide polymorphisms (SNPs), now allow many of these mutations to be detected before the patient initiates therapy, thus allowing alternative treatments (10).

The most important limitation of HAART, however, is that it does not provide a cure. Although some persons may have viral loads below detectable levels for many years, discontinuation of HAART will result in reappearance of HIV in the system. Another major limitation to HAART, in addition to antiviral resistance, is noncompliance. The reason that compliance is difficult for many patients is that HAART requires a lifetime commitment and often necessitates daily ingestion of multiple medications, avoidance of certain foods, and constant awareness of the potential of negative interactions with other medications. An unexpected consequence of the success of HAART is that many high-risk individuals have become complacent about AIDS. Because they know of the availability of HAART and do not see large numbers of AIDS patients suffering horrible deaths due to HIV in industrialized countries, many younger individuals are returning to unprotected sex, intravenous drugs, etc.

With more than 20 antiretroviral drugs currently available and many more in clinical trials, many questions remain to be answered, such as

- What is the best combination of antiretroviral agents?
- When is the best time to start therapy?
- What is the optimal sequence in which to use the antiretroviral agents?
- What parameters should be used to define the success or failure of HAART?

Whereas the best antiretroviral agents usually depend on multiple factors, such as the HIV strain involved and the individual patient's potential for adverse reactions to a given drug, it was recently confirmed that the efficacy of antiretroviral drugs depends on how they are combined (11). Robbins et al. (12) determined that the combination of zidovudine, lamivudine, and efavirenz was superior to other antiretroviral combinations used in the study. This combination not only works longer and better, but is also easier to take and suppresses HIV more quickly. In previous studies, a combination of three antiretroviral drugs was superior to two agents, and a combination of two agents was better than one. Shafer et al. (13) reported, however, that a four-drug regimen was not significantly different from two consecutive three-drug regimens.

The best time to initiate therapy depends on many factors and is currently debated among HIV experts. Until recently, the standard of care was to start therapy at a low-plasma HIV RNA level and when the CD4 cell count decreased to below 500/mm^3. In 2004, however, most clinicians are advocating initiation of therapy when the CD4 cell count falls below 350/mm^3 or if the plasma HIV RNA level raises above 55,000 copies/ml. If symptoms of HIV and/or an opportunistic infection develop, however, therapy should be initiated before these laboratory landmarks are reached. Another factor is patients' potential to be compliant with the medication. If they are not prepared to adhere to therapy, drug resistance can develop. In fact, some studies suggest that missing even 5% of antiretroviral medication can hasten drug resistance. In vitro resistance testing of the virus and pharmacogenetics can help prevent the use of antiretrovirals that may be resisted. New classes of medication, such as the fusion inhibitors, have allowed new regimens to be initiated, if resistance develops. Although new drugs are rapidly appearing on the market, new classes of drugs are developed more slowly. These new categories of antiretroviral agents include viral adsorption inhibitors, viral entry inhibitors, viral assembly and disassembly inhibitors, integrase inhibitors, and inhibitors of viral mRNA transcription (transactivation) processes (14).

The most important criteria for successful antiretroviral therapy are the clinical parameters of reductions in morbidity and mortality. Improvements in morbidity may be measured by reductions in opportunistic infections or lessened drug toxicities. Laboratory changes, such as increasing CD4 cell counts and/or decreasing viral loads, usually correlate with clinical improvements.

While the treatment of hepatitis A is symptomatic, a safe and effective vaccine exists and is recommended for persons at high risk for this virus. The risk of hepatitis A is dependent on the quality of food preparation procedures and on the sanitary habits of food service workers. Many persons are therefore unaware of their risk of hepatitis A. This fact became obvious when 555 persons became ill with hepatitis A and three died in November, 2003, after ingesting green onions at a restaurant in Pennsylvania (15).

The vaccine to prevent hepatitis B was the first recombinant vaccine and is recommended for health care personnel as well as for anyone at high risk for infection with this virus. Because of the severe health consequences of hepatitis B infection, it is now given to neonates as part of their recommended childhood vaccines (www.cdc.gov/nip). A series of three injections is needed for vaccination against hepatitis B, and a series of two injections is needed for hepatitis A. For persons who have not been vaccinated against either virus, however, a simpler alternative to five injections is to receive the combination of vaccines against both viruses, which only requires three shots. Approved therapies for hepatitis B include interferon alpha, lamivudine, and adefovir, although a number of other treatments are under study.

Hepatitis C is a major cause of morbidity and mortality in many parts of the world and infections are increasing rapidly. Unfortunately, because of the rapid mutation rate of this virus, vaccine development is progressing relatively slowly. Therapy for hepatitis C was only moderately effective with interferon alpha monotherapy, but improved with the addition of ribavirin. Most recently, clinical and virological results have been significantly better with pegylated interferon combined with ribavirin.

Other hepatitis viruses (i.e., D, E, and G) have no specific antiviral therapies or vaccines. The first line of defense against all these viruses, including those for which a vaccine is available, continues to be good public health procedures.

Although antiviral drugs and vaccines are widely used, the third classification of medical intervention—passive immunity via immunoglobulins—is generally less common. Immunoglobulins (IG) are difficult to produce in large qualities, have the potential of microbial contamination, and have only transient benefits. In certain cases, the use of IGs has largely been replaced by specific vaccines that provide lifelong immunity (e.g., hepatitis A vaccine). Virus-specific IGs are given to unvaccinated persons exposed to hepatitis B or rabies. Varicella-zoster IG (VZIG) is given to susceptible persons exposed to varicella who have a high risk for complications (e.g., immunocompromised patients and neonates). Cytomegalovirus IG is administered to seronegative transplant recipients of an organ from a CMV-positive donor. Vaccinia IG is indicated for the therapy of eczema vaccinatum, but this IG is in very limited supply. Nonspecific IG is given to unvaccinated, high-risk persons exposed to measles, hepatitis A, rubella, or varicella (if VZIG is not available). Perhaps the most widely used IG is the specific monoclonal antibody against respiratory syncytical virus, which is used as prophylaxis in high-risk infants (e.g., those with bronchopulmonary dysplasia or prematurity).

Although approval of agents against other families of viruses (e.g., rhinoviruses) is expected in the near future, most advances are being made in antiretroviral drugs. Today, one-half of all antiviral agents are antiretrovirals, but greater understanding of how to interfere with replication of retroviruses will aid in the development of antiviral agents against other families of viruses.

Vaccines for a number of emerging viral diseases are in development and include vaccines for West Nile virus, Ebola virus, and the coronavirus responsible for severe acute respiratory syndrome (SARS). Development of a Dengue vaccine is a particular challenge because a person with antibodies to one strain of Dengue usually develops more severe clinical manifestations when subsequently exposed to a different strain. The analogous situation could arise if the antibodies to the first strain originated from vaccination. Therefore, the ideal vaccine against Dengue would elicit antibodies to all four common strains.

Development of future antiviral agents and vaccines will require enhanced knowledge of viral immunology and pharmacogenetics. Studies that led to the first safe and effective herpes simplex vaccine revealed at least two surprises:

1. Neither studies of circulating antibodies to the recombinant gD2 glycoproteins nor investigations of peripheral blood mononuclear cells in vaccinees were predictive of the clinical efficacy of the vaccine; and
2. Women seronegative for HSV-1 and HSV-2 were protected by the vaccine, but men were not (3).

Because of the fact that in over two centuries of vaccine development, there have been no previous reports of one gender being protected by a vaccine that did not protect the other, current studies involving the herpes simplex vaccine are focusing on the component of immunity that may play a greater role in protecting a woman against an STD than a man, i.e., mucosal immunity. In addition to understanding this component of viral immunity, development of future vaccines and antiviral agents will need to focus on persons' genetic ability to respond, i.e., on the field of pharmacogenetics. Just as some persons are more susceptible to infection than others, some individuals are genetically more able to respond to prophylaxis or therapy than others. One method used to distinguish the smallest possible genetic differences between individuals and thus identify those who could best benefit from a drug or a vaccine is the SNP. Alternatively, SNPs can also be used to determine who will suffer an adverse effect of a drug, as is already being done in HIV therapy. For example, SNPs are used to detect the 5% of the population who inherit a predisposition to a potentially fatal side effect of abacavir. Ultimately, future vaccines and drugs may be designed for a specific patient and against a specific virus.

The future development of drugs and vaccines, however, will be increasingly expensive. According to one study, the average investment required to get one drug approved by the FDA and marketed in the United States has risen to approximately $1.7 billion if one extrapolates from spending by pharmaceutical companies on the various stages of research and development during the 2000–2002 period. This figure is an increase from $1.1 billion from 1995–2000, when clinical trials cost less and drug companies were more productive in drug discovery. A 2001 study, however, placed the cost of bringing a new drug to market at $802 million, but this study did not include such commercialization costs as preparing marketing materials. For every 13 drugs that start out in animal testing, only one reached the market in 2003–2004, in contrast to one in eight during the 1995–2000 period.

In summary, public health measures should remain the first line of defense against viral diseases, and should be combined with antiviral vaccines when available. Antiviral drugs and passive immunity with IGs provide a second line of defense, but are usually more expensive than vaccines and public health measures, and provide shorter duration of protection. Although many more antiviral drugs will become available in the 21st century, the greatest need is for safe and effective vaccines against HIV, HPV, HSV, Dengue, rotaviruses, Ebola, West Nile virus, SARS, coronavirus, etc. (16).

REFERENCES

1. Hull, H.F. 1998. Perspectives from the global poliomyelitis eradication initiative. *Global Disease Elimination and Eradication as Public Health Strategies.* Bulletin of the World Health Organization 76 (Suppl. 2): 42–46.

2. De Quadros, C.A. 1998. Measles eradication: experience in the Americas. *Global Disease Elimination and Eradication as Public Health Strategies.* Bulletin of the World Health Organization 76 (Suppl. 2): 47–52.

3. Stanberry, L.R., S.L. Spruance, L. Cunningham, D. I. Bernstein, A. Mindel, S. Sacks, S.K. Tyring, F.Y. Aoki, M. Slaoui, M. Denis, P. Vandepapeliere, and G. Dubin. 2002. Glycoprotein D adjuvant vaccine to prevent genital herpes. *N Engl. J. Med.* 347: 1652–1661.

4. Koutsky, L.A., K.A. Ault, C.M. Wheeler, D.R. Brown, E. Barr, F.B. Alvarez, L.M. Chiacchierini, K.U. Jansen, and Proof of Principle Study Investigators. 2002. A controlled trial of a human papillomavirus type-16 vaccine. *N Engl J Med* 347: 1645–1651.

5. Warzecha, H., H.S. Mason, C. Lane, A. Tryggvesson, E. Rybicki, A. Williamson, J.D. Clements, and R.C. Rose. 2003. Oral immunogenicity of human papillomavirus-like particles expressed in potato. *J Virol* 77: 8702–8711.

6. Eisenberg J.N., B.L. Lewis, T.C. Porco, A.H. Hubbard, and J.M. Colford, Jr. 2003. Bias due to secondary transmission in estimation of attributable risk from intervention trials. *Epidemiology* 14: 442–450.

7. Wald, A., L. Corey, R. Cone, A. Hobson, G. Davis, and J. Zeh. 1997. Frequent genital herpes simplex virus 2 shedding in

immunocompetent women: effect of acyclovir treatment. *J Clin Invest* 99: 1092–1097.

8. Corey L., A. Wald, R. Patel, S.L. Sacks, S.K. Tyring, T. Warren, et al. 2004. Once-daily valacyclovir to reduce the risk of transmission of genital herpes. *N Engl J Med* 350: 11–20.

9. Mansur, C.P. 2002. Human papillomaviruses. *Mucocutaneous Manifestations of Viral Diseases* (S.K. Tyring, ed.) Marcel Dekker, pp. 247–294.

10. Clavel, F., and A.J. Hance. 2004. HIV drug resistance. *N Engl J Med* 350: 1023–1035.

11. Skolnik, P.R. 2003. "HIV therapy—what do we know, and when do we know it?" *N Engl J Med* 349: 2351–2352.

12. Robbins, G.K., V. De Gruttola, R.W. Shafer, L.M. Smeaton, S.W. Snyder, and C. Pettinelli. 2003. "Comparison of sequential three-drug regimens as initial therapy for HIV-1 infection." *N Engl J Med* 349: 2293–2303.

13. Shafer R.W., L.M. Smeaton, G.K. Robbins, V. De Gruttola, S.W. Snyder, and R. D'Aquila. 2003. "Comparison of four-drug regimens and pairs of sequential three-drug regimens as initial therapy for HIV-1 infection." *N Engl J Med* 349: 2304–2315.

14. De Clercq, E. 2002. New anti-HIV agents and targets. *Med Res Reviews* 22: 531–565.

15. Anonymous. 2003. "Hepatitis A outbreak associated with green onions at a restaurant—Monaca, Pennsylvania, 2003." *MMWR* 52: 1155–1157.

16. Enserink, M. 2003. "New vaccine and treatment excite Ebola researchers." *Science* 302: 1141–1142.

Chapter 2

Antiretroviral Drugs to Treat Human Immunodeficiency Virus Infections

INTRODUCTION

In less than two decades, human immunodeficiency virus (HIV) has dramatically progressed from a little-known or understood infection to the cause of a major global epidemic. In 1998, 36 million people were infected worldwide (1). Today, more than 46 million people are infected worldwide, with 16,000 new infections occurring in the world each day. Ninety-five percent of the HIV-infected population lives in the undeveloped-to-developing world where adequate treatment and prevention programs are lacking. For instance, the majority of new HIV infections in 2003 occurred in sub-Saharan Africa, where even monotherapy for HIV is lacking.

While the rate of new infections in the United States has been stabilizing overall in past years, this infection is becoming disproportionately concentrated in the lower socioeconomic class as well as the African-American community. Currently, African Americans are more than eight times as likely as whites to be infected with HIV, and AIDS is now the leading cause of death in black males between the ages of 25 and 44 (1).

Prior to the availability of highly active antiretroviral therapy (HAART), more than 90% of HIV-infected patients developed cutaneous manifestations at some time during the course of disease (2). In some of these individuals, disorders of the skin are the first presenting sign of HIV infection (3). A wide variety of skin conditions may arise in this immunosuppressed population, such as molluscum contagiosum (4), bacillary angiomatosis (5,6), Kaposi's sarcoma (7), eosinophilic folliculitis (8), candidiasis (7), mycobacterial infections (9–11), and a litany of others.

Because health care workers, in addition to those specializing in infectious diseases, will increasingly be involved in the collaborative management of these patients, it is imperative that we become familiar not only with the clinical manifestations of HIV, associated opportunistic infections, and their treatments, but also with the general antiviral therapies used for HIV infection. In addition, due to the rapid development of new antiretroviral drugs (Figure 2.1) and the need for

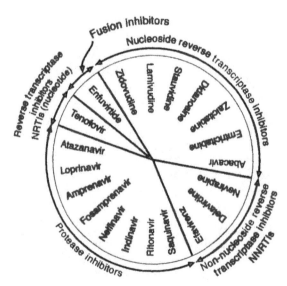

Fig. 2.1   Current antiretrovirals approved by the FDA (2004).

multiple medications in these patients, a plethora of drug interactions and adverse effects have complicated the issues of treatment Table 2.1. The goals of antiretroviral therapy are to decrease morbidity and mortality via suppression of viral load and maintenance of CD4(+) cell counts. Other objectives are to prevent the emergence of viral resistance, to capitalize on complementary drug actions, and to attack the virus in activated and in resting immune cells. Furthermore, antiretroviral treatment should attack HIV at multiple stages of reproduction, target viral compartments (e.g., lymph nodes), minimize side effects, and maximize patient compliance.

HUMAN IMMUNODEFICIENCY VIRUS

Antriretroviral drugs are used primarily to treat the patients with HIV infection which has become a major global scourge with little relief in sight for developing nations. The virus is transmitted through exposure to infected semen, cervical or vaginal secretions, or infected blood. Intravenous drug users who share contaminated needles are most at risk for contracting HIV. Unprotected sex between partners is a worldwide cause of transmission. Children born to HIV-infected women contract the disease during pregnancy through cross-contamination with the mother's body secretions or blood during delivery, or during breast-feeding.

When initially infected, patients usually have normal CD4 cell numbers, a low viral load, and an immunological response that indicates a prevalence of Th 1 lymphocytes. With advanced infection, CD4 levels fall, viral loads rise, and Th 2 lymphocytes are predominant. The Th 2 lymphocytes enhance humoral immunity and produce IL-4, IL-5, IL-10, and allergic responses. As CD4 levels fall, patients are bombarded with a variety of organisms as immunological responses decline. Many patients develop previously "rare" diseases due to viruses, bacteria, parasites, and fungi as well as neoplastic and other noninfectious disorders.

Interventions for HIV. Mechanistic analyses of the replication of HIV infection within a patient have revealed several

Table 2.1 Adverse Effects and Drug Interactions of Antiretroviral Agents

Antiretroviral drug	Mucocutaneous side effects	Nondermatologic side effects	Concomitant drugs to avoid
Zidovudine AZT	Longitudinal melonychia; skin pigmentation, macules, papules, pruritis, urticaria	Bone marrow suppression (anemia, neutropenia); gastrointestinal upset (nausea); neuropathy, hepatotoxicity, myopathy, myositis	Any that suppress bone marrow
Didanosine ddI	Erythema, macules, papules; oral and esophageal ulcers; Ofuji papuloerythroderma	Pancreatitis; peripheral neuropathy; fever; malaise	Any that cause pancreatitis; quinolone antibiotics and azole antifungals must not be given within 2 hours before or within 6 hours after ddI
Stavudine D4T	Erythema, macules, papules; esophageal ulcers	Peripheral neuropathy; lactic acidosis; hepatomegaly with steatosis	Same as for AZT
Zalcitabine ddc	Macules, papules, oral ulcers, esophageal ulcers	Peripheral neuropathy, severe pancreatitis, severe lactic acidosis, severe hepatomegaly with steatosis	Cimetidine, metoclopramide, Al and Mg OH antacid preparations; probenacid
Lamivudine 3TC	Alopecia, erythema, macules, papules, pruritis, urticaria	Peripheral neuropathy, nausea/ vomiting, anorexia, headache, malaise, neutropenia, pancreatitis	Any that cause pancreatitis

Abacavir ABC	Hypersensitivity reaction; macules, papules, urticaria	Hypersensitivity reaction; Fever, fatigue, malaise, nausea, vomiting, diarrhea, abdominal pain, arthralgias, cough, dyspnea	Alcohol
Emtricitabine	Hyperpigmentation	Headache, abdominal pain, diarrhea, nausea, vomiting, fatigue	
Nevirapine NVP	Erythematous macules and papular eruption; Stevens-Johnson syndrome	Hepatic reaction	Ketoconazole and oral contraceptives, dose adjustments for other drugs metabolized by cytochrome P450 system (especially isozyme (CYP3A) (e.g. protease inhibitors and rifampin)
Delavirdine DLV	Erythematous macular and papular exanthem +/- pruritis; Stevens-Johnson syndrome, erythema multiforme	Fever, arthralgias	Drugs metabolized by CYP3A pathway (clarithromycin, cisopride, terfenadine, astemazole, warfarin, protease inhibitors, certain benzodiazepines, certain calcium channel blockers, certain anticonvulsants and antimycobacterial agents, high fat meals, antacids, certain H_2-receptor antagonists

(Continued)

Table 2.2 *(Continued)*

Antiretroviral drug	Mucocutaneous side effects	Nondermatologic side effects	Concomitant drugs to avoid
Efavirenz EFV	Morbilliform or macular and papular eruptions; Less common: blistering, desquamation, ulceration; Rare: Stevens-Johnson syndrome; erythema mutliforme	Central nervous system or psychiatric symptoms: dizziness, somnolence, insomnia, confusion, impaired concentration, amnesia, agitation, euphoria, hallucinations, abnormal dreaming, abnormal thinking	Drugs metabolized by CYP3A pathway: astemizole, cisapride, midazolam, triazalam, clarithromycin, ergot derivatives, rifampin, phenobarbital
Tenofovir		Nausea, vomiting, diarrhea, flatulence, osteopenia, lipodystrophy, renal toxicity	Any that decrease renal function
Saquinavir SQV	Fat redistribution, wasting appearance, protease pouch, buffalo hump, crix belly	Lipodystrophy syndrome, hyperlipidemia, hyperglycemia, probable coronary artery disease, new onset diabetes mellitus, diarrhea, nausea, abdominal discomfort, dyspepsia	Vitamin A supplements; drugs metabolized by CYP3A enzymes; terfenadine, cisapride, triazolam, midazolam, ergot derivatives
Ritonavir RTV	Macules, papules and others listed under SQV	Nausea/vomiting, fever, diarrhea, circumoral paresthesias, peripheral paresthesias, taste perversion, hepatitis, hypermenorrhea and others listed under SQV	Drugs metabolized by cytochrome P450 system (e.g., astemizole; certain antiarrythmics as quinidine, amiodarone, encainide, flecainide; certain sedative/hypnotics as diazepam and flurazepam) as well as others listed under SQV

Drug			
Indinavir IDV	Erythematous macules and papules, dry skin, alopecia, paronychia, pyogenic granulomas and others listed under SQV; rare: Stevens-Johnson syndrome	Nephrolithiasis, renal insufficiency or renal failure; pharyngitis, gastrointestinal upset, anemia, hepatitis and other listed under SQV and RTV	Same as listed under SQV and RTV
Nelfinavir NFV	Same as listed under SQV	Diarrhea and other as listed under SQV and RTV	Same as listed under SQV and RTV
Amprenavir APV	Macules and papules +/– pruritis; Rare: Stevens-Johnson syndrome; others as listed under SQV	Perioral paraesthesias, diarrhea, headache, nausea/vomiting and others listed under SQV and RTV	As listed under SQV and RTV
Lopinavir	As listed under SQV	Diarrhea and others listed under SQV and RTV	As listed under SQV and RTV
Fosamprenavir GW 433908	"Rash" 1% develop Stevens-Johnson syndrome	Nausea, diarrhea	Sulfonamide, lovastatin, simavastatin, triazolam, midazolam, ergot-based drugs, cisapride, pimozole
Atazanavir BMS–232632		Diarrhea, jaundice	
Enfuviritide ENF, T-20	Injection site reactions	Allergic reactions, pain or numbness in feet or legs, decreased appetite, weakness, constipation, pancreatitits	

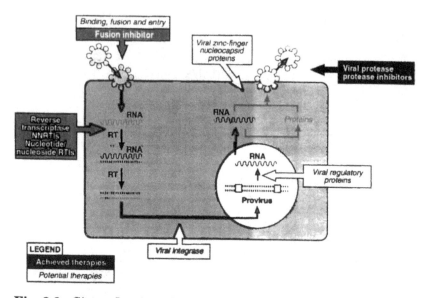

Fig. 2.2 Sites of action of antiretroviral drugs. Nucleoside, nucleotide and non-nucleoside reverse transcriptase (RT) inhibitors act at the same step in the replication of HIV. Nucleoside analogues, when phosphorylated, competitively inhibit RT by acting as an alternative substrate for the enzyme. Non-nucleoside analogues do not require phosphorylation but noncompetitively bind directly to the active site of RT. Protease inhibitors prevent the cleavage of viral polyproteins in the final stage of viral protein processing, thus preventing the assembly of mature HIV virions. Fusion inhibitors prevent binding to the surface of the cell and subsequent infection of the cell.

avenues for therapy. These include inhibitors that are active during the binding, fusion, and entry of the viral capsid into the cell. Then, during RNA replication, reverse transcriptase drugs interfere with RNA replication. Viral integrase drugs (of which there are none approved at this writing) interfere with entry into the nucleus. Another potential, but not yet having any approved drugs, target would be the viral zinc-finger nucleocapsid proteins. Finally, viral protease inhibitors attack the virus as it leaves the cell to infect other cells. (See Fig. 2.2)

Treatments for HIV. There is no known "cure" for HIV disease. The initial regimen programs for HIV began with nucleoside reverse transcriptase inhibitors (NRTIs) in 1987 and therapy was with one drug, zidovudine Over time, it became obvious that as HIV replicated, it also mutated. This meant that therapy began to fail. Progress (rising CD4+ counts and lowered HIV RNA levels) began to unravel. Other drugs, administered individually, were no better. However, combinations of antiretroviral drugs provided a "cocktail" that attacked the virus at multiple points (12). This HAART became the standard of care in 1996 in developed countries where insurance or government health care pays for the nearly $20,000 bill for drugs prescribed for a patient each year. In developing countries, however, monotherapy may be the only option, if any antiretroviral therapy is available. Figures 2.1 and 2.2 illustrate the available therapies that can be used in HAART and their sites of action.

Typically HAART consists of two nucleoside analogues and a protease inhibitor (PI) or a non-nucleoside reverse transcriptase inhibitor (NNRTI). Today there is an armada of antiretrovirals in the arsenal with many more being developed (Fig. 2.2). Nucleotide and nucleoside reverse transcriptase inhibitors, PIs, and NNRTIs have been joined by fusion inhibitors. Selecting the appropriate therapy, however, is no longer a simple matter.

There have been several suggested therapy cocktails consisting of three or even four antiretrovirals taken concurrently. The "original combination therapy" called for two NRTIs administered with one NNRTI or a PI. (13,14)

Recent studies indicate that a combination of three antivirals appears most efficacious and that efavirenz, lamivudine, and zidovudine provide the best combination for patients receiving their first HIV medication. At this time, lamivudine and zidovudine are available as a combination pill (Combivir®). This combination drug, administered with efavirenz, means patients take only three pills/day with a concomitant increase in patient compliance.

If resistance is detected, the patient and doctor must consider other antiretroviral drugs as alternative therapy. The options may appear numerous, but many factors enter into the picture. Once resistance occurs, other related drugs may demonstrate cross-resistance. Allergies to one drug usually transfer to other drugs in the same category. Concomitant non-antiretroviral drugs also must be considered. For example, prescribing a drug known to cause hepatic toxicity might prove to be risky to a patient with any type of hepatitis. Likewise, any drug that affects liver metabolism must be used with extreme care if given along with other agents metabolized by the liver.

Controversy still exists regarding the optimal time to initiate therapy due to the cost of treatment, the side effects, and the difficulty with compliance which results in potential resistance. Newly revised guidelines on treating adults and adolescents with HIV and AIDS provide suggestions for regimens that are more definitive. The guidelines were prepared by the Panel on Clinical Practices for Treatment of HIV Infection, convened by the Department of Health and Human Services. For the first time, the guidelines include lists of "preferred" and "alternative" regimens. These lists are available at http://aidsinfo.nih.gov; the document also lists regimens or components that should never be offered.

The preferred regimen based on NNRTIs calls for a combination of efavirenz, lamivudine, and zidovudine, tenofovir or stavudine, except for women who are pregnant or may become pregnant. Patients on this regimen take three to five pills per day.

The preferred regimen based on PIs calls for a combinatioin of lopinavir/ritonavir (coformulated as Kaletra®) together with lamivudine and either zidovudine or stavudine. Patients on this regimen take 8 to 10 pills per day.

Triple NRTI regimens should be used only when an NNRTI- or PI-based regimen cannot be used as first-line therapy. The panel's preferred triple-NRTI regimen calls for a combination of abacavir, lamivudine, and either zidovudine or stavudine. Patients on this regimen take two to six pills per day. Regimens listed as "alternative" in the guidelines, however, may actually be the preferred regimen for a specific patient.

The panel listed 12 regimens or components that should never be offered. Several, including monotherapy and dual nucleoside therapy, had been listed as contraindicated in previous versions of the guidelines. The newly listed contraindicated regimens are a three-NRTI regimen with abacavir, tenofovir, and lamivudine (because of early virologic nonresponse); a three-NRTI regimen with didanosine, tenofovir, and lamivudine (because of a high rate of virologic failure); the combination of didanosine and stavudine (because of a high incidence of toxicities, including several deaths); the combination of atazanavir and indinavir (both of which can cause high-grade hyperbilirubinemia and jaundice); and emtricitabine plus lamivudine as a two-NRTI backbone (since both drugs have similar resistance profiles and minimal additive antiviral activity).

The guidelines found at www.hivatis.org recommend initiation of treatment for all HIV-infected persons who have symptoms of HIV infection, a rapidly declining CD4 count, a CD4 count <200–350 cells/mm^3, or a viral load >30,000 RNA copies/ml (bDNA assay) or 55,000 RNA copies ml (RT-PCR assay) (regardless of the CD4 count) (15).

Guidelines are less established for pediatric patients, but it is generally recommended that therapy be initiated in children with clinical symptoms of HIV infection or evidence of immunosuppression, regardless of viral load. However, any child with HIV RNA levels >100,000 copies/ml is at a high risk for mortality, and antiretroviral therapy should be started. Others recommended starting therapy in children at HIV RNA levels >10,000–20,000 copies/ml. Zidovudine (AZT) monotherapy is indicated only for infants of indeterminate HIV status during the first six weeks of life to prevent perinatal HIV transmission (16).

Even combination therapy has many side effects that HIV-infected persons must tolerate. Side effects and the required number of pills to be taken daily affect patient compliance. Even missing 5% of one's pills may put a patient at risk for drug resistance. These factors have led to the development of more potent and safer antiretroviral agents. Although resistance is less likely with HAART than with monotherapy, it remains a problem.

Combination therapies. To address the need for fewer pills, pharmaceutical companies have begun to market combination therapies. Three of these are currently marketed. Zidovudine and lamivudine are marketed as Combivir. A combination of abacavir, zidovudine, and lamivudine is marketed as Trizivir®. Lopinavir, which was approved only as a combination drug with ritonavir, is marketed in this combination as Kaletra.

Maintenance therapy after combination therapy. One study of maintenance therapy of HIV infection (after an initial response to combination therapy) showed that suppression of plasma HIV RNA was better sustained with a combination of indinavir, zidovudine, and lamivudine than either indinavir alone or zidovudine and lamvudine (17). A similar study also found that three-drug therapy (zidovudine, lamivudine, and indinavir) was more effective than two-drug maintenance therapy (zidovudine plus lamivudine or zidovudine plus indinavir) in sustaining a reduced viral load in HIV-1–infected patients after three months of induction therapy (18).

These studies and others have led to the current therapeutic approach to HIV, which involves HAART. These treatment guidelines suggest early and aggressive drug therapy with three antiretroviral drugs from different classes of drugs. In previously untreated patients, this approach is expected to reduce the plasma HIV virus levels to levels below the limits of detection (19). However, studies have shown that even with effective HAART therapy and undetectable plasma HIV virus levels, virus is still present in lymph nodes, semen, or possibly elsewhere. Furtado et al. (20) showed that despite treatment with potent antiretroviral drugs and suppression of plasma HIV-1 RNA, HIV transcription was actively present in peripheral blood mononuclear cells. Zhang et al. (21) found that several HIV-1–infected men on HAART therapy continued to have virus present in seminal cells, which may still allow for sexual transmission of the virus. Moreover, combination antiretrovirals appear to suppress HIV-1 replication in some, but not all, patients (22).

Regardless of these dilemmas, the leading problem with HAART therapy is its cost and availability. With the extremely high expense of daily combination treatment (i.e., $15,000 to $20,000 per year), more than 95% of the 46 million HIV-infected people worldwide cannot afford it. Further progress in the battle against HIV will require a more economic and accessible means of treatment that can reach the population in the developing world.

Prophylactic antiretroviral drugs. Another advance in the treatment of HIV is the potential to administer prophylactic antiretroviral drugs to exposed individuals in order to decrease the risk of acquiring infection. Although large-scale, placebo-controlled clinical trials are not logistically possible, one study has found that zidovudine prophylaxis reduced HIV seroconversion after percutaneous exposure (23,24). Current basic recommendations for postexposure prophylaxis (PEP) include a four-week regimen of zidovudine and lamivudine, begun as soon as possible after exposure (25). For occupational HIV exposure with additional risk for transmission (e.g., higher virus titers or larger blood exposure), indinavir or nelfinavir is added to the basic regimen.

Zidovudine chemoprophylaxis is also effective in the reduction of perinatal transmission, in some studies decreasing the risk of vertical transmission from mother to child by 66 to nearly 70% (26,27). This regimen consists of daily oral zidovudine given during the last six weeks of pregnancy, followed by intravenous zidovudine during labor (28). Thereafter, the newborn is given oral zidovudine for the first six weeks of life. Implementation of this regimen in the United States and Europe has dropped the rate of perinatal transmission to 6% or less (29). However, the high expense of treatment is cost-prohibitive for developing countries. Three recent studies have evaluated the efficacy of short-term zidovudine in decreasing the risk of HIV-1 perinatal transmission. The trial regimens generally consisted of oral zidovudine given during the last four weeks of pregnancy, some with additional doses during labor. Results revealed a 37 to 38% decrease in vertical transmission of HIV-1 in subjects who breastfed (30,31). In a similar study without breastfeeding, the reduction in the rate of transmission was 50% (32). While a shorter course of zidovudine is considerably cheaper, ($50 for the shorter course vs. $800 for the longer course), the cost of therapy remains too high for most developing countries. Musoke et al. (33) found that a single dose of nevirapine administered to HIV-positive women during labor and another dose given to their infants during the first week of life may be a safe and well-tolerated treatment that is helpful in reducing perinatal transmission of HIV. This treatment would be a low-cost and accessible alternative for poor and developing countries with high rates of HIV infection and limited funds for treatment.

Guidelines for therapy. The National Institutes of Health has defined general principles for the therapy of HIV (34). Both plasma HIV RNA levels (viral load) and CD4+ T cell counts should be followed for monitoring of response to treatment. The combination of these values has been determined to be a more accurate assessment of prognosis (35). In addition, they are a useful tool in determining the efficacy of antiretroviral treatment while the patient is awaiting clinical response. CD4+ counts indicate the extent of immune system damage and the risk for opportunistic infections. Although HIV RNA levels are more predictive of the risk for disease progression, CD4+ counts are a more accurate measurement of the effect of antiretroviral therapy.

HIV RNA levels should begin to decline within days of effective treatment and ideally should progressively fall to below the limits of detection within eight weeks, although complete suppression is seen in a maximum of only 60–80% of previously untreated patients. A more realistic eight-week target is a one-log reduction of the viral load. Rebound of viral load levels during consistent treatment may indicate resistant HIV variants and may likely require changes in the current antiretroviral regimen. It should be noted that if one of the drugs in the antiretroviral regimen must be stopped, they all should be stopped and that a single-drug substitution can be made only if the patient's viral load is completely suppressed.

NUCLEOSIDE REVERSE TRANSCRIPTASE INHIBITORS

Nucleoside analogs were the first line of defense for the treatment of HIV infection in 1987 (36). Subsequent studies of various combination therapies of indinavir, zidovudine, and lamivudine led to the beginnings of general combination therapy and the refinement of HAART combination therapy. These early studies suggested that a prompt and aggressive drug therapy with three or more antiviral drugs from two or three classes of drugs might be more effective. HAART can reduce the plasma HIV virus levels to levels below the existing limits of detection (17).

Mechanisms of action. Nucleoside analogues are dideoxynucleoside analogues which are phosphorylated intracellularly into active triphosphate metabolites. The active form then competitively inhibits HIV reverse transcriptase by acting as an alternate substrate for the enzyme. This family of compounds lacks the 3'-hydroxyl group, which leads to chain termination once the active metabolite is incorporated into the developing DNA strand. Figure 2.2 depicts the site of action of the existing and new antiretroviral drugs.

Zidovudine [AZT] (Retrovir®)

Zidovudine is the most extensively studied drug of all the antiretrovirals. It is no longer used as monotherapy, except in parts of the world where other antiretroviral drugs are not available. It has been widely prescribed by practitioners after early studies revealed improved survival rates and delayed declines in CD4 counts in patients with HIV infection (36–38). As a result of monotherapy with zidovudine, resistant HIV strains have developed, which have limited the efficacy of this treatment. After six months of therapy with zidovudine alone, HIV isolates with reduced susceptibility can be recovered (39,40). The quantity and frequency of resistant strains progressively increases over time with monotherapy. As HIV-1 strains develop resistance to zidovudine therapy, those resistant strains have been proven to be transmittable to other persons (41–45). There are studies underway to develop a

Generic Name	Structure	Viral Diseases Treated
Zidovudine **Brand Name** Retrovir Combivir (zidovudine + lamivudine) Trizivir (abacavir + lamivudine + zidovudine) Other Name(s) AZT	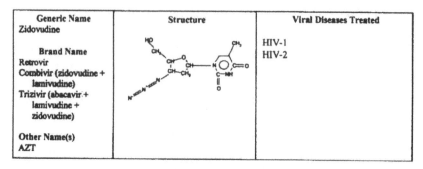	HIV-1 HIV-2

Fig. 2.3 Trade names, structure, and uses of Zidovudine.

quantitative method to validate zidovudine resistance (46). There is a report that Korean red ginseng delays the development of resistance to zidovudine (47). The nucleoside analogue drugs are closely related and have similar mechanisms of action; there is cross-resistance among these compounds, but they have different side effect profiles (48). The structure of zidovudine, its brand names, and its approved usage are shown in Fig. 2.3. Zidovudine monotherapy is used for infants of indeterminate HIV status during the first six weeks of life to prevent HIV transmission (16).

Adverse Events

Phosphorylation of zidovudine. Poor phosphorylation of zidovudine has been implicated in the intracellular accumulation of zidovudine monophosphate. This accumulation is associated with cytotoxicity as mediated through mitochondrial damage (49).

Bone marrow suppression. The most frequently seen adverse effect of zidovudine is bone marrow suppression, with severe anemia and/or neutropenia.

Coadministration with other drugs. Coadministration with other drugs which may potentially suppress the bone marrow should be done cautiously, with frequent monitoring of hematologic parameters.

Gastrointestinal upset and/or nausea.

Hematoticity. Zidovudine may directly induce apoptosis by a hematotoxic mechanism and may be discontinued to restore T-cell levels and reduce apoptosis (50).

Neuropathy. Peripheral neuropathy with lactic acidosis and coproporphyria has been reported in a patient with human T-cell leukemia virus (HTLV)-1–associated T-cell leukemia (51).

Hepatotoxicity. There is one report of death from hepatitis with lactic acidosis occurring in an individual who had discontinued zidovudine (due to nucleoside-induced acute hepatitis and lactic acidaemia) 18 months previously (52).

Myopathy or myositis.

Longitudinal melonychia. The most common cutaneous manifestation of AZT use is longitudinal melonychia which is usually noted after 2–6 weeks of therapy (53). The color of the affected nails has been described as "dark bluish or brownish."

Other dermatologic manifestations. Skin pigmentation, nonspecific macules and papules, pruritis, and urticaria are rarely reported.

Psoriasis. Patients with HIV infection may develop psoriasis which is very difficult to treat using conventional therapy. An open-label study to determine the safety and efficacy of AZT in HIV-associated psoriasis demonstrated that 90% of 19 evaluable patients had partial (58%) or complete (32%) improvement of their psoriasis (54). Other studies demonstrated that clinical improvement of HIV-associated psoriasis parallels a reduction of HIV viral load (55). Interestingly, AZT has also been given to HIV-negative patients with psoriasis. In a pilot study, 33% of these persons showed improvement in their psoriasis, but no complete remissions occurred (56).

Special Considerations

Pancreatitis. When compared with didanosine, stauvidine, and hydroxyurea, zidovudine causes the fewest cases of pancreatitis (57).

Pregnancy. Zidovudine has been shown to reduce perinatal transmission. However, many women who are HIV-positive have reservations about taking the drug. Concerns revolve around fear of toxic effects on the mother, fear of toxic effects on the baby, fear of drug resistance, the belief that "healthy" women don't need zidovudine, and having given birth to a healthy baby without using zidovudine. Clearly, additional educational interventions are needed to increase the use of zidovudine during pregnancy to reduce perinatal transmission (58).

Pediatric patients. To reduce mother-to-child transmission of HIV, zidovudine is often prescribed. The treatment is not without complications. Lactic acid levels in the plasma often rise and these are associated with possible mitochondrial dysfunction (59). Not only is zidovudine-resistance transferred from mothers to children, but also there is evidence that zidovudine-resistance develops in newborns almost immediately (60).

Didanosine [ddI] (Videx®)

Didanosine (ddI) is indicated for patients with HIV who are either unable to tolerate zidovudine or those who have became refractory to its effects. The structure, brand names, and approved usage of didanosine areshown in Fig. 2.4. In 1993, a partially randomized study compared zidovudine alone versus

Generic Name Didanosine Brand Name Videx Other Name(s) DDI, ddi, Dideoxyinosine	Structure	Viral Diseases Treated HIV-1 HIV-2

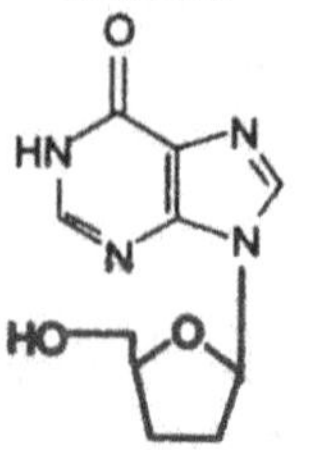

Fig. 2.4 Trade names, structure, and uses of Didanosine.

different combination regimens of zidovudine and didanosine. The results showed more sustained increases in CD4-positive cell counts and more frequent decreases in plasma HIV-1 RNA titers among all combination regimens when compared with zidovudine alone (61). In cases of HIV-1-associated myelopathy, didanosine combined with zidovudine effected significant neurological improvement (62).

Adverse Events

Pancreatitis. The most serious side effect is pancreatitis which occurs in 7% of treated patients, with some fatalities reported. The use of hydroxyurea to potentiate the antiviral activity of didanosine yields a four-fold higher risk of pancreatitis (57).

Hyperamylasemia. Hyperamylasemia occurs in 20% of treated patients (63).

Coadministration with other drugs at risk to cause pancreatitis. Extreme caution should be used in prescribing concomitant drugs that may cause pancreatitis, and only if necessary. If pancreatitis develops, it is usually reversible with prompt cessation of therapy.

Peripheral neuropathy. This occurs in 15% of treated patients and is related to the dose of didanosine, stage of disease, and combination therapy (64).

Fever and malaise. Fever and malaise are rare.

Ulcers. Oral and esophageal ulcers are rarely seen with ddI (65). One report notes Ofuji papuloerythroderma associated with ddI (66).

Special Considerations

Antacid and antibiotic coadministration. Didanosine is an acid-labile compound which is formulated with an antacid buffer. It should be taken on an empty stomach, at least 30 minutes prior to or 2 hours after a meal, in order to avoid an unfavorable acidic environment. The quinolone antibiotics (e.g., ciprofloxacin) and certain antifungals, such as ketoconazole and itraconazole, require an acidic environment for absorption, and will be affected if administered with the antacid buffer found in didanosine. These drugs should be given at least 2 hours prior to or 6 hours after a dose of didanosine.

Coadministration with ribavirin. Coadministration of ribavirin with didanosine promotes mitochondrial toxicity. More studies need to be completed to determine if reducing the dose of didanosine (when coadministered with ribavirin), changing the modalities of prescriptions, or avoiding concomitant prescriptions can avoid mitochondrial toxicity (67–69).

Stavudine [d4T] (Zerit®)

Stavudine (d4T) is indicated for AIDS patients in the later stages of disease who have proven either intolerant or unresponsive to the other antiretroviral drugs which are more commonly used. The structure, brand names, and approved usage of stavudine are shown in Fig. 2.5. When the effect of stavudine was studied in patients on therapy, the median virus titers in peripheral blood mononuclear cells were decreased by 1–2 logs and the plasma RNA content was reduced approximately 0.5 log from baseline median values at both 10 weeks and 52 weeks (70). Stavudine is administered orally as a capsule or in an oral solution. For adults and preadults weighing at least 132 pounds or more, 40 mg should be taken every 12 hours. For adults and

Generic Name Stavudine Brand Name Zerit Other Name(s) D4T	Structure	Viral Diseases Treated
		HIV-1 HIV-2

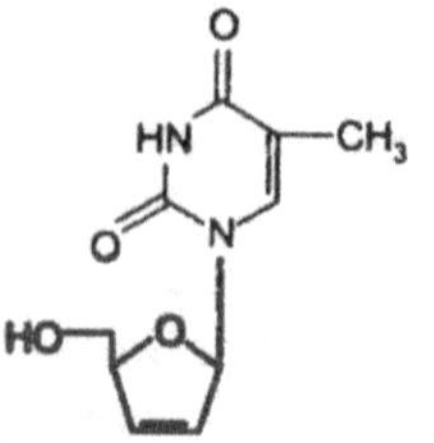

Fig. 2.5 Trade names, structure, and uses of Stavudine.

preadults weighing at least 66 but not more than 132 pounds, 30 mg should be taken every 12 hours. For children less than 66 pounds, 1 mg for every kg (0.45 mg per pound) of body weight should be given every 12 hours. For those patients with only one mutation conferring viral resistance to zidovudine, stavudine may be a reasonable alternative. The more mutations that are present, the less effective the stavudine will be as a replacement therapy (71).

Adverse Events.

The side effect profile of stavudine is similar to that of zidovudine.

> **Peripheral neuropathy.** The major side effect of stavudine is a dose-related peripheral neuropathy, affecting 20% of patients. Peripheral neuropathy is characterized by a tingling, burning, numbness or pain in the hands or feet.
>
> **Lactic acidosis and severe hepatomegaly with steatosis.** These adverse events have been reported in patients using certain nucleoside analogues, such as stavudine and didanosine. Renal tubular dysfunction has occurred in at least one patient (72).
>
> **Mucocutaneous responses.** Occasional erythema, macules, and papules have been observed in patients taking d4T (65). Esophageal ulcers are also rarely seen.
>
> **Lipoatrophy.** Lipoatrophy is associated with mitochondrial toxicity, lactic acidemia, and insulin resistance. Switching from stavudine or zidovudine to abacavir can lead to modest increases in limb fat, but clinical lipoatrophy does not resolve (73–75).
>
> **Neuromuscular weakness/respiratory failure.** Hyperlactatemia, a common stavudine adverse effect, is associated with a Guillain-Barre syndrome mimic. Twenty-two cases with seven deaths were reported. Should severe hyperlactatemia or motor weakness develop, the patient should be removed from the drug and supportive care supplied, including ventilation, as needed. If symptoms, such as fatigue, weight loss,

abdominal pain, nausea, vomiting, or dyspepsia, occur, the patient's lactate levels should be monitored to prevent fatal lactic acidosis (76).

Zalcitabine [ddC] (Hivid®)

Zalcitabine (ddC), another synthetic nucleoside analogue, has minimal efficacy when used alone, but is useful for combination therapy in HIV patients. The structure, brand names, and approved usage for zalcitabine are shown in Fig. 2.6. Zalcitabine is a reverse transcriptase inhibitor. It is indicated, along with zidovudine, for patients with deteriorating HIV infection according to both clinical and immunological parameters (CD4 <300 /ml). The oral dosage is 0.75 three times daily. Most formulations are as 0.375-mg or 0.75-mg tablets. When zalcitabine was taken with nelfinavir and zidovudine as combination therapy, viral replication was suppressed, CD4 counts increased, and the quality of life improved for Nigerian patients with HIV (77). Triple therapy of saquinavir/stavudine/zalcitabine is reasonably well-tolerated with a rapid reduction in viral load and immunological improvement. It is considered to be an additional therapeutic option that is favorable when compared with other triple therapy regimens (78). Saquinavir, zidovudine, and zalcitabine combination therapy is considered successful with some synergistic effect between saquinavir and zalcitabine (79,80). The opposite has been

Generic Name Zalcitabine Brand Name HIVID Other Name(s) ddC Dideoxycitidine	Structure	Viral Diseases Treated
		HIV-1 HIV-2

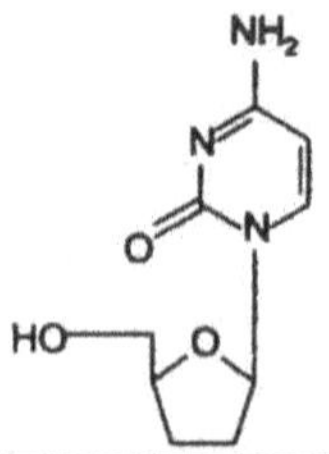

Fig. 2.6 Trade names, structure, and uses of Zalcitabine.

reported for zalcitabine combined with zidovudine (81). Zalcitabine combined with saquinavir alone was not sufficient to increase significantly the CD4 count even though there was a 79% clinical improvement in the patients (82). Zalcitabine is often coadministered with foscarnet, an antiviral used to treat cytomegalovirus infection, with no apparaent negative or positive pharmacokinetic interaction (83).

Adverse Events

Zalcitabine may contribute more to mitochondrial toxicity than lamivudine in that the exonuclease has more difficulty removing zalcitabine from the DNA chain (84).

Peripheral neuropathy. Peripheral neuropathy occurs in 17 to 30% of patients.

Pancreatitis. Severe pancreatitis may occur due to swelling of the pancreas.

Lactic acidosis. Lactic acidosis without hypoxemia may occur.

Hepatomegaly with steatosis. Hepatomegaly with steatosis may be severe.

Anemia, leucopenia, fatigue, and headache.

Coadministration with metoclopramide, and with aluminum and magnesium hydroxide preparations (e.g., Maalox or Mylanta). These combinations administered with zalcitabine cause a decrease in the bioavailability of zalcitabine.

Coadministration with probenicid or cimetidine. Coadministration with probenicid or cimetidine results in a 50% increase in zalcitabine exposure as these drugs decrease elimination of zalcitabine and may increase chances for toxicity.

Cutaneous eruptions. Macular and papular eruptions have been reported to develop in 14 of 20 (70%) patients treated with zalcitabine (85). This eruption usually presented on day 10 or 11 of therapy.

Oral ulcers. Oral ulcers developed in nine of 14 patients on days four to six of treatment.

Esophageal ulcers. Esophageal ulcers have also been reported in 2–4% of patients treated with ddC (86). The eruption and ulcers usually resolve with continual ddC treatment.

Special Considerations

Pregnancy and neonates. Pregnancy is not recommended either before or during administration of zalcitabine. The effect of zalcitabine on a developing fetus is unknown. In pigtailed macaque monkeys, administration of zalcitabine during the pregnancy did not affect the pharmacokinetics of the drug. In infant macaques, it appears that smaller and less frequent dosing in HIV-infected neonates is warranted than in older children and adults (87).

Renal impairment. Clearance of zalcitabine decreases in patients with renal impairment. Dosage adjustments may have to be made, especially in those with severe renal impairment (88).

Lamivudine [3TC] (Epivir®)

Lamivudine (3TC) is a synthetic nucleoside analogue that is FDA-approved for the treatment of HIV and chronic hepatitis B virus infections (See chapter 3 for a description of Hepatitis B infection). Combination therapy of lamivudine-interferon (IFN) to treat chronic hepatitis B has been suggested (89). Fig. 2.7

Generic Name	Structure	Viral Diseases Treated
Lamivudine	NH$_2$	HIV-1
Brand Name		HIV-2
Epivir		Hepatitis B virus (HBV)
Combivir (lamivudine + zidovudine)		
Trizivir (lamivudine + abacavir + zidovudine)		
Other Name(s)		
3TC		

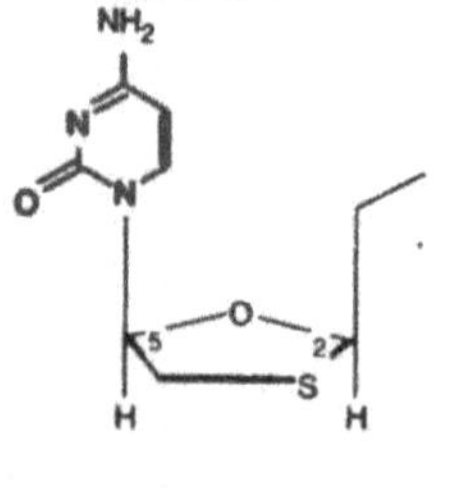

Fig. 2.7 Trade names, structure, and uses of Lamivudine.

highlights the molecular structure and brand names of lamivudine. Recently, it was found that HIV-infected patients who received initial therapy with regimens including either stavudine or lamivudine had significantly lower mortality and longer AIDS-free survival than those receiving initial therapies with regimens limited to zidovudine, didanosine, and zalcitabine (90). A combination of lamivudine and zidovudine (Combivir) has also been FDA-approved for the treatment of HIV infection. However, there are reports of recurrent hypersensitivity to Combivir (91). Lamivudine appears to have little or no genotoxicity (92). Lamivudine has greater efficacy in treating Chinese patients with chronic hepatits B infection than does famciclovir (93).

Lamivudine has been incorporated into main-line prescriptions for HAART therapy. Lamivudine is often combined with zidovudine (Combivir) and abacavir with successful results regarding CD4 counts and general tolerance for the therapy (94).

Adverse Events

Hepatotoxicity. In one rare case, an elderly man treated with lamivudine developed hepatic decompensation (95). Hepatic necrosis can also occur (96).

Peripheral neuropathy.

Nausea/vomiting.

Anorexia.

Headache.

Malaise.

Neutropenia.

Cutaneous responses. Alopecia, erythema, macules, papules, pruritis, and urticaria have been seen rarely with lamivudine (65).

Special Considerations

Pediatric patients. In pediatric clinical trials, 14% of children on monotherapy and 15% of those on combination therapy with lamivudine developed pancreatitis.

Mucocutaneous manifestations. When mucocutaneous manifestations are seen with Combivir, there appears to be an equal chance that zidovudine or lamivudine may be responsible.

Lamivudine resistance. One of the concerns of lamivudine use for the treatment of chonic hepatitis B is the emergence of a variety of genotypes for lamivudine resistance, particularly in HIV-1/HBV–coinfected patients (97–99).

Abacavir [ABC] (Ziagen®)

Abacavir (ABC) is a second-generation NRTI given accelerated FDA approval for use in multi-drug cocktails. It is a synthetic carboxycyclic nucleoside with a 6-cyclopropylamino modification. The structure, brand names, and approved usage are shown in Fig. 2.8. Abacavir is the most powerful nucleoside analogue and one of the most powerful antiretroviral drugs currently available. Its use results in reduction in viral loads and increases in CD4 counts which are unparalleled by any other nucleoside analogue and are similar to most potent PIs (100). Abacavir is normally administered as 300-mg doses twice daily although there is some indication that a 600-mg dose once daily is equally effective (101). In one study, abacavir plus zidovudine and lamivudine raised CD4 counts and lowered plasma HIV RNA to undetectable levels in two-thirds of previously untreated patients (102). In addition, abacavir plus a PI lowered HIV viral loads in the majority of previously

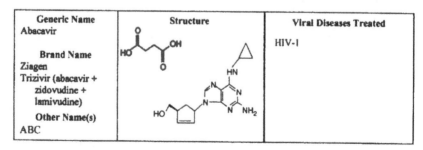

Generic Name	Structure	Viral Diseases Treated
Abacavir		HIV-1
Brand Name Ziagen Trizivir (abacavir + zidovudine + lamivudine)		
Other Name(s) ABC		

Fig. 2.8 Trade names, structure, and uses of Abacavir.

untreated patients to undetectable levels (103,104). However, it should be noted that resistance to zidovudine and lamivudine gives cross-resistance to abacavir (105). In patients with lipoatrophy caused by stavudine or zidovudine sensitivity, abacavir results in modest increases in limb fat over 24 weeks (73). In patients who have previously been heavily treated with other nucleoside analogues, the addition of abacavir would be ineffective. Abacavir combined with zidovudine and lamivudine is now marketed as Trizivir for HAART therapy.

Adverse Events

Hypersensitivity reactions. A serious and potentially lethal hypersensitivity reaction to abacavir is seen in 2–5% of patients (106–110). Clinical presentation includes fever to 39–40°C, macules, papules, and urticaria, fatigue, malaise, nausea, vomiting, diarrhea, abdominal pain, arthralgias, cough, and/or dyspnea. These clinical presentations may be associated with increased creatine phosphokinase (CPK), elevated liver function tests, and lymphopenia. These findings usually occur within the first six weeks of therapy. The hypersensitivity reaction usually resolves with cessation of abacavir, but a rechallenge of the drug after this reaction can be fatal. All physicians and patients should be aware of this potentially serous side effect. Therefore, patients taking ABC who develop a skin eruption associated with fever, gastrointestinal symptoms, cough, dyspnea, and constitutional symptoms should be instructed to promptly contact their physician or, if severe, go to the nearest emergency room. Prednisolone may not be effective in treating hypersensitivity from drug toxicity (111).

Vertigo. Many HIV-positive patients report symptoms and signs of inner ear disease. Vertigo can cause significant morbidity and prevent patients from living a normal life. The appearance of vertigo with the introduction and removal of abacavir therapy implies that it may be a causative agent, with mitochondrial toxicity being the suspected mechanism (112).

Agranulocytosis after rash resolution. Several weeks after resolution of a slight rash, one patient developed a fever, sore throat, ulcerated lips, diarrhea, and abdominal pain, probably the result of drug-related antibodies (113).

Hypersensitivity. Hypersensitivity includes not only rash, as described earlier, but anaphylactic shock (114–116). Many severe reactions seem to occur when abacavir is reintroduced after a previous cessation of treatment for hypersensitivity.

Emtricitabine (Emtriva, Coviracil, FTC)

Emtricitabine is a deoxycytidine nucleoside approved for use in combination with other antiretroviral agents (Fig. 2.9). It was tested in combination with didanosine and efavirenz against a stavudine, didanosine, and efavirenz combination. After 24 and 48 weeks, patients receiving the emtricitabine had significantly higher rates of virologic suppression and elevated CD4 levels than the combination recipients. The dosage recommendation at this printing is one daily dose of 200 mg.

Adverse Events

Mirochondrial toxicity. Mitochondrial toxicity is often associated with the use of NRTIs. To manage the tissue and drug-related toxicities (i.e., myopathy, peripheral neuropathy, lactic acidosis), interruption of NRTI

Generic Name Emtricitabine Brand Name Emtriva Other Name(s)	Structure	Viral Diseases Treated
		HIV-1

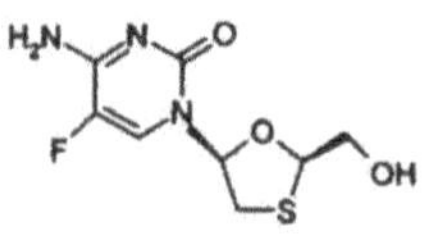

Fig. 2.9 Trade names, structure, and uses of Emtricitabine.

therapy with a better-tolerated substitute should be considered (117).

The most common side effects during combination therapy involving emitricitabine include:

Headache.

Abdominal pain and/or diarrhea.

Nausea and vomiting.

Fatigue.

Other side effects:

Skin discoloration. Hyperpigmentation of soles of feet and/or palms of hands may occur. In most cases this has been mild and asymptomatic.

Special Considerations

Reproductive profile. A reproductive profile has not been done on humans. However, in mice and rabbits, there were no increased numbers of malformations in embryofetal toxicology studies. Emtricitabine did not appear to affect fertility, sperm count, or early embryonic development. Thus far, emtricitabine has a favorable reproductive safety profile (118).

Lamivudine resistance. The mutations associated with emtricitabine resistance are nearly identical to those that confer lamivudine resistance. Therefore, emtricitabine most likely will not be beneficial to patients who need to change treatment because of lamivudine resistance. Because of the high tendency for HIV to develop resistance to emtricitabine, it should be used only in regimens that normally fully suppress viral replication.

Hepatitis B. Although not currently FDA-approved for this indication, emtricitabine is active against hepatitis B infection (119,120), as are interferon alpha and nucleoside analogs (121).

NON-NUCLEOSIDE REVERSE TRANSCRIPTASE INHIBITORS

The class of NNRTIs is a chemically heterogeneous group of compounds that are entirely unrelated to nucleosides. They inhibit HIV replication at the same stage as nucleoside analogues, but they noncompetitively bind directly to the active site of reverse transcriptase (122). (See Fig. 2.2 for the site of action.) These drugs are not substrates for the reverse transcriptase enzyme and are not incorporated into the developing viral DNA chain. They are also active in their native state and do not require phosphorylation to become an active metabolite (123). The NNRTIs are highly active for HIV-1, but have no activity against HIV-2. Resistance is a significant problem with mono-therapy (124) and cross-resistance occurs among members of this class (125). However, there is no cross-resistance with nucleoside analogues (126). The NNRTIs are a suitable addi-tion for combination therapy, as they have in vitro synergistic activity with nucleoside analogues and PIs.

Nevirapine [NVP] (Viramune®)

In 1996, nevirapine was the first NNRTI to become available. The structure, brand names, and FDA-approved usage for nevirapine are shown in Fig. 2.10. After binding to the HIV reverse transcriptase, this compound specifically blocks RNA- and DNA-dependent DNA polymerase activities by disrupting the catalytic site of the viral enzyme. Nevirapine is indicated for use in combination with nucleoside analogues in individuals with HIV-1 who have experienced clinical and/or immunologic deterioration while on an initial therapeutic regimen. Nevi-rapine has been found to be cost-effective when administered to sub-Saharan African women to prevent vertical HIV trans-mission to their fetuses/infants. Nevirapine is taken at the

Generic Name Nevirapine Brand Name Viramune Other Name(s) NVP	Structure	Viral Diseases Treated
		HIV-1

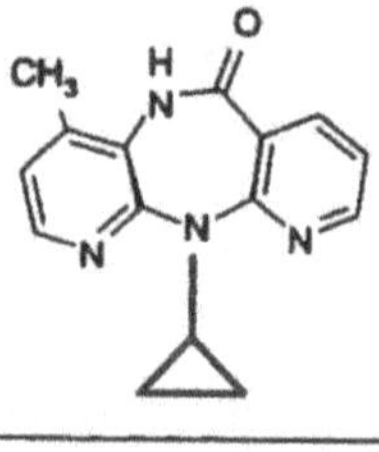

Fig. 2.10 Trade names, structure, and uses of Nevirapine.

onset of labor and an infant dose is administered just after delivery (127). Resistance to nevirapine can develop quickly (128), and it is recommended that therapy be discontinued if no clinical benefits are seen with its addition. When HAART combinations of nevirapine, stavudine, and didanosine are administered, elevated triglyceride and low-density lipoprotein (LDL) levels may indicate a potential increased risk of coronary artery disease (129).

Adverse Events

> **Induction of CYP3A enzymes.** Nevirapine is extensively metabolized by the cytochrome P450 system, particularly by the isozyme CYP3A family. Because it leads to induction of CYP3A enzymes, other drugs that are similarly metabolized (i.e., PIs and rifampin) may have lower plasma concentrations, and dosage adjustments may be necessary.
>
> **Coadministration with Ketoconazole.** Ketoconazole, an imidazole derivative used as a broad-spectrum antifungal agent, should not be coadministered with nevirapine.
>
> **Oral contraceptives.** Oral contraceptives are contraindicated with nevirapine therapy because of significant reductions in their plasma concentrations.
>
> **Rash.** The most common toxicity reported with nevirapine is rash which is seen in at least 17% of patients and can be associated with a life-threatening hepatic reaction. Others report that a transient, self-limited rash develops in almost half of patients on nevirapine (124,130), typically within one to eight weeks of initiation of therapy. This eruption is usually erythematous and maculopapular and can be mild or moderately severe. It is typically located on the trunk, face, and extremities, and may have associated pruritus. The eruption appears to be more prevalent in women (131) and can be associated with eosinophilia and systemic symptoms (132). The rash becomes severe in 6 to 20% of patients, some of whom develop Stevens-Johnson

syndrome (133). Short-term prednisone administration does not prevent nevirapine rash and may actually increase the incidence (134).

Stevens-Johnson syndrome. This syndrome may be diagnosed prior to mucous membrane lesions by complaints of pain and/or tingling of the mucous membranes. Nevirapine should be stopped if this occurs. Intravenous immunoglobulin may abort Stevens-Johnson syndrome if given early (135,136). A dose escalation schedule for nevirapine is recommended during initiation of therapy to reduce the risk of rash (137). If a patient on nevirapine develops a skin eruption, the dosage should not be increased until the rash resolves. If the rash is moist or extensive, is associated with fever, or involves the mucous membranes, prompt and permanent cessation of nevirapine is indicated (138).

Special Considerations

Coadministration with St. John's wort. Herbal extracts of St. John's wort (*Hypericum perforatum*) are often taken as an antidepressant. These extracts often contain inducers of hepatic enzymes and may cause clinically relevant drug interactions. With concomitant use of St John's wort and nevirapine, nevirapine plasma concentration levels are lower and the efficacy of the drug may be affected (139).

Delavirdine [DLV] (Rescriptor®)

In 1997, delavirdine (DLV) was the second NNRTI to gain FDA approval (Fig. 2.11). It is indicated for combination therapy of HIV-1, but its specific function in the current management of HIV has yet to be completely determined. In one study, delavirdine was added to combination therapy in patients for whom multiple drug treatment had failed (140,141). Results showed a rapid and sustained decrease in the mean plasma HIV-1 RNA as well as a 66 to 90% increase in CD4-positive cells. Additional studies of the use of delavirdine in combination regimens are ongoing. Delavirdine is prescribed for adults as 400 mg three

Generic Name	Structure	Viral Diseases Treated
Delavirdine **Brand Name** Rescriptor Other Name(s) DLV	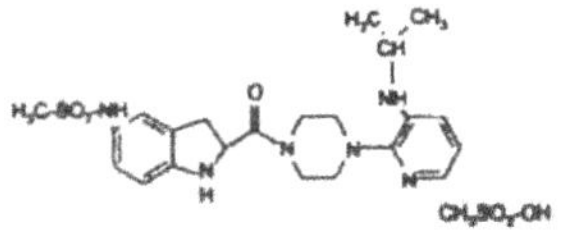	HIV-1

Fig. 2.11   Trade names, structure, and uses of Delavirdine.

times a day. For children younger than 16 years, the use and dosage is determined by the physician. For patients with low levels and concentrations of stomach acid, delavirdine may be taken with orange or cranberry juice. Delavirdine may be taken with or without food but should be taken the same way for each dose. Delavirdine comes in tablet form and some patients may have trouble swallowing all the tablets. By dissolving the tablets in at least three ounces of water, the suspension can be mixed and swallowed immediately. For ritonavir-boosted PIs delavirdine increases drug exposure levels (142).

Adverse Events

> **Hepatotoxicity.** Hepatotoxicity has been associated with all NNRTIs, especially nevirapine (143,144). A retrospective study of the incidence of NNRTI hepatotoxicity indicates that there is no significant difference among nevirapine, efavirenz, and delavirdine when treating HIV-positive patients coinfected with HBV and HCV (145).
>
> **Inhibition of enzymatic metabolism.** Delavirdine is metabolized in the liver by cytochrome CYP3A enzymes. Unlike nevirapine's induction of these enzymes, delavirdine inhibits the enzymatic metabolism of itself and other affected drugs. This results in increased plasma levels of drugs which are metabolized by this enzymatic pathway.
>
> **Coadministration with other CYP3A enzymatic pathway drugs.** Clarithromycin, cisapride, terfenadine,

astemizole, warfarin, PIs, certain benzodiazepines, and certain calcium channel blockers share the same enzymatic pathway (146). Coadministration of delavirdine with these drugs and others may result in significant and potentially life-threatening adverse effects.

Coadministration with anticonvulsants and antimycobacterial agents. Certain anticonvulsants and antimycobacterial agents are not recommended due to the decrease in plasma delavirdine levels. Certain H_2 receptor antagonists reduce the gastrointestinal absorption of delavirdine.

Coadministration of statins and protease inhibitors. HIV-positive patients with hypercholesterolemia must be careful as to which statins are used when taking PIs such as delavirdine. For example, pravastatin and atorvastatin are recommended while lovastatin and simvastatin should be avoided. Although atorvastatin and delavirdine were coadministered as recommended, a case of rhabdomyolysis with acute renal failure has been reported (147).

Rash. The most frequent and significant adverse effect with delavirdine is a rash, which occurred in 18% of clinical trial participants (138,140). The rash is typically a diffuse, erythematous, maculopapular exanthem on the upper body and proximal arms, with or without pruritus. It usually arises within one to three weeks of treatment initiation, and resolves between 3 to 14 days after onset and usually does not require dose reduction or discontinuation (after interrupted treatment). A severe rash (requiring discontinuation of drug) was reported in 3.6% of subjects in the clinical trials (146). Delavirdine should be promptly discontinued if the rash is associated with fever, mucous membrane involvement, swelling, or arthralgias.

Erythema multiforme. Erythema multiforme occurs in approximately one of 1000 patients taking delavirdine.

Stevens–Johnson syndrome. Stevens–Johnson syndrome has been reported in one of 1000 patients taking delavirdine (148).

Special Considerations

Coadministration with antacids. Patients should wait at least one hour between taking an antacid and delavirdine for maximum efficacy.

Pregnancy and breast-feeding. Delavirdine has not been studied in pregnant women although it has been shown to cause birth defects in animal studies. It is not known if delavirdine passes into the breast milk.

Efavirenz [EFV] (Sustiva®)

Efavirenz (EFV) is the most recently FDA-approved NNRTI. The structure, brand names, and approved uses are shown in Fig. 2.12. It is a potent drug that is well-tolerated and can be given once daily (138). As in the case of all NNRTIs, resistant viruses emerge rapidly when efavirenz is used as monotherapy. Thus, it cannot be used as a single agent to treat HIV-1 or added on as a sole agent to a failing regimen. It must be administered with a PI and/or an NRTI. The guidelines for the treatment of pediatric HIV infection have been altered to allow efavirenz to be substituted for the PI in the preferred regimen of two nucleoside analogues and a PI.

Efavirenz appears to have some unique characteristics. For example, in vitro studies indicate that high-level resistance will develop more slowly as it requires two mutations to occur before viral resistance is effective. Efavirenz, used in combination with zidovudine and lamivudine, resulted in complete remission of Kaposi's sarcoma in an AIDS patient

Generic Name	Structure	Viral Diseases Treated
Efavirenz		HIV-1
Brand Name Sustiva		
Other Name(s) EFV		

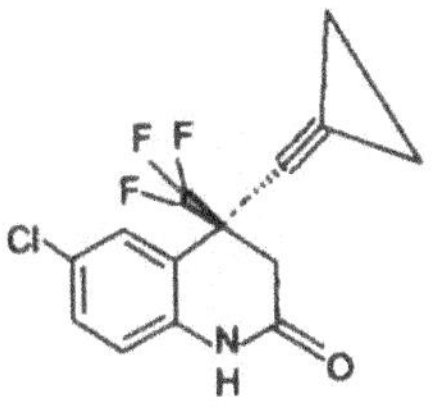

Fig. 2.12   Trade names, structure, and uses of Efavirenz.

(149). Hepatotxicity, commonly reported with nevirapine, has not been reported with efavirenz (150). Although transmission of HIV can occur during antiretroviral therapy, there is some indication that efavirenz is present in the seminal plasma and could have antiviral activity within the male genital tract (151). Efavirenz has been substituted for PIs with the thought that persistent dyslipidemia from the PIs could be reduced. This has met with some success (152).

Adverse Events

Metabolism inhibition. Efavirenz also competes for the CYP3A enzyme system, which results in the inhibition of the metabolism of certain drugs, leading to increases in their plasma concentrations.

Coadministration with astemizole, cisapride, midazolam, triazolam, clarithromycin, or ergot derivatives. Life-threatening adverse events could result (e.g., cardiac arrhythmias, prolonged sedation, or respiratory depression).

Coadministration with rifampin and phenobarbital. Other drugs that induce CYP3A activity, such as rifampin and phenobarbital, may lead to increased clearance of efavirenz and lower plasma concentrations.

Central nervous system or psychiatric symptoms. In clinical trials, 52% of patients receiving efavirenz reported central nervous system (CNS) or psychiatric symptoms. Most of these adverse effects were mild in severity and included the following symptoms: dizziness, somnolence, insomnia, confusion, impaired concentration, amnesia, agitation, hallucinations, euphoria, abnormal dreaming, and abnormal thinking. Patients with high plasma levels of efavirenz (>4000 ug/l) were three times more likely to develop CNS toxicity. In some cases, the dosage may be reduced from 600 mg once a day to 400 mg once a day, particularly if the patient has low body weight (153,154). Insomnia has been reported and may require a dosage adjustment (155).

Delusions and inappropriate behavior. There have been reports of delusions and inappropriate behavior in patients treated with efavirenz, predominantly in those with a history of mental illness or substance abuse. Manic syndrome is also associated with efavirenz overdose (156).

Skin rash. Approximately 27% of patients treated with efavirenz in clinical trials developed a rash, typically described as morbilliform or maculopapular. The rash can be mild to moderate, occurs within the first two weeks of therapy and usually requires discontinuation of drug in only 2% of patients. A rash associated with blistering of the face, trunk, and extremities, moist desquamation, or an ulceration occurred in only 1% of participants, requiring discontinuation of therapy (157). There is a report of one person developing a skin eruption after a single dose of efavirenz (158). A regimen to desensitize a patient against efavirenz-induced skin eruptions has been described (159).

Cutaneous vasculitis. Leukocytoclastis vasculitis has developed in at least two patients soon after beginning treatment with efavirenz (160).

Stevens-Johnson syndrome and erythema multiforme. One case each of erythema multiforme and Stevens-Johnson syndrome has been reported (i.e., one of 2200 recipients of EFV).

Severe skin rash. In patients without severe skin eruptions, treatment can be continued, with resolution of the rash typically within one month. If therapy must be discontinued because of a rash, it can later be reinitiated, with appropriate antihistamines and/or corticosteroids recommended during retreatment. Photoallergic dermatitis may occur after ultraviolet exposure to patients using efavirenz (161).

Pulmonary hypersensitivity. Efavirenz has been reported to cause severe pulmonary hypersensitivity (162).

Monitoring of blood cholesterol levels. Cholesterol should be monitored in efavirenz-treated patients.

Gynecomastia. Gynecomastia without lipodystrophy has been reported in HIV-infected men treated with efavirenz (163).

Diabetic ketoacidosis. Diabetes mellitus and diabetic ketoacidosis can occur in patients taking PIs. In these cases, efavirenz may be substituted. Metformin may be useful in increasing the sensitivity of the peripheral tissues to the insulin (164).

Special Considerations

Pregnancy. Pregnancy should be avoided in women receiving efavirenz, as malformations have been observed in fetuses from efavirenz-treated monkeys (165). In women of child-bearing potential, a barrier method of contraception must always be used in combination with another method, such as oral contraceptives. A pregnancy test prior to the initiation of efavirenz is also necessary. At least one case of myelomeningocele has been reported in a newborn (166).

NUCLEOTIDE REVERSE TRANSCRIPTASE INHIBITORS

Tenofovir Disoproxil Fumerate (Viread®)

Tenofovir is a nucleotide analog reverse transcriptase inhibitor. The best-known nucleotide analogues are the antivirals, adefovir (Hepsera) and cidofovir (Vistide), used for the treatment of hepatitis B and cytomegalovirus infections. Adefovir was discontinued as an HIV therapy due to proximal renal tubular dysfunction. See Fig. 2.13 for names, structure, and approved uses of tenofovir. It is FDA-approved for the treatment of HIV infection in combination with other anti-HIV therapies. The recommended dosage for tenofovir is 300 mg taken orally once each day. The lower number of dosages per day increases the probability that the patient will exercise medication compliance (167). The medication is in tablet form and may be taken with or without food. If patients have a decreased kidney function, the medication may need to be taken less frequently. Tenofovir resistance occurs and may be

Generic Name	Structure	Viral Diseases Treated
Tenofovir		HIV-1
Brand Name		HIV-2
Viread		
Other Name(s)		

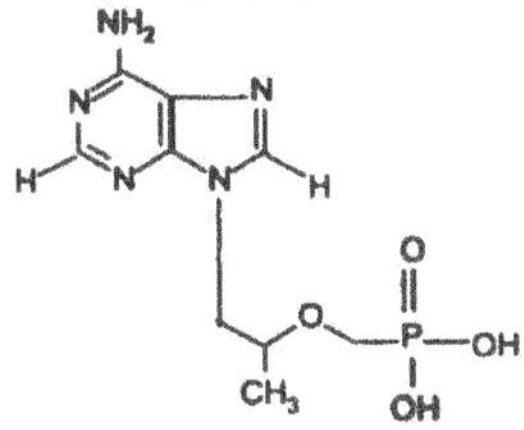

Fig. 2.13 Trade names, structure, and uses of Tenofovir.

the result of several resistant mutations (168,169). However, there are reports that tenofovir can be used to treat HIV-1 strains that are nucleoside-resistant (170). Tenofovir is also active against hepatitis B virus. In one case, an HIV-positive patient with liver cirrhosis secondary to chronic hepatitis B and resistance to lamivudine was treated with tenofovir with significant virologic and histopathologic improvements. This case was so successful that the patient was removed from the liver transplant program and has not had any further hepatic complications (171). Long-term administration of tenofovir (96 weeks), combined with exisiting antiretroviral therapy for patients with preexisting resistance mutations, showed significant and durable reductions in HIV-1 RNA levels (172).

Adverse Events

> **Gastric reactions.** Nausea, vomiting, diarrhea, and flatulence are the most common short-term events of tenofovir (173).
>
> **Osteopenia.** When taken with efavirenz and lamivudine, tenofovir was more likely to cause bone mineral density decreases than stavudine taken with efavirenz and lamivudine. Over time, this could lead to osteoporosis with bone breakage of the hip, spine, wrist, or other small bones.
>
> **Lipodystrophy.** Redistribution, loss, or accumulation of body fat and/or increases in cholesterol, triglycerides, or other blood lipids may occur with any patient receiving anti-HIV therapy.

Kidney toxicity. Numerous studies have reported kidney toxicity (and some cases of renal acidosis) with use of tenofovir (174–178). One of the risk factors associated with tenofovir renal toxicity is the prior proximal renal tubular acidosis reported during adefovir therapy (179). Factors that increase the risk for developing hypophosphotemia include: patients receiving HAART, length of time on HAART, concurrent use of lopinavir-ritonavir, increased time since HIV diagnosis, and a history of nephrotoxic agents. Tenofovir is not associated with mitochondrial toxicity or cytotoxicity (180,181).

Special Considerations

Coadministration of tenofovir with didanosine and lamivudine and other triple-NRTI therapies. This combination is not recommended when considering a new treatment regimen for therapy-naïve or experienced patients with HIV infection. A 91% virological failure occurred, as defined by a <2 log reduction in plasma HIV RNA levels, by week 12 of a clinical study. Patients treated with this combination of therapies should be considered for treatment modification (182). Other triple-NRTI therapies have had suboptimal response. These include: 1) abacavir/lamivudine/zidovudine (183); 2) abacavir/didanosine/stavudine (184); and 3) abacavir/lamivudine/tenofovir (185–187).

Reduction in lipid side effects. When patients receiving stavudine switched to tenofovir because of stavudine-induced side effects, most patients experienced a rapid and significant decrease in triglyceride levels after the switch.

Coadministration with didanosine. Coadministration with didanosine is not recommended except in closely monitored cases (188). Plasma concentrations of didanosine will increase with coadministration of tenofovir. Coadministration is not recommended for patients who weigh less than 60 kg, already have renal impairment, or are receiving current therapy with lopinavir-ritonavir, as pancreatitis may occur (189). Adjusting the didanosine dosage may be all that is needed to accommodate the systemic drug interaction (190,191).

HIV PROTEASE INHIBITORS

The PIs were introduced in 1995 as a promising new category of antiretrovirals that work by a different mechanism than the reverse transcriptase inhibitors (192). These compounds block a separate virus-specific enzyme known as HIV protease.

Mechanism of action. Inhibition of the protease enzyme prevents the cleavage of viral polyproteins in the final stage of viral protein processing (See Fig. 2.2 for site of action.). Without the HIV protease activity, mature HIV virions cannot be assembled and released from infected cells, which results in the production of defective, noninfectious viral particles (193). While the reverse transcriptase inhibitors prevent replication only in newly infected cells, PIs block enzyme activity in both newly infected and chronically infected cells (194).

Adverse events. When compared to the nucleoside analogues, the PIs are more potent in reducing viral load (126,195), but are associated with the major morbidity of lipodystrophy as well as possible increased mortality secondary to coronary artery disease (48). All of the PIs have been shown to be associated with increases in weight and body mass index as well as an improved quality of life. Unfortunately, the chemical structures of these drugs are remarkably complex and are difficult to synthesize on a large-scale basis, resulting in high costs (126).

Enzymatic inhibition. Protease inhibitors are all metabolized by hepatic microsomal enzymes (i.e., P450) to a certain degree that may cause significant drug interactions with some of these compounds. Since the list of such drugs that are contraindicated with PIs is constantly evolving, a comprehensive resource such as www.hivatis.org should be consulted before initiating any drug with hepatic metabolism concomitantly with PIs or NNRTIs. Furthermore, none of the PIs adequately penetrate into the CNS.

Cross resistance. Cross-resistance commonly occurs among several of the PIs (196), and these drugs should be used only in combination with the reverse transcriptase inhibitors.

Specific observations. Protease inhibitor use is associated with fat redistribution, hyperlipidemia, hyperglycemia with insulin resistance, and probable increases in coronary artery disease with variable frequency (197–201). These changes may occur as isolated observations or they may occur together. Similar observations have been reported in HIV-infected patients not receiving PIs, but the incidence in persons receiving PI-containing HAART regimens appears to be increasing (202–204).

Lipodystrophy syndrome. Fat distribution abnormalities result in a "wasting" appearance ("slim disease") and abnormal fat accumulation in localized areas ("protease pouch," "buffalo hump," and "crix belly") (205–220). Some studies have shown that saquinavir, ritonavir, and nelfinavir all reduce the development of fat cells from stem cells in vitro. In addition, they increase the metabolic destruction of fat in existing fat cells. It is postulated that loss of deposited fat in the body could lead to high levels of LDL, cholesterol, and triglycerides. An alternative mechanism could involve retinoids (221). When retinoids are combined with PIs, complex reactions occur in certain genes. It is postulated that indinavir may cause some effects resembling lipodystrophy by changing retinoid signaling. Therefore, patients taking PIs may be advised to avoid vitamin A supplements. Still another hypothesis suggests that PIs, which show approximately 60% homology with lipoprotein receptor-related protein and cytoplasmic retinoic acid-binding-protein type I, may bind to lipoprotein receptor-related proteins and result in hypertriglyceridemia and lipodystrophy (222).

Abnormal adipose distribution. Human aspartic proteases playing a role in adipose regulation may be downregulated by PIs, resulting in abnormal adipose deposition (223).

Insulin resistance and associated cardiovascular risk. Metformin reduces insulin resistance and related cardiovascular risk parameters in patients with lipodystrophy (224).

Surgical interventions. Liposuction, reduction mammoplasty, fat transfer to cheeks, and other forms of cosmetic surgery have been used to treat the lipodystrophy syndrome with varying success (225,226).

Saquinavir [SQV] (Invirase®: Hard Gel; Fortovase®: Soft Gel)

Saquinavir (SQV) was the first PI to be approved for the treatment of HIV-1 and HIV-2. It is a synthetic, transition-state peptidomimetic which inhibits the HIV protease and prevents the infectivity of the viral particle. When given as the original hard gel form (Invirase), saquinavir is limited by extremely poor absorption. After reformulation as a soft gel cap (Fortovase), saquinavir was predicted to have a five-fold increased bioavailability (205) and greater viral load reduction (206). This would make it more useful in potent triple-combination therapies (227). However, the increase in bioavailability was not as high as predicted. The uptake of saquinavir may improve with high-fat meals and/or administration with grapefruit juice (228), but this may cause plasma concentrations to be too low for good antiviral activity. Saquinavir can be combined with ritonavir for better efficacy and availability (229). "Average" doses for saquinavir are 600 mg three times a day for adults for oral capsules. The soft gelatin capsules require 1200 mg three times per day. The capsules and the soft gelatin capsules are not interchangeable. In both cases, children's (under the age of 16 years) dosages must be calculated based on the body mass of the child and other factors. The structure, brand names, and approved uses for saquinavir are shown in Fig. 2.14. Saquinavir competes for CYP3A enzymes and inhibits the metabolism of similarly metabolized drugs.

Adverse Events

Rare events include a burning or prickling sensation, confusion, dehydration, dry or itchy skin, fruity mouth odor, increased hunger, increased thirst, increased urination, nausea, skin rash, unusual tiredness, and weight loss.

Less common or rare side effects include:

Diarrhea.
Nausea.

Generic Name	Structure	Viral Diseases Treated
Saquinavir		
		HIV-1
Brand Name		HIV-2
Fortovase		
Invirase		
Other Name(s)		
SQV		

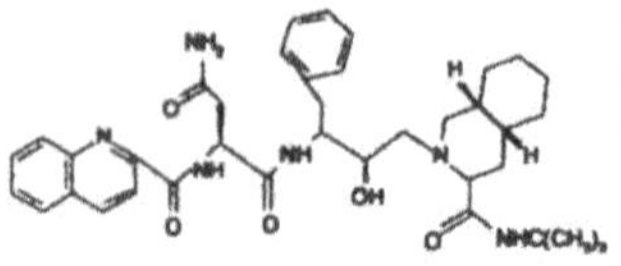

Fig. 2.14 Trade names, structure, and uses of Saquinavir.

Abdominal discomfort.

Dyspepsia.

Blood sugar levels. New-onset diabetes mellitus and hyperglycemia have been reported with all of the PI drugs (207).

Special Considerations

Liver disease. Saquinavir may be more potent in patients with liver disease because of slower removal of medicine from the body. Dosage adjustments may be necessary

Coadministration with terfenadine, cisapide, triazolam, midazolam, or ergot derivatives. Coadministration with terfenadine, cisapride, triazolam, midazolam, or ergot derivatives may cause potentially serious reactions. Several other drug interactions occur that may increase or decrease drug plasma concentrations of either compound, requiring dosage adjustments.

Ritonavir [RTV] (Norvir®)

In March 1996, ritonavir (RTV) was the second PI to receive FDA approval. Brand names, chemical structure, and uses are shown in Fig. 2.15. In a randomized, double-blind, placebo-controlled trial, ritonavir was added to the previous treatment regimens (with up to two nucleoside drugs) in patients with advanced HIV-1 disease (230). Results revealed that the addition of ritonavir lowered the complications of AIDS and

Generic Name	Structure	Viral Diseases Treated
Ritonavir **Brand Name** Norvir Kaletra (ritonavir + lopinavir) **Other Name(s)** ABT-538 RTV	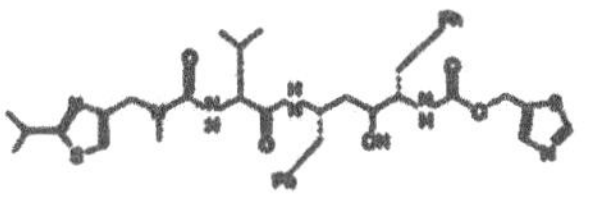	HIV-1 HIV-2

Fig. 2.15 Trade names, structure, and uses of Ritonavir.

prolonged survival in these patients, although earlier intervention would likely have been much more effective. Coadministration of ritonavir with amprenavir results in a synergistic relationship between the two (231). Indinavir and ritonavir combinations have improved pharmacokinetic properties with twice-daily dosing with food (232). Ritonavir is taken orally as a capsule or in an oral solution. Adults take 600 mg two times a day in capsule form. For the oral solution, adults take 600 mg two times a day. Children's dosages are to be determined by the physician, but the capsules are not normally used for children. Ritonavir is often used to boost HIV PI combinations to reduce pill burden and improve the pharmacokinetic profile of other PIs but with mixed results (233).

Adverse Events

Hepatotoxicity. Ritonavir is associated with higher rates of severe hepatotoxicity in HIV/HCV-coinfected patients when compared with other protease inhibitors. Hepatotoxicity also is prevalent in patients with alcohol abuse or intravenous drug use (234).

Gastric upsets. The most common adverse effects seen with ritonavir include significant nausea/vomiting and diarrhea. It is recommended that this drug be taken with a large meal to decrease diarrhea and cramping.

Circumoral paresthesias and peripheral paresthesias. Other less frequent side effects include circumoral paresthesias (for up to five weeks), peripheral paresthesias, taste perversion, and hepatitis.

Hypermenorrhea. Four cases of hypermenorrhea associated with the use of ritonavir have been reported (235).

Hypertriglyceridemia and pancreatitis. Pancreatitis due to a ritonavir-induced hypertriglyceridemia in a HIV-patient has been reported (236).

Maculopapular eruption and fever. Occasionally, a few days after treatment was initiated, maculopapular eruption and fever have been reported (237). In some cases clinical improvement occurred despite continuation of therapy, while in others treatment was stopped.

Ingrown toenails. Ingrown toenails are associated with indinavir/ritonavir combination therapy (238).

Hyperparathyroidism, osteopenia, and bone pain. Ritonavir has been implicated in in vitro studies in which ritonavir, nelfinavir, and indinavir have an effect on vitamin D metabolism and differentiation of osteocytes (239). Extreme bone pain has been reported, possibly as an idiosyncratic reaction to ritonavir (240). Calcium inhibition has been reported by others and may result in children on ritanovir experiencing impaired growth (241,242).

Special Considerations

Drug interactions. Ritonavir is associated with numerous drug interactions and adverse effects, which have limited its widespread use. It is a considerably strong inhibitor of the cytochrome P450 system, which leads to increased serum levels of other hepatically metabolized drugs. Therefore, coadministration with carbamazepines should not occur. Ritonavir has been associated with carbamazepine toxicity (243).

Coadministration with cisapride, terfenadine, astemizole, antiarrythmics (e.g., quinidine, amiodarone, encainide, and flecainide), and certain sedative/hypnotics. Because of potential serious and life-threatening reactions, the use of ritonavir is contraindicated with the following: cisapride, terfenadine, astemizole, certain antiarrythmics (e.g., quinidine, amiodarone, encainide, and flecainide), and certain sedative/hypnotics (e.g., midazolam, diazepam, triazolam, and flurazepam).

Coadministration with the tuberculosis drugs rifampin and rifabutin. Rifampin decreases the blood plasma levels of protease inhibitors by 80%. Rifabutin is expected to decrease the level of interaction by only 32%. Patients taking tuberculosis drugs concomitantly with ritanovir should be monitored for liver function as both drugs have a tendency to cause severe liver toxicity (244).

Coadministration of budesonide and ritonavir. Budesonide is metabolized by cytochrome P-450 3A and is 90% eliminated by first-pass hepatic clearance. When combined with ritanovir, the metabolism of budesonide is reduced as the cytochrome P-450 3A is inhibited by ritanovir. This might cause bedesonide to accumulate and cause acute hepatitis, as has been reported in one patient (245).

Sexual dysfunction. Ritonavir is significantly associated with sexual dysfunction in men when compared with indinavir, nelfinavir, and saquinavir. The latter three were also associated with sexual dysfunction but were not statistically significant (246).

Patient compliance and virologic potency. Conventional dosing of ritonavir (400–600 mg twice daily) can result in high rates of intolerance. A study of lower doses of ritonavir supports the use of low-dose ritonavir to improve the activity of current PIs in twice-daily regimens. The relative efficacy of ritonavir combined with other PIs has not been profiled (247).

Indinavir [IDV] (Crixivan®)

Also approved in March 1996, indinavir (IDV) (when combined with zidovudine and lamivudine) reduces viral loads to undetectable levels after 16 weeks of therapy in approximately 90% of patients (248). The structure of indinavir, brand names, and uses are shown in Fig. 2.16. Indinavir is taken

Generic Name Indinavir Brand Name Crixivan Other Name(s) IDV	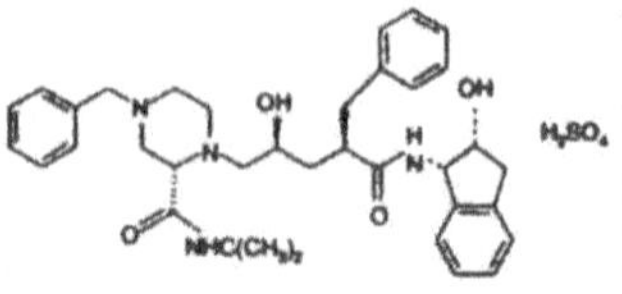 Structure	Viral Diseases Treated HIV-1 HIV-2

Fig. 2.16   Trade names, structure, and uses of Indinavir.

orally on an empty stomach, either one hour before a meal or two hours after a meal with at least eight ounces of water. For those who experience a stomach upset with indinavir, it may be taken with a light meal, but grapefruit juice should not be coadministered. Patients should drink at least 48 ounces of water or other liquids every 24 hours. Indinavir has a significant number of adverse effects associated with it. For example, the administration of combination antiretroviral prophylaxis for healthy individuals with nonoccupational exposure to HIV resulted in those receiving zidovudine and lamivudine with indinavir being more likely to experience nausea, rash, anorexia, insomnia, and abdominal pain. Two of the 16 patients experienced nephrolithiasis or toxic hepatitis (249).

Adverse Events

Like ritonavir, saquinavir, nelfinavir, and delavirdine, indinavir is a potent inhibitor of the cytochrome P450 pathway, resulting in similar drug interactions and contraindications.

Nephrolithiasis. Due to the poor solubility of indinavir in urine, nephrolithiasis was reported in 9% of clinical trial subjects on indinavir (48). In some cases, renal insufficiency or acute renal failure have developed. Individuals at greater risk for nephrolithiasis include those with a low body mass index or those receiving trimethoprim/sulfamethoxazole prophylaxis (250). The risk for all patients can be minimized by adequate oral hydration.

Lipodystrophy. Women are more at risk to develop lipodystrophy than men, and this risk increases with age and increasing exposure to antiretroviral therapy. The duration of indinavir use, in particular, may represent an additional contribution for the development of lipodystrophy with a tendency for central obesity (251).

Crystalluria. Patients treated with indinavir are often prone to precipitate and form deposits inside cortical and medullary ducts with later development of kidney stones in 4 to 12% of patients. This may be alleviated by reducing the drug dosage or by drug withdrawal. Crystalluria may be used as a monitor for the risk of urolithiasis. Crytalluria is found in 20–67% of indinavir-treated patients (252).

Homocysteinemia. Protease-inhibitors tend to cause homocysteinaemia which can be an increased risk for cardiovascular risk and for accelerated atherosclerosis (253).

Diabetes and hyperglycemia. Blood glucose levels may rise in patients who are prescribed PIs (254). The prevalence of fat atrophy and fat accumulation can be characterized by using several signs of body fat loss or gain. For the fat atrophy group these are: fat loss in the extremities, fat loss in the hips/buttocks, and sunken cheeks. Signs for the fat accumulation group are: enlarged abdomen, other facial structure changes, and presence of a dorsal cervical fat pad (255).

Renal atrophy. Hanabusa et al. reported two cases of HIV-positive patients on prolonged indinavir treatment who developed renal atrophy (256).

Pharyngitis.

Gastrointestinal upset.

Hemolytic anemia. Reported rarely.

Hyperbilirubinemia. Indinavir therapy is associated with a 6–25% incidence of asymptomatic, unconjugated hyperbilirubinemia (257,258). Mechanistic studies in rats indicate that hyperbilirubinemia is due to indinavir-mediated impairment of bilirubin-conjugating activity (259).

Gilbert's syndrome. Gilbert's syndrome is a benign, inherited condition of deficient bilirubin conjugation, occurring in 5 to 10% of the general population. Gilbert's genotype is associated with a 50% reduction in bilirubin-conjugation activity in homozygotes (260).

Rash. An erythematous, maculopapular skin eruption frequently occurs within two weeks of initiating therapy with indinavir. The rash usually begins in a localized area and then spreads to other regions of the body, often with associated pruritus. Most patients are able to continue therapy despite this skin eruption.

Paronychia of the large toes. Bouscarat et al. (261) have also described 42 HIV-infected patients on indinavir who developed hypertrophic paronychia of the great toes, many with pyogenic granuloma-like lesions. This number represented 4% of their total patients on indinavir therapy.

Xerosis and alopecia. Other cutaneous side effects of indinavir include xerosis and alopecia (262).

Stevens-Johnson syndrome. There has been one report of Stevens-Johnson syndrome caused by indinavir (263).

Erectile dysfunction. Homosexuality, CD4 cell count, viral load, and indinavir treatment are independent variables predictive of erectile dysfunction. Indinavir has been associated with peripheral neuropathy causing erectile dysfunction (264).

Special Considerations

Coadministration with acyclovir. Concomitant acyclovir nearly doubles the risk of indinavir-associated renal complications. In one study, events occurred in nearly 26% of the cases, many of which could have been avoided. Careful monitoring should be done if acyclovir is prescribed with indinavir (265).

Coadministration with other drugs. Many drugs either increase or decrease the amount of indinavir in the body and care must be taken to adjust dosages. Physicians should consult the available literature when prescribing PIs. Cannabinoids do not have any effect on antiretroviral efficacy (266).

Nelfinavir [NFV] (Viracept®)

FDA-approved in March 1997, nelfinavir (NFV) is a powerful and well-tolerated drug which is indicated in initial combination regimens for HIV therapy. The actual effect and mechanism of action for nelfinavir on the clinical progression of HIV infection have not been determined. The structure and brand names are given in Fig. 2.17. NFV causes potent and durable suppression of viral replication (like indinavir and ritonavir) when used in combination with two nucleoside analogues (267). If salvage antiretroviral treatment (when insufficient drug potency occurs, resistance develops, pharmacological issues arise, or poor adherence to other therapies occurs) is needed, a possible replacement for indinavir and ritonavir is nelfinavir combined with two nucleoside analogs (268). Nelfinavir is either a tablet or a powder to be taken orally, usually three times a day with a meal or a light snack. The powder can be added to a variety of liquids, including water, milk, formula, soy milk, or dietary supplements. All of the liquid must be consumed to obtain the maximum effect of the drug. Children can be given the oral powder with physicians determining the dosage for children under 2 years of age. Children 2–13 years of age are given doses of 20–30 mg/kg of body

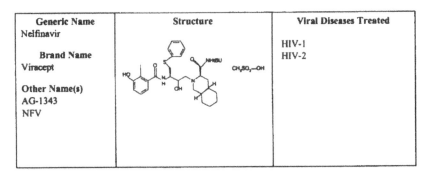

Generic Name Nelfinavir Brand Name Viracept Other Name(s) AG-1343 NFV	Structure	Viral Diseases Treated HIV-1 HIV-2

Fig. 2.17 Trade names, structure, and uses of Nelfinavir.

weight (9–13.6 mg/lb of body weight) three times a day with food. Adults and teenagers are usually given 750-mg tablets three times a day with food (269). Both nelfinavir and indinavir have no effect on accelerated bone loss (270).

Adverse Events

When compared with other PIs, nelfinavir has a more favorable side effect profile (138). The majority of its adverse effects are of mild intensity.

> **Diarrhea.** Diarrhea is the most common side effect, occurring in 13 to 20% of treated patients (138). This may be controlled symptomatically with the use of pancrelipase enzyme preparations.
>
> **Upset stomach, gas, or stomach pain.** These are usually mild symptoms, but patients may complain of severe symptoms or symptoms that do not go away.
>
> **Levels of blood sugar.** As with the other PIs, new-onset diabetes mellitus, hyperglycemia, and hypertriglyceridemia have been reported. Patients should be aware that more frequent urination, increased thirst, weakness, dizziness, and headaches may be a sign of developing diabetes. Nelfinavir may induce insulin resistance and activate basal lipolysis to contribute to the development of diabetes (271). Even with all the negative reports of nelfinavir usage on blood sugar levels, nelfinavir or nelfinavir/saquinavir combination therapy can used to replace ritonavir with the likelihood that lipid markers will improve over time. Cholesterol levels do not improve significantly and high-density lipoprotein (HDL) cholesterol may rise, but the most significant results are seen in the lowering of triglyceride levels (272).
>
> **Lipodystrophy syndrome and gynecomastia.** Changes in body fat are caused by a spectrum of clinical and metabolic abnormalities. These changes may also be responsible for gynecomastia and female breast hypertrophy. These two emerging effects of antiretroviral therapy may cause less adherence to drug therapy due

to cosmetic and psychological problems in patients (273). Bone marrow fat decreases with nelfinavir usage during antiretroviral therapy (274).

Hyperlipidemia. In children treated with protease inhibitors, hyperlipidemia has not been shown to increase the risk for development of cardiovascular disease (275).

Adhesive capsulitis of the shoulder. Adhesive capsulitis, occurring in the shoulder, can be one side-effect of nelfinavir therapy. This has been successfully treated by analgesic therapy with calcitonine and physiotherapy for passive mobilization of the shoulders (276).

Special Considerations

Coadministration with terfenadine, astemizole, cisapride, triazolam, and midazolam. Caution should be taken with coadministration with terfenadine, astemizole, cisapride, triazolam, and midazolam, because life-threatening arrhythmia or prolonged sedation may occur due to the inhibition of the cytochrome P450 pathway.

Genetic resistance. The primary mutation D30N was thought to be the main cause of nelfinavir resistance. In one study, 26 of 38 of patients who were nelfinavir-resistant had secondary mutations that affected nelfinavir resistance. The remaining two had only one direct mutational substitution (D30N) (277).

Although delta-9-tetrahydrocannabinol (THC) is administered orally as dronabinol to treat anorexia in AIDS patients, many patients elect to smoke marijuana for easier titration and, perhaps, better effect. Most patients use a cannabinoid to stimulate appetite and manage other antiretroviral side effects. Neither dronabinol nor marijuana is likely to impact PI antiretroviral efficacy (266).

Amprenavir [APV] (Agenerase®)

Amprenavir (APV) received FDA approval in April 1999 and is indicated for use in combination regimens with other

Generic Name Amprenavir Brand Name Agenerase Other Name(s) APV	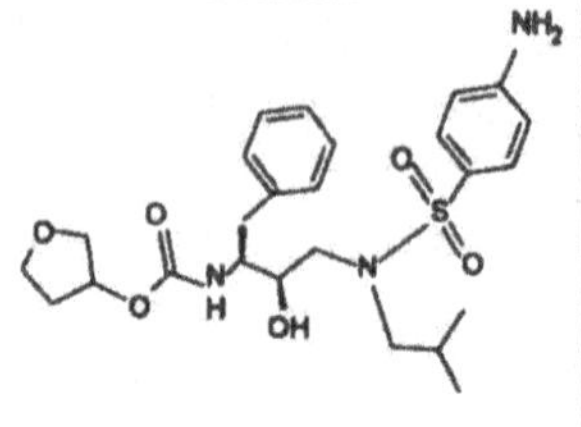 Structure	Viral Diseases Treated HIV-1 HIV-2

Fig. 2.18 Trade names, structure, and uses of Amprenavir.

antiretroviral agents. The chemical structure, brand names, and approved uses are shown in Fig. 2.18. Interestingly, amprenavir has been shown to lower virus levels in semen as well as in plasma. In addition, treatment in combination with two nucleoside analogues reduced viral loads to less than 400 copies/ml in 15 of 37 treated pediatric patients in phase III clinical trials. Researchers at the University of Texas Southwest Medical Center have found that HIV-infected patients taking PIs spend fewer days in the hospital and have lower overall health care costs, despite the high cost of PI treatment (278). Amprenavir has a long half-life which permits twice-daily dosing. It can be taken with or without food and does not require a liquid carrier. Amprenavir should be taken one hour before or one hour after taking antacids or didanosine. For adults, the dosage is 1200 mg twice daily. For patients who weigh less than 50 kg, the dosage is prescribed at 20 mg/kg twice daily for solid formulation or 1.5 ml/kg twice daily for the liquid formulation. The simplicity of dosage may be helpful in increasing patient compliance in taking the antiretroviral regimen. Preclinical and clinical data indicate that amprenavir is unlikely to cause metabolic disturbances such as lipid and glucose abnormalities and fat redistribution. In addition, there is a distinct resistance profile that permits both naïve and experienced PI users to take amprenavir (279).

Adverse Events

Grade four toxicity levels occurred for elevated serum creatine phosphokinase levels in 2.8% of patients; elevated triglycerides in 2.4% of patients; and neutropenia in 2.2% of patients. These are low numbers when compared with other antiretrovirals, and amprenavir is considered to have an acceptable safety profile and is generally well-tolerated with other antiretroviral regimens (279). Patients should not drink alcoholic beverages when taking oral amprenavir.

The other chief side effects of amprenavir are usually mild to moderate in intensity and include:

> **Perioral paresthesias.** Some patients experience a tingling sensation around the mouth.
> **Diarrhea.** Up to 9% of patients reported diarrhea (279).
> **Headache.**
> **Nausea/vomiting.** Up to 13% of patients reported nausea; 6.7% reported vomiting (279).
> **Blood sugar levels.** Like other PIs, amprenavir has been associated with diabetes mellitus and hyperglycemia. Five percent of treated individuals developed grade three toxicity levels for elevated triglycerides.
> **Acute hemolytic anemia.**
> **Rash.** A maculopapular rash develops in 28% of patients, with or without pruritus.
> **Stevens-Johnson syndrome.** Severe skin reactions, such as Stevens-Johnson syndrome, have occurred in 1% of treated patients.
> **Neutropenia.** Grade three toxicity occurred in 3–4% of patients with grade three toxicity for neutropenia.

Special Considerations

> **Central nervous system toxicity.** Physicians should monitor patients who receive the oral solution of amprenavir for possible effects, including stupor, seizures, tachycardia, hemolysis, renal problems, and lactic acidosis. The liquid formulation of amprenavir is 55% propylene glycol that is used to achieve solubility of amprenavir, whereas the solid form only contains 5% propylene glycol. The liquid form should be used only when the amprenavir capsules or other PIs will not work with specific patients (280). There has been one reported case of

an HIV-positive patient who developed hallucinations, disorientation, buzzing in the ears, and vertigo when switching from indinavir/ritonavir therapy to amprenavir oral solution. Once removed from the therapy, he returned to normal (281).

Coadministration with grapefruit juice. Coadministration of amprenavir with grapefruit juice can reduce the maximum concentration of the drug when compared with administration with water. However, the concentration curve is not significantly challenged so the grapefruit juice does not clinically affect amprenavir pharmacokinetics (282).

Young children and pregnant women. Children under 4 years of age and pregnant women should not take amprenavir liquid.

Liver and kidney disease. Those patients with liver or kidney failure should not take liquid amprenavir.

Coadministration with disulfiram (Antabuse) or metronidazole (Flagyl). Oral amprenavir should not be prescribed for patients taking disulfiram or metronidazole.

Erectile dysfunction. Use of amprenavir with sildenafil (Viagra) may increase the retention of sildenafil in the body. This could result in low blood pressure, changes in vision, and penile erection lasting more than 4 hours.

Fosamprenavir (Lexiva, GW 433908)

Fosamprenavir is a water-soluble, calcium phosphate ester prodrug of amprenavir. It was approved by the FDA on October 20, 2003. The water solubility permits a reduction in pill size and count when compared with the parent compound, amprenavir. Fig. 2.19 shows the structure, nomenclature, and approved usage. By reducing the pill number and size, it is hoped that patient compliance will improve (283). Fosamprenavir combined with ritonavir is not inferior to lopinavir/ritonavir (Kaletra) in protease inhibitor-experienced patients and achieved viral loads below the limits of detection, even in

Generic Name	Structure	Viral Diseases Treated
Fosamprenavir **Brand Name** Lexiva Other Name(s) GW 433908	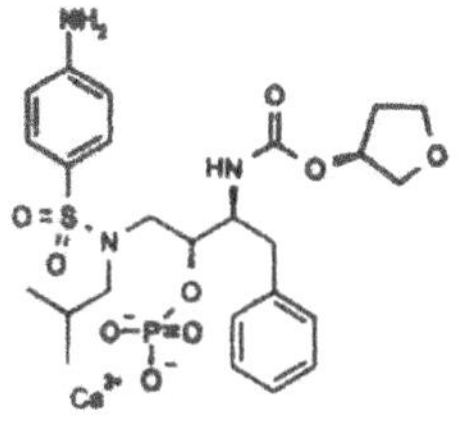	HIV-1

Fig. 2.19   Trade names, structure, and uses of Fosamprenavir.

patients with high viral RNA levels or low CD4+ counts (284). In treatment of naïve patients, fosamprenavir achieved better viral suppression than nelfinavir. Fosamprenavir appears to be suitable for first-line use as there is no indication that it is cross-resistant with other PIs (except amprenavir). Fosamprenavir is administered as 700-mg tablets. There are three recommended dosages for fosamprenavir: 1) 1400 mg twice daily for those not using ritonavir; 2) 1400 mg once daily plus ritonavir 200 mg daily; or 3) 700 mg daily plus ritonavir 100 mg daily. For protease inhibitor-experienced patients, the recommendation is 700 mg twice daily plus 100 mg of ritonavir twice daily. An additional 100 mg/day of ritonavir is recommended when efavirenz is administered with fosamprenavir/ritonavir once daily. The drug is rapidly hydrolyzed by cellular phosphatases in the gut epithelium during absorption. The absolute oral bioavailability of amprenavir from fosamprenavir administration has not been established. It has been proposed, however, that the development of water-soluble prodrugs of HIV-1 PIs have the potential to control the conversion time to the parent drug and to improve gastrointestinal absorption (285). Treatment-naïve HIV patients taking fosamprenavir once daily may have favorable increases in HDL cholesterol levels (286).

Adverse Events

Patients with known sulfonamide allergy or any patient who has demonstrated significant hypersensitivity to amprenavir should not use fosamprenavir. Most adverse events were moderate to mild during clinical studies and included:

Nausea. Nausea occurs in 61% of patients on amprenavir. For low and high doses of fosamprenavir, the occurrence was 31% and 55%, respectively.

Diarrhea. The frequency of diarrhea was nearly equal in both low and high dose treatments.

Rash. Nineteen percent of fosamprenavir patients experienced a rash. Most rashes are of moderate to mild intensity. Fewer than 1% developed severe or life threatening rash, including Stevens-Johnson syndrome. Medication should be discontinued in case of severe or life-threatening rash or moderate rash with accompanying systemic reactions.

Special Considerations

Fosamprenavir is contraindicated or should not be coadministered with a number of different types of drugs. Most of these recommendations are based upon prior severe events, known biochemical composition, and mechanisms of action of amprenavir and other related drugs.

Coadministration with amiodarone, systemic lidocaine, tricyclic antidepressants, and quinidine. Drug concentrations should be monitored if any of these are coadministered with fosamprenavir.

Coadministration with lovastatin or simvastatin. Fosamprenavir should not be used concomitantly with either lovastatin or simavastatin as the increased concentrations of statins may increase the risk of myopathy or rhabomyolysis. Other drugs that are dependent upon the CYP3A4 clearance pathway or may be associated with increased plasma concentrations that cause severe events should be avoided. These include the numerous ergot-based drugs, cisapride, pimozole, midazolam, and triazolam.

Coadministration with products containing St. John's wort. St John's wort is expected to substantially reduce drug plasma levels. This, in turn, may lead to loss of viral response to fosamprenavir and contribute to viral resistance to amprenavir or other PIs.

Coadministration with rifampin. Rifampin may reduce plasma concentrations of amprenavir by 90% when coadministered with fosamprenavir.

Fosamprenavir combined with ritonavir. Neither flecainide nor propafenone may be coadministered if ritonavir is coadministered with fosamprenavir.

Coadministration with sildenafil. Coadministration of any protease inhibitor with sildenafil will increase sildenafil concentrations which may cause hypotension, visual changes, and priapism.

Atazanavir (Reyataz, BMS-232632)

Atazanavir has been approved for use with two NRTIs to clinically reduce HIV viral load. Atazanavir is a novel azapeptide PI that specifically attacks and acts against the HIV-1 protease. It specifically inhibits the P450 hepatic cytochrome enzymes and interacts with several drugs. Figure 2.20 shows the nomenclature, structure, and usage of atazanavir. A benefit has been shown to last at least 48 weeks with no adverse effect on total cholesterol, LDL cholesterol or triglyceride levels after 108 weeks. In some cases, the lipid profile improved over the first 48 weeks of treatment (287–289). Atazanavir is administered once-daily orally (290).

Generic Name	Structure	Viral Diseases Treated
Atazanavir sulfate		HIV-1
Brand Name Reyataz		
Other Name(s) BMS-232632		

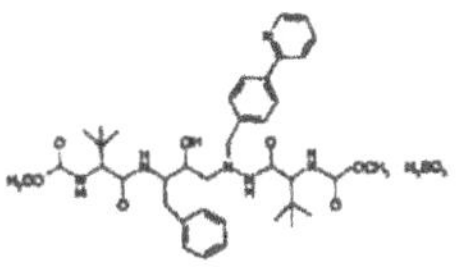

Fig. 2.20   Trade names, structure, and uses of Atazanavir.

Adverse Effects.

Atazanavir was recently released and there are few reports of concerns or events from individual physicians.

Diarrhea. Diarrhea occurs in 23–30% of patients who take atazanavir as compared with 60% of patients who take nelfinavir.

Jaundice. Jaundice can occur in those who take atazanavir.

Lopinavir + Ritonavir [ABT-378/r] (Kaletra®)

On September 18, 2000, the FDA approved the combination coformulation of two PIs, ritonavir and lopinavir (Kaletra®), also know as ABT-378/r, for the treatment of HIV infection in adults and children 6 months and older in combination with other antiretroviral medications. The antiviral activity of ABT-378/r is mostly attributable to lopinavir, not ritonavir. Figure. 2.21 shows the nomenclature, structure, and approved usage for lopinavir. ABT-378/r takes advantage of the ability of ritonavir to boost the levels of other PIs, creating a potent anti-HIV combination. ABT-378/r is to be used in conjunction with other antiretrovirals for the treatment of HIV infection. ABT-378/r is available in capsules and solution. A 400/100 mg/5 ml lopinavir/ritonavir solution should be given twice daily. The capsules contain 133.3/33.3 mg lopinavir/ritonavir, and three capsules should be taken twice a day.

Generic Name Lopinavir Brand Name Kaletra (lopinavir + ritonavir) Other Name(s) ABT-378/r Aluviran	Structure	Viral Diseases Treated
		HIV-1 HIV-2

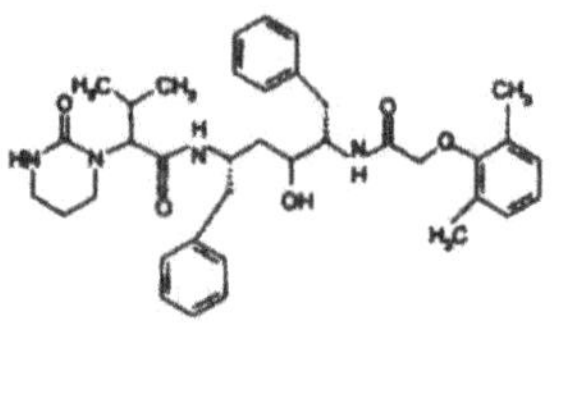

Fig. 2.21   Trade names, structure, and uses of Lopinavir.

Adverse Events

Multiple severe toxicities involving the kidney have been reported in persons taking Kaletra, tenofovir, and didanosine concurrently (291).

The most common adverse effects are gastrointestinal.

Diarrhea. Diarrhea is described as usually moderately severe in 10–20% of patients.

Triglyceride and cholesterol levels. Significant increases in triglyceride and cholesterol levels have been seen in 12–14% of patients receiving ABT-378/r.

Cutaneous side effects. Cutaneous side effects have yet to be reported.

Special Considerations

Coadministration of Kaletra and phenytoin. Phenytoin (dilantin) and Kaletra levels are reduced by one another. In PI-experienced patients, the dosage of Kaletra may need to be increased (292).

FUSION INHIBITORS

Fusion inhibitors are included in the general group of entry inhibitors. Entry inhibitors bind to specific proteins and prevent HIV from entering otherwise healthy cells. A diagram of this mechanism is shown in Fig. 2.2. The currently approved fusion inhibitor, enfuvirtide, appears to interact with biological membranes, based on the molecular sequence and the eventual arrangement in an alpha helix. Enfuvirtide, however, does not form the alpha helix when binding to membranes. Instead, it remains in a random-coil conformation when inserted into the membranes. Enfuviritide enters the external layer of the plasmalemma and cannot translocate due to the negatively charged lipids of the inner layer. When HIV tries to enter the cell, the virus lipidic membrane cannot remove the enfuvirtide from the outer cell surface. The high cholesterol content and the concentration of

enfuvirtide effect a barrier to penetration by the HIV particle (293,294).

Fusion inhibitors have an advantage over the other anti-
HIV drugs in that many patients develop resistance to PIs,
NRTIs, and/or NNRTIs. Because entry inhibitors are a different class of drugs, it is thought that this type of resistance will
not develop in entry inhibitors. It is predicted in the future
that optimal treatment of HIV infection will require various
combinations of drugs that attack novel stages of HIV-1 entry
and replication (295–297).

Enfuvirtide (ENF, T-20, pentafuside, Fuzeon)

Enfuvirtide blocks the ability of HIV to infect healthy CD4
cells. When used with other antiretrovirals, the amount of
HIV RNA in the blood lowers and the number of CD4 cells
increases (298). Enfuvirtide protects CD4 T cells from envelope presentation and therefore inhibits virus replication
and blocks HIV-1 envelope-induced cell death. This protection could lead to a better immune restoration of HIV-1-
infected patients treated with enfuvirtide (299). Figure 2.22
shows the structure, brand name, and usage for enfuvirtide.
Enfuvirtide is not approved for use by itself—it must be combined with other antiretrovirals and the choice of these antivirals is between the patient and physician, based on each

Generic Name Enfuvirtide	Structure	Viral Diseases Treated
Brand Name Fuzeon		HIV-1
Other Name(s) ENF, T-20		

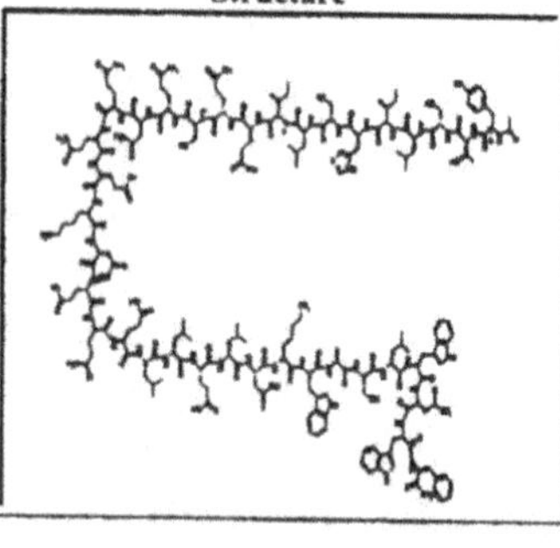

Fig. 2.22 Trade names, structure, and uses of Enfuvirtide.

individual patient's circumstances. Enfuvirtide will most likely be used as "salvage" therapy, replacements for other antiretrovirals to which the HIV has become resistant. Because resistance in one class of drugs does not equate to resistance in another class of drugs, enfuvirtide has been heralded as a great breakthrough in HIV/AIDS therapy. However, relegation of the drug to "salvage" therapy is probably not the best approach in that it is least likely to work with seriously immunocompromised individuals. Instead, the drug should become a replacement therapy earlier in the drug regimen process, probably combined with an NNRTI, one or two PIs, and nucleoside/nucleotide analogs, based on susceptibility (300). Enfuvirtide provides significant viral suppression and immunologic benefit over a 24-week period in HIV-infected patients who had previously received multiple antiretroviral drugs (301,302). In one laboratory study, all viral isolates known to provide genetic resistance to more common antiretrovirals were sensitive to enfuvirtide (303). For clinical trials, enfuvirtide was injected or delivered intravenously with the intermittent injections being superior to continuous infusions (304). In some patients, the benefit was short-lived, suggesting the development of resistance (305). Pharmacokinetics studies indicate that the absorption process is complex and that enfuvirtide is completely absorbed when subcutaneously injected abdominally (306). In that enfurvirtide is newly approved, many side effects have not yet been documented.

Adverse Events

Injection site reactions. Minor injection site reactions are frequent, but are rarely treatment limiting and include redness, itching, hardened skin, tenderness, bruising, and swelling (307).

Serious allergic reactions. For those who may be allergic to any of the ingredients in enfuvirtide, serious allergic reactions can occur. These include difficulty breathing, fever with vomiting, hematuria, and swelling of feet. Patients should seek immediate medical help if any of these symptoms occur.

Special Considerations

Patient compliance. Acceptance of enfuvirtide by patients appears to be low because of the two abdominal injections/day for administration of the drug and the high cost of the drug per patient per year ($\sim$\$14,000–\$20,000)(308). Auto-injection devices are being explored as are multidose vials to serve as near-term modifications. An oral enfuvirtide is years from becoming a reality (309). Patient issues with injections may be resolved through better training of nurses for better patient comprehension and an effective nurse-patient relationship (310,311).

Other side effects. Some of the other side effects of enfuvirtide include: pain or numbness in feet or legs, loss of sleep, depression, decreased appetite, weakness or loss of strength, muscle pain, constipation, and pancreatitis.

Bacterial pneumonia. Although bacterial pneumonia is not common among patients taking enfuvirtide, more patients on enfuvirtide developed bacterial pneumonia than those who were not on enfuvirtide (312).

INVESTIGATIONAL DRUGS

At the time of this writing, there are 23 new antiretroviral agents under current development and study. Five nucleoside analogues, six NNRTIs and seven PIs show promise based on early study results. New classes of antiretroviral drugs are currently under investigation, with possible alternative mechanisms for effective therapy against HIV. Zintevir (AR177) is the main compound under development as an integrase inhibitor (313). In vitro, this compound is a potent inhibitor of the HIV integrase enzyme, but its in vivo actions have yet to be confirmed.

Four different fusion inhibitor compounds are currently undergoing evaluation.

CONCLUSION

As the population of HIV-infected individuals increases, the need for better access to antiretroviral therapy becomes more critical. In countries where HAART is available, however, the role of the physician has expanded from therapy of HIV and associated opportunistic infections to include the adverse effects of antiretroviral therapy, drug resistance, and noncompliance. Not only will it be necessary to be aware of these limitations of HAART, it will also be necessary to be knowledgeable of drugs that are incompatible with antiretroviral agents. Since there are now more than 20 FDA-approved antiretroviral drugs, many available in combination tablets and capsules, and many more antiretroviral drugs in clinical trials, therapy of HIV disease is constantly in evolution. Therefore, it is imperative that physicians be aware of the following Web sites for HIV treatment information: www.medscape.com; www.iasusa.org; www.hivatis.org; www.retroconference.org; www.hopkins-aids. edu; and http://aidsinfo. nih.gov.

The collection of antiretroviral medications is in a constantly changing state, due to the rapid and exciting advances in HIV therapy. While five classes of antiretroviral drugs are now the mainstay of therapy, new groups of drugs are currently under development and investigation in order to inhibit HIV through additional mechanisms. Combination therapy regimens using drugs from two or more separate classes have proven to be more effective in delaying both the progression of HIV infection and the development of resistant viruses.

Although antiretroviral drugs have led to decreased morbidity and mortality for the less than 5% of the world that can afford them, they have produced no cures. Hope for control of the epidemic lies in public health measures such as abstinence/safer sex, condoms, testing of blood products, elimination of sharing of needles, education, and the development of vaccines to prevent HIV infection.

REFERENCES

1. AIDS epidemic update, December 2003, WHO/UNAIDS. Available at http://www.unaids.org/wac/2000/wad00/files/WAD_epidemic_report.html. Accessed January 5, 2003.

2. Coldiron, B.M., and P.R. Bergstresser. 1988. Prevalence and clinical spectrum of skin disease in patients infected with human immunodeficiency virus. *Arch. Dermatol.* 125:357–361.

3. Tschachler, E., P.R. Bergstresser, and G. Stingl. 1996. HIV-related skin diseases. *Lancet* 348:659–663.

4. Schwartz, J.J., and P.L. Myskowski. 1992. Molluscum contagiosum in patients with human immunodeficiency virus infection: A review of twenty-seven patients. *J. Am. Acad. Dermatol.* 27:583–588.

5. Cockerell, C.J., and P.E. LeBoit. 1990. Bacillary angiomatosis: A newly characterized, pseudoneoplastic, infectious, cutaneous vascular disorder. *J. Am. Acad. Dermatol.* 22:501–512.

6. Cockerell, C.J., M.A. Whitlow, G.F. Webster, and A.E. Friedman. 1987. Epithelioid angiomatosis: A distinct vascular disorder in patients with the acquired immunodeficiency syndrome or AIDS-related complex. *Lancet* 2:654–656.

7. Ray, M.C., and L.E. Gately, III. 1994. Dermatologic manifestations of HIV infection and AIDS. *Infect. Dis. Clin. N. Am.* 8:583–605.

8. Rosenthal, D., P.E. LeBoit, L. Klumpp, and T.G. Berger. 1991. Human immunodeficiency virus-associated eosinophilic folliculitis: A unique dermatosis associated with advanced human immunodeficiency virus infection. *Arch. Dermatol.* 127:206–209.

9. Sack, J.B. 1990. Disseminated infection due to *Mycobacterium fortuitum* in a patient with AIDS. *Rev. Infect. Dis.* 12:961–963.

10. Stack, R.J., L.K. Bickley, and I.G. Coppel. 1990. Miliary tuberculosis presenting as skin lesions in a patient with the acquired immune deficiency syndrome. *J. Am. Acad. Dermatol.* 23:1031–1035.

11. Straus, W.L., S.M. Ostroff, D.B. Jernigan, T.E. Kiehn, E.M. Sordillo, D. Armstrong, N. Boone, N. Schneider, J.O. Kilburn, V.A. Silcox, et al. 1994. Clinical and epidemiologic characteristics of *Mycobacterium haemophilum*, an emerging pathogen in immunocompromised patients. *Ann. Intern. Med.* 120:118–25.

12. Detels, R., A. Munoz, G. McFarlane, L.A. Kingsley, J.B. Margolick, J. Giorgi, L.K. Schrager, and J.P. Phair. 1998. Effectiveness of potent antiretroviral therapy on time to AIDS and death in men with known HIV infection duration. Multicenter AIDS Cohort Study Investigators. *J.A.M.A.* 280:1497–1503.

13. Shafer, R.W., L.M. Smeaton, G.K. Robbins, V. De Gruttola, S.W. Snyder, R. D'Aquila, et al. 2003. Comparison of four-drug regimens and pairs of sequential three-drug regimens as initial therapy for HIV-1 infection. *N. Engl. J. Med.* 349:2304–2315.

14. Robbins, G.K., V. De Gruttola, R.W. Shafer, L.M. Smeaton, S.W. Snyder, C. Pettinelli, et al. 2003. Comparison of sequential three-drug regimens as initial therapy for HIV-1 infection. *N. Engl. J. Med.* 349:2293–2303.

15. Carpenter, C.C., M.A. Fischl, S.M. Hammer, M.S. Hirsch, D.M. Jacobsen, D.A. Katzenstein, J.S. Montaner, D.D. Richman, M.S. Saag, R.T. Schooley, M.A. Thompson, S. Vella, P.G. Yeni, and P.A. Volberding. 1997. Antiretroviral therapy for HIV infection in 1997: Updated recommendations of the International AIDS Society—USA panel. *J.A.M.A.* 277:1962–1969.

16. Rosenthal, T. 1999. Efavirenz added to treatment guidelines for children. *Infect. Dis. Child.* 12:11–13.

17. Havlir, D.V., I.C. Marschner, M.S. Hirsch, A.C. Collier, P. Tebas, R.L. Bassett, J.P. Ioannidis, M.K. Holohan, R. Leavitt, G. Boone, and D.D. Richman. 1998. Maintenance antiretroviral therapies in HIV infected patients with undetectable plasma HIV RNA after triple-drug therapy. AIDS Clinical Trials Group Study 343 Team. *N. Engl. J. Med.* 339:1261–1268.

18. Pialoux, G., F. Raffi, F. Brun-Vezinet, V. Meiffredy, P. Flandre, J.A. Gastaut, P. Dellamonica, P. Yeni, J.F. Delfraissy, and J.P. Aboulker. 1998. A randomized trial of three maintenance regimens given after three months of induction therapy with zidovudine, lamivudine, and indinavir in previously untreated HIV-1 infected patients. Trilege (Agence Nationale de Recherches sur le SIDA 072) Study Team. *N. Engl. J. Med.* 339: 1269–1276.

19. Shafer, R.W., and D.A. Vuitton. 1999. Highly active antiretroviral therapy (HAART) for the treatment of infection with human immunodeficiency virus type 1. *Biomed. Pharmacother.* 53:73–86.

20. Furtado, M.R., D.S. Callaway, J.P. Phair, K.J. Kunstman, J.L. Stanton, C.A. Macken, A.S. Perelson, and S.M. Wolinsky. 1990 Persistence of HIV-1 transcription in peripheral-blood mono-nuclear cells in patients receiving potent antiretroviral activity. *N. Engl. J. Med.* 340:1614–1622.

21. Zhang, H., G. Dornadula, M. Beumont, L. Livornese, Jr., B. Van Uitert, K. Henning, and R.J. Pomerantz. 1998. Human immu-nodeficiency virus type 1 in the semen of men receiving highly active antiretroviral therapy. *N. Engl. J. Med.* 339:1803–1809.

22. Zhang, L., B. Ramratnam, K. Tenner-Racz, Y. He, M. Vesanen, S. Lewin, A. Talal, P. Racz, A.S. Perelson, B.T. Korber, M. Markowitz, and D.D. Ho. 1999. Quantifying residual HIV-1 replication in patients receiving combination antiretroviral therapy. *N. Engl. J. Med.* 340:1605–1613.

23. Cardo, D.M., D.H. Culver, C.A. Ciesielski, P.U. Srivastava, R. Marcus, D. Abiteboul, J. Heptonstall, G. Ippolito, F. Lot, P.S. McKibben, and D.M. Bell. 1997. A case-control study of HIV seroconversion in health care workers after percutane-ous exposure. Centers for Disease Control and Prevention Needlestick Surveillance Group. *N. Engl. J. Med.* 337:1485–1490.

24. Centers for Disease Control and Prevention. 1995. Case-control study of HIV seroconversion in health-care workers after per-cutaneous exposure to HIV-infected blood—France, United Kingdom, and United States, January 1988–August 1994. *M.M.W.R.* 44:929–933.

25. Centers for Disease Control and Prevention. 1998. Public Health Service Guidelines for the Management of Health-Care Worker Exposures to HIV and Recommendations for Postexpo-sure Prophylaxis. *M.M.W.R.* 47(No. RR-7):1–28.

26. Connor, E.M., R.S. Sperli.ng, R. Gelber, P. Kiselev, G. Scott, M.J. O'Sullivan, R. VanDyke, M. Bey, W. Shearer, R.L. Jacobson, et al. 1994. Reduction of maternal-infant transmission of human immunodeficiency virus type 1 with zidovudine treatment. *N. Engl. J. Med.* 331:1173–1180.

27. Sperling, R.S., D.E. Shapiro, R.W. Coombs, J.A. Todd, S.A. Herman, G.D. McSherry, M.J. O'Sullivan, R.B. Van Dyke, E. Jimenez, C. Rouzioux, P.M. Flynn, and J.L. Sullivan. 1996. Maternal viral load, zidovudine treatment, and the risk of

transmission of human immunodeficiency virus type 1 from mother to infant. Pediatric AIDS Clinical Trials Group Protocol 076 Study Group. *N. Engl. J. Med.* 335:1621–1629.

28. Centers for Disease Control and Prevention. 1998. Public Health Service task force recommendations for the use of antiretroviral drugs in pregnant women infected with HIV-1 for maternal health and for reducing perinatal HIV-1 transmission in the United States. *M.M.W.R.* 47(No. RR-2):1–30.

29. Mofenson, L.M. 1999. Short-course zidovudine for prevention of perinatal infection [commentary]. *Lancet* 353:766–777.

30. Wiktor, S.Z., E. Ekpini, J.M. Karon, J. Nkengasong, C. Maurice, S.T. Severin, T.H. Roels, M.K. Kouassi, E.M. Lackritz, I.M. Coulibaly, and A.E. Greenberg. 1999. Short-course oral zidovudine for prevention of mother-to-child transmission of HIV-1 in Abidjan, Cote d'Ivoire: A randomised trial. *Lancet* 353:781–785.

31. Dabis, F., P. Msellati, N. Meda, C. Welffens-Ekra, B. You, O. Manigart, V. Leroy, A. Simonon, M. Cartoux, P. Combe, A. Ouangre, R. Ramon, O. Ky-Zerbo, C. Montcho, R. Salamon, C. Rouzioux, P. Van de Perre, and L. Mandelbrot. 1999. Six-month efficacy, tolerance, and acceptability of a short regimen of oral zidovudine to reduce vertical transmission of HIV in breastfed children in Cote d'Ivoire and Burkina Faso: A double-blind placebo-controlled multicentre trial. *Lancet* 353:786–792.

32. Shaffer, N., R. Chuachoowong, P.A. Mock, C. Bhadrakom, W. Siriwasin, N.L. Young, T. Chotpitayasunondh, S. Chearskul, A. Roongpisuthipong, P. Chinayon, J. Karon, T.D. Mastro, and R.J. Simonds. 1999. Short-course zidovudine for perinatal transmission in Bangkok, Thailand: A randomised controlled trial. *Lancet* 353:773–780.

33. Musoke, P., L.A. Guay, D. Bagenda, M. Mirochnick, C. Nakabiito, T. Fleming, T. Elliott, S. Horton, K. Dransfield, J.W. Pav, A. Murarka, M. Allen, M.G. Fowler, L. Mofenson, D. Hom, F. Mmiro, and J.B. Jackson. 1999. Phase I/II study of the safety and pharmacokinetics of nevirapine in HIV-1-infected pregnant Ugandan women and their neonates (HIVNET006). *AIDS* 13:479–486.

34. Centers for Disease Control and Prevention. 1998. Report of the NIH Panel to define principles of therapy of HIV Infection and guidelines for the use of antiretroviral agents in HIV-infected adults and adolescents. *M.M.W.R.* 47(No. RR-5):1–32.

35. Mellors, J.W., A. Muñoz, J.V. Giorgi, J.B. Margolick, C.J. Tassoni, P. Gupta, L.A. Kingsley, J.A. Todd, A.J. Saah, R. Detels, J.P. Phair, and C.R. Rinaldo Jr. 1997. Plasma viral load and CD4+ lymphocytes as prognostic markers of HIV-1 infection. *Ann. Intern. Med.* 126:946–954.

36. Fischl, M.A., D.D. Richman, M.H. Grieco, M.S. Gottlieb, P.A. Volberding, O.L. Laskin, J.M. Leedom, J.E. Groopman, D. Mildvan, R.T. Schooley, et al. 1987. The efficacy of azidothymidine (AZT) in the treatment of patients with AIDS and AIDS-related complex. A double-blind, placebo-controlled trial. *N. Engl. J. Med.* 317:185–191.

37. Fischl, M.A., D.D. Richman, N. Hansen, A.C. Collier, J.T. Carey, M.F. Para, W.D. Hardy, R. Dolin, W.G. Powderly, J.D. Allan, et al. 1990. The safety and efficacy of zidovudine (AZT) in the treatment of subjects with mildly symptomatic human immunodeficiency virus type 1 (HIV) infection. A double-blind, placebo-controlled trial. The AIDS Clinical Trials Group. *Ann. Intern. Med.* 112:727–737.

38. Volberding, P.A., S.W. Lagakos, M.A. Koch, C. Pettinelli, M.W. Myers, D.K. Booth, H.H. Balfour, Jr., R.C. Reichman, J.A. Bartlett, M.S. Hirsch, et al. 1990. Zidovudine in asymptomatic human immunodeficiency virus infection: A controlled trial in persons with fewer than 500 CD4-positive cells per cubic millimeter. The AIDS Clinical Trials Group of the National Institute of Allergy and Infectious Diseases. *N. Engl. J. Med.* 322:941–949.

39. Larder, B.A., and S.D. Kemp. 1989. Multiple mutations in HIV-1 reverse transcriptase confer high-level resistance to zidovudine (AZT). *Science* 246:1155–1158.

40. Richman, D.D. 1993. Resistance of clinical isolates of human immunodeficiency virus to antiretroviral agents. *Antimicrob. Agents Chemother.* 37:1207–1213.

41. Blower, S. 2001. Transmission of zidovudine resistant strains of HIV-1: The first wave. *AIDS* 15:2317–2318.

42. Goudsmit, J., G.J. Weverling, L. Vanderoeek, A. deRonde, F. Miedema, R.A. Coutinho, J.M.A. Lang, and M.C. Boerlijst. 2001. Carrier rate of zidovudine-resistant HIV-1: The impact of failing therapy on transmission of resistant strains. *AIDS* 15:2293–2301.

43. Garcia-Lerma, J.G., S. Nidtha, K. Blumoff, H. Weinstock, and W. Heneine. 2001. Increased ability for selection of zidovudine resistance in a distinct class of wild-type HIV-1 from drug-naïve persons. *Proc. Natl. Acad. Sci. USA* 98:13907–13912.

44. Geretti, A.M., M. Smith, N. Osner, S. O'Shea, I. Chrystie, P. Easterbrook, and M. Zuckerman. 2001. Prevalence of antiretroviral resistance in a South London cohort of treatment-naïve HIV-1 infected patients. *AIDS* 15:1082–1084.

45. Briones, C., M. Perez-Olmeda, C. Rodriguez, J. del Romero, K. Hertogs, and V. Soriano. 2001. Primary genotypic and phenotypic HIV-1 drug resistance in recent seroconverters in Madrid. *J. AIDS* 26:145–150.

46. Kyriakides, T.C., and R.R. Heimer. 2001. Development and application of a genotypic AZT resistance assay. *J. AIDS* 28: 211–230.

47. Cho, Y.K., H. Sung, J.H. Lee, C.H. Joo, and G.J. Cho. 2001. Long-term intake of Korean red ginseng in HIV-1-infected patients: Development of resistance mutation to zidovudine is delayed. *Int. Immunopharmacol.* 1:1295–1305.

48. Chaudry, M.N., and D.H. Shepp. 1997. Antiretroviral agents: Current usage. *Dermatol. Clin.* 15:319–329.

49. Sales, S.D., P.G. Hoggard, D. Sunderland, S. Khoo, C.A. Hart, and D.J. Back. 2001. Zidovudine phosphorylation and mitochondrial toxicity in vitro. *Toxicol. Appl. Pharmacol.* 177:54–58.

50. Benveniste, O., J. Estaquier, J.D. Lelievre, J.L. Vilde, J.C. Ameisen, and C. Leport. 2001. Possible mechanism of toxicity of zidovudine by induction of apoptosis of CD4+ and CD8+ T-cells in vivo. *Eur. J. Clin. Microbiol. Infect. Dis.* 20:896– 897.

51. Aramideh, M., R.P. Koopmans, J.H.T.M. Koelman, and J. Stam. 2001. Rapidly progressing peripheral neuropathy with lactic acidosis and coproporphyria in a patient with HTLV-1 associated T-cell leukemia treated with zidovudine. *J. Neurol.* 248:621–622.

52. Carr, A., A. Morey, P. Mallon, D. Williams, and D.R. Thorburn, 2001. Fatal portal hypertension, liver failure, and mitochondrial dysfunction after HIV-1 nucleoside analogue-induced hepatitis and lactic acidaemia. *Lancet* 357:1412–1413.

53. Daniel, C.R. 1997. Pigmentation abnormalities. In: Scher, R.K., Daniel, C.R., eds. *Nails: Therapy, Diagnosis, Surgery,* 2nd ed. Philadelphia:W.B. Saunders, pp. 205, 257.

54. Duvic, M., M.M. Crane, M. Conant, S.E. Mahoney, J.D. Reveille, and S.N. Lehrman. 1994. Zidovudine improves psoriasis in human immunodeficiency virus-positive males. *Arch. Dermatol.* 130:447–451.

55. Fischer, T., H. Schworer, C. Vente, K. Reich, and G. Ramadori. 1999. Clinical improvement of HIV-associated psoriasis parallels a reduction of HIV viral load induced by effective antiretroviral therapy. *AIDS* 13:628–629.

56. Townsend, B.L., P.R. Cohen, and M. Duvic. 1995. Zidovudine for the treatment of HIV-negative patients with psoriasis: A pilot study. *J. Am. Acad. Dermatol.* 32:994–999.

57. Moore, R.D., J.C. Keruly, and R.E. Chaisson. 2001. Incidence of pancreatitis in HIV-infected patients receiving nucleoside reverse transcriptase inhibitor drugs. *AIDS* 15:617–620.

58. Siegel, K., H.-M. Lekas, E.W. Schrimshaw, and J.K. Johnson. 2001. Factors associated with HIV-infected women's use or intention to use AZT during pregnancy. *AIDS Educ. Prev.* 13:189–206.

59. Giaquinto, C.I., A. De Romeo, V. Giacomet, O. Rampon, E. Ruga, A. Burlina, A. De Rossi, M. Sturkenboom, and R. D'Elia. 2001. Lactic acid levels in children perinatally treated with antiretroviral agents to prevent HIV transmission. *AIDS* 15:1074– 1075.

60. Masquelier, B., M.L. Chaix, M. Burgard, J. Lechenadec, A. Doussin, F. Simon, J. Cottalorda, J. Izopet, C. Tamalet, D. Douard, H. Fleury, M.J. Mayaux, S. Blanche, and C. Rouzioux. 2001. Zidovudine genotypic resistance in HIV-1 infected newborns in the French perinatal cohort. French Pediatric HIV Infection Study Group. *J. AIDS* 27:99–104.

61. Collier, A.C., R.W. Coombs, M.A. Fischl, P.R. Skolnik, D. Northfelt, P. Boutin, C.J. Hooper, L.D. Kaplan, P.A. Volberding, L.G. Davis, et al. 1993. Combination therapy with zidovudine and didanosine compared with zidovudine alone in HIV-1 infection. *Ann. Intern. Med.* 119:786–793.

62. Eyer-Silva, W.A., I. Auto, J.F.C. Pinto, and C.A. Morais-de-Sa. 2001. Myelopathy in a previously asymptomatic HIV-1 infected patient. *Infection* 29:99–101.

63. Kahn, J.O., S.W. Lagakos, D.D. Richman, A. Cross, C. Pettinelli, S.H. Liou, M. Brown, P.A. Volberding, C.S. Crumpacker, G. Beall, et al. 1992. A controlled trial comparing continued zidovudine with didanosine in human immunodeficiency virus infection. The NIAID AIDS Clinical Trials Group. *N. Engl. J. Med.* 327:581–587.

64. Dalakas, M.C. 2001. Peripheral neuropathy and antiretroviral drugs. *J. Peripher. Nerv. Syst.* 6:14–20.

65. *Physicians' Desk Reference,* 57th ed. 2003. Montvale, NJ: Medical Economics/Thomson Healthcare.

66. Just, M., J.M. Carrascosa, M. Ribera, I. Bielsa, and C. Ferrandiz. 1997. Dideoxyinosine-associated Ofuji papuloerythroderma in an HIV infected patient. *Dermatology* 195:410–411.

67. Lafeuillade, K.A., G. Hittinger, and S. Chadapaud. 2001. Increased mitochondrial toxicity with ribavirin in HIV/HCV coinfection. *Lancet* 357:280–281.

68. Salmon-Ceron, D., L. Chauvelot-Moachon, S. Abad, B. Silbermann, and P. Sogni. 2001. Mitochondrial toxic effects and ribavirin [response]. *Lancet* 357:1802.

69. Kakuda, T.N., and K. Brinkman. 2001. Mitochondrial toxic effects and ribavirin. *Lancet* 357:1802–1803.

70. Griffith, B.P., H. Brett-Smith, G. Kim, J.W. Mellors, T.M. Chacko, R.B. Garner, Y.C. Cheng, P. Alcabes, and G. Friedland. 1996. Effect of stavudine on human immunodeficiency virus type 1 virus load as measured by quantitative mononuclear cell culture, plasmsa RNA, and immune complex-dissociated antigenemia. *J. Infect. Dis.* 173:1252–1255.

71. Shulman, N.S., R.A. Machekano, R.W. Shafer, M.A. Winters, A.R. Zolopa, S.H. Liou, M. Hughes, and D.A. Katzenstein. 2001. Genotypic correlates of a virologic response to stavudine after zidovudine monotherapy. AIDS Clinical Trials Group 302 Study Team. *J. AIDS* 27:377–380.

72. Morris, A.A.M., S.V. Baudouin, and M.H. Snow. 2001. Renal tubular acidosis and hypophosphataemia after treatment with nucleoside reverse transcriptase inhibitors. *AIDS* 15:140–141.

73. Carr, A., C. Workman, D.E. Smith, J. Hoy, J. Hudson, N. Doong, A. Martin, J. Amin, J. Freund, M. Law, and D. Cooper. 2002.

(for the Mitochondrial Toxicity (MITOX) Study Group. Abacavir substitution for nucleoside analogs in patients with HIV lipoatrophy. *J.A.M.A.* 288:207–215.

74. Mikhail, N. 2002. Insulin resistance and HIV-related lipoatrophy. Letter to the Editor. *J.A.M.A.* 288:1716.

75. Carr, A., and J. Amin. 2002. Reply. *J.A.M.A.* 288:1716.

76. Wooltorton, E. 2002. HIV drug stavudine (Zerit, d4T) and symptoms mimicking Guillain-Barre syndrome. *C.M.A.J.* 166:1067.

77. Idoko, J.A., L. Akinsete, A.D. Abalaka, L.B. Keshinro, L. Dutse, B. Onyenekwe, A. Lhekwaba, O.S. Njoku, M.O. Kehinde, and C.O. Wambebe. 2002. A multicentre study to determine the efficacy and tolerability of a combination of nelfinavir (VIRA-CEPT), zalcitabine (HIVID) and zidovudine in the treatment of HIV infected Nigerian patients. *West Afr. J. Med.* 21:83–86.

78. Katlama, C., J.L. Pellegrin, D. Lacoste, C. Aquilina, F. Raffi, G. Pialoux, D. Vittecoq, G. Raguin, O. Lantz, M. Mouroux, V. Calvez, A. Trylesinski, F. Montestruc, E. Dohin, J.M. Goehrs, and J.F. Delfraissy. 2001. MIKADO: A multicentre, open-label pilot study to evaluate the antiretroviral activity and safety of saquinavir with stavudine and zalcitabine. *HIV Med.* 2:20.

79. Vanhove, G.F., J.-M. Gries, D. Verotta, L.B. Sheiner, R. Coombs, A.C. Collier, and T.R. Blaschke. 1997. Exposure-response relationships for saquinavir, zidovudine, and zalcitabine in combination therapy. *Antimicrob. Agents Chemother.* 41:2433–2438.

80. Collier, A.C., R.W. Coombs, D.A. Schoenfeld, R.l. Bassett, J. Timpone, A. Baruch, M. Jones, K. Facey, C. Whitacre, V.J. McAuliffe, H.M. Friedman, T.C. Merigan, R.C. Reichman, C. Hooper, and L. Corey. 1996. Treatment of human immunodeficiency virus infection with saquinavir, zidovudine, and zalcitabine. AIDS Clinical Trials Group. *N. Engl. J. Med.* 334:1011–1017.

81. Gries, J.M., I.F. Troconiz, D. Verotta, M. Jacobson, and L.B. Sheiner. 1997. A pooled analysis of CD4 response to zidovudine and zalcitabine treatment in patients with AIDS and AIDS-related complex. *Clin. Pharmacol. Ther.* 61:70–82.

82. Akinsete, I., O.S. Njoku, C.C. Okanny, C.M. Chukwuani, and A.S. Akanmu. 2000. Management of HIV infection in Nigeria with zalcitabine in combination with saquinavir mesylate:

Preliminary findings. Hivid/Inverase Compassionate Programme Investigation Team. *West Afr. J. Med.* 19:265–268.

83. Aweeka, F.T., S.R. Brody, M. Jacobson, K. Botwin, and S. Martin-Munley. 1998. Is there a pharmacokinetic interaction between foscarnet and zalcitabine during comcomitant administration? *Clin. Ther.* 20:232–243.

84. Feng, J.F., A.A. Johnson, K.A. Johnson, and K.S. Anderson. 2001. Insights into the molecular mechanism of mitochondrial toxicity by AIDS Drugs. *J. Biol. Chem.* 276:23832–23837.

85. McNeely, M.C., R. Yarchoan, S. Broder, and T.J. Lawley. 1989. Dermatologic complications associated with administration of 2',3'-dideoxycytidine in patients with human immunodeficiency virus infection. *J. Am. Acad. Dermatol.* 21:1213–1217.

86. Indorf, A.S., and P.S. Pegram. 1992. Esophageal ulceration related to zalcitabine (ddC). *Ann. Intern. Med.* 117:133–134.

87. Tuntland, T., C. Nosbisch, and J.D. Unadkat. 1997. Effect of pregnancy, mode of administration and neonatal age on the pharmacokinetics of zalcitabine (2',3'-dideoxycytidine) in the pigtailed macaque (*Macaca nemestrina*). *J. Antimicrob. Chemother.* 40:687–693.

88. Bazunga, M., H.T. Tran, H. Kertland, M.S. Chow, and J. Masarella. 1998. The effects of renal impairment on the pharmacokinetics of zalcitabine. *J. Clin. Pharmacol.* 38:28–33.

89. van Nunen, A.B., H.L.A. Janssen, L.M.M. Wolters, H.G.M. Niesters, R.A deMan, and S.W. Schalm. 2001. Is combination therapy with lamivudine and interferon-alpha superior to monotherapy with either drug? *Antiviral Res.* 52:139–146.

90. Hogg, R.S., K.V. Heath, B. Yip, K.J. Craib, M.V. O'Shaughnessy, M.T. Schechter, and J.S. Montaner. 1998. Improved survival among HIV-infected individuals following initiation of antiretroviral therapy. *J.A.M.A.* 279:450–454.

91. Winston, A., and K. McLean. 2002. Recurrent hypersensitivity to combivir. *Int. J. STD AIDS* 13:213–214.

92. Wutzler, P., and R. Thust. 2001. Genetic risks of antiviral nucleoside analogues: A survey. *Antiviral Res.* 49:55–74.

93. Lai, C.L., M.F. Yuen, C.K. Hui, S. Garrido-Lestache, C.T. Cheng, and Y.P. Lai. 2002. Comparison of the efficacy of lamivudine and famciclovir in Asian patients with chronic hepatitis B: Results of 24 weeks of therapy. *J. Med. Virol.* 67:334–338.

94. Henry, K., R.J. Wallace, P.C. Bellman, D. Norris, R.L. Fisher, L.L. Ross, Q. Liao, and M.S. Shaefer. 2001. Twice-daily triple nucleoside intensification treatment with lamivudine-zidovudine plus abacavir sustains suppression of human deficiency virus type 1: Results of the TARGET group. TARGET Study Team. *J. Infect. Dis.* 183:571–178.

95. Ormseth, E.J., K.C. Holtzmuller, Z.D. Goodman, J.O. Colonna, D.S. Batty, and M.H. Sjogren. 2001. Hepatic decompensation associated with lamivudine: A case report and review of lamivudine-induced hepatotoxicity. *Am. J. Gastroenterol.* 96:1619–1622.

96. Kim, J.W., H.S. Lee, G.H. Woo, J.H. Yoon, J.J. Jang, J.G. Chi, and C.Y. Kim. 2001. Fatal submassive hepatic necrosis associated with tyrosine-muthionine-aspartate, aspartate-motif mutation of hepatitis B virus after long-term lamivudine therapy. *Clin. Infect. Dis.* 33:403–405.

97. Benhamou, Y., M. Bochet, V. Thibault, V. Calvez, M.H. Fievet, P. Vig, C.S. Gibbs, C. Brosgart, J. Fry, H. Namini, and C. Katlama. 2001. Safety and efficacy of adefovir dipivoxil in patients co-infected with HIV-1 and lamivudine-resistant hepatitis B virus: An open-label study. *Lancet* 358:718–723.

98. Kao, J.H., C.J. Liu, and D.S. Chen. 2002. Hepatitis B viral genotypes and lamivudine resistance. *J. Hepatol.* 36:303–305.

99. Petrelli, E., M. Balducci, C. Pierette, M.B.L. Rocchi, M. Clementi, and A. Manzin. 2001. Lamivudine treatment failure in preventing fatal outcome of de novo severe acute hepatitis B in patients with haematological diseases. *J. Hepatol.* 35: 823–826.

100. Paluge, S.M., S.S. Good, and W.H. Miller. 1998. Abacavir (1592), a second generation nucleoside HIV reverse transcriptase inhibitor. *Intl. Antiviral News* 6:7.

101. Harris, M., D. Back, S. Kewn, S. Jutha, R. Marina, and J.S.G. Montaner. 2002. Intracellular carbovir triphosphate levels in patients taking abacavir once a day. *AIDS* 16:1196–1197.

102. Fischl, M., F. Greenberg, N. Clumeck, B. Peters, R. Rubio, J. Gould, G. Boone, M. West, B. Spreen, and S. Lafon. 1999. Ziagen combined with 3TC and ZDV is highly effective and durable through 48 weeks in HIV-1 infected antiretroviral-therapy-naive subjects (CNAA3003). In: 6th International Conference on Retroviruses and Opportunistic Infections; Chicago, Illinois, January 31–February 4, 1999, #19, p. 70.

103. Kellener, K., J. Mellors, M. Lederman, et al. 1998. Activity of abacavir (1592) combined with protease inhibitors in therapy naïve patients. In: 12th World AIDS Conference; Geneva, Switzerland, June 28–July 3, 1998, #12210, p. 58.

104. Mellors, J., M. Lederman, D. Haas, J. Horton, R. Haubrich, J. Stanford, E. Cooney, S. Lafon, and D. Kelleher. 1999. Durable activity of Ziagen (abacavir, ABC) combined with protease inhibitors (PI) in therapy naïve adults. In: 6th Conference on Retroviruses and Opportunistic Infections; Chicago, Illinois, January 31–February 4, 1999, #625, p. 185.

105. Walter, H., B. Schmidt, M. Werwein, E. Schwingel, and K. Korn. 2002. Prediction of abacavir resistance from genotypic data: Impact of zidovudine and lamivudine resistance in vitro and in vivo. *Antimicrob. Agents Chemother.* 46:89–94.

106. Loeliger, A.E., H. Steel, S. McGuirk, W.S. Powell, and S.V. Hetherington. 2001. The abacavir hypersensitivity reaction and interruption in therapy. *AIDS* 15:1325.

107. Shapiro, M., K.M. Ward, and J.J. Stern. 2001. A near-fatal hypersensitivity reaction to abacavir: Case report and literature review. *AIDS* 11:222–226.

108. Hervey, P.S., and C.M. Perry. 2000. Abacavir: A review of its clinical potential in patients with HIV infection. *Drugs* 60:447–479.

109. Escaut, L., J.Y. Liotier, E. Albengres, N. Cheminot, and D. Vittecoq. 1999. Abacavir rechallenge has to be avoided in case of hypersensitivity reaction. *AIDS* 13:1419–1420.

110. Frissen, P.H., J. de Vries, H.M. Weigel, and K. Brinkman. 2001. Severe anaphylactic shock after rechallenge with abacavir without preceding hypersensitivity. *AIDS* 15:289.

111. Wit, F.W.N.M., R. Wood, A. Horban, M. Beniowski, R.E. Schmidt, G. Gray, A. Lazzarin, A. Lafeuillade, D. Paes, H. Carlier, L. van Wert, C. de Vries, R. van Leeuwen, and J.M.A.

Lange. 2001. Prednisolone does not prevent hypersensitivity reactions in antiretroviral drug regimens containing abacavir with or without nevirapine. *AIDS* 15:2423–2429.

112. Fantry, L.E., and H. Staecker. 2002. Vertigo and Abacavir (Case Report). *AIDS Patient Care STDs* 16:5–7.

113. Sankatsing, S.U.C., and J.M. Prins. 2001. Agranulocytosis and fever seven weeks after starting abacavir. *AIDS* 15:2464–2465.

114. Peyriere, H., J. Nocolas, M. Siffert, P. Demoly, D. Hillaire-Buys, and J. Reynes. 2001. Hypersensitivity related to abacavir in two members of a family. *Ann. Pharmacother.* 35:1291–1292.

115. Frissen, P.H.J., J. deVries, H.M. Weigel, and K. Brinkman. 2001. Severe anaphylactic shock after rechallenge with abacavir without preceding hypersensitivity. *AIDS* 15:289–292.

116. Loeliger, A.E., H. Steel, S. McGuirk, W.S. Powell, and S.V. Hetherington. 2001. The abacavir hypersensitivity reaction and interruptions in therapy. *AIDS* 15:1325.

117. Moyle, G. 2000. Clinical manifestations and management of antiretroviral nucleoside analog-related mitochondrial toxicity. *Clin. Ther.* 22:911–936.

118. Szczech, G.M., L.H. Wang, J.P. Walsh, and F.S. Rousseau. 2003. Reproductive toxicology profile of emtricitabine in mice and rabbits. *Reprod. Toxicol.* 17:95–108.

119. Sykes, A., C. Wakeford, F. Rousseau, A. Rigney, and E. Mondou. 2002. Antiviral efficacy and rate of development of resistance in patiented treated 1 year for chronic HBV infection with FTC. In: 9th Conference on Retroviruses and Opportunistic Infections; Seattle, WA, February 24–28. Abstract 674-M.

120. Gish, R.G., N.W. Leung, T.L. Wright, H. Trinh, W. Lang, H.A. Kessler, L. Fang, L.H. Wang, J. Delehanty, A. Rigney, E. Mondou, A. Snow, and F. Rousseau. 2002. Dose range study of pharmacokinetics, safety, and preliminary antiviral actrivity of emtricitabine in adults with hepatitis B virus infection. *Antimicrob. Agents Chemother.* 46:1734–1740.

121. Darque, A., G. Valette, F. Rousseau, L.H. Wang, J.P. Sommadossi, and X.J. Zhou. 1999. Quantitation of intracellular triphosphate of emtricitabine in peripheral blood mononuclear cells from

human immunodeficiency virus-infected patients. *Antimicrob. Agents Chemother.* 43:2245–2250.

122. Holodniy, M., D.A. Katzenstein, S. Sengupta, A.M. Wang, C. Casipit, D.H. Schwartz, M. Konrad, E. Groves, and T.C. Merigan. 1991. Detection and quantification of human immunodeficiency virus RNA in patient serum by use of the polymerase chain reaction. *J. Infect. Dis.* 163:862–866.

123. Smerdon, S.J., J. Jager, J. Wang, L.A. Kohlstaedt, A.J. Chirino, J.M. Friedman, P.A. Rice, and T.A. Steitz. 1994. Structure of the binding site for nonnucleoside inhibitors of the reverse transcriptase of human immunodeficiency virus type 1. *Proc. Natl. Acad. Sci. USA* 26:3911–3915.

124. Havlir, D., S.H. Cheeseman, M. McLaughlin, R. Murphy, A. Erice, S.A. Spector, T.C. Greenough, J.L. Sullivan, D. Hall, M. Myers, et al. 1995. High-dose nevirapine: Safety, pharmacokinetics, and antiviral effect in patients with human immunodeficiency virus infection. *J. Infect. Dis.* 171:537–545.

125. Nunberg, J.H., W.A. Schleif, E.J. Boots, J.A. O'Brien, J.C. Quintero, J.M. Hoffman, E.A. Emini, and M.E. Goldman. 1991. Viral resistance to human immunodeficiency virus type 1: Specific pyridinone reverse transcriptase inhibitors. *J. Virol.* 65:4887–4892.

126. Schmit, J.C., and B. Weber. 1997. Recent advances in antiretroviral therapy and HIV infection monitoring. *Intervirology* 40:304–321.

127. Stringer, J.S., D.J. Rouse, S.H. Vermund, R.L. Goldenberg, M. Sinkala, and A.A. Stinnett. 2000. Cost-effective use of nevirapine to prevent vertical HIV transmission in sub-Saharan Africa. *J. AIDS* 24:369–377.

128. Richman, D., D. Havlir, J. Corbeil, D. Looney, C. Ignacio, S.A. Spector, J. Sullivan, S. Cheeseman, K. Barringer, D. Pauletti, C.-K. Shih, M. Myers, and J. Griffin. 1994. Nevirapine resistance mutations of human immunodeficiency virus type 1 selected during therapy. *J. Virol.* 68:1660–1666.

129. van der Valk, M., J.J.P. Kastelein, R.L. Murphy, F. van Leth, C. Katlama, A. Horban, M. Glesby, G. Behrens, B. Clotet, R.K. Stellato, H.O.F. Molhuizen, and P. Reiss. 2001. Nevirapine-containing antiretroviral therapy in HIV-1 infected patients

results in an anti-atherogenic lipid profile. Atlantic Study Team. *AIDS* 15:2407–2414.

130. Barner, A., and M. Myers. 1998. Nevirapine and rashes. *Lancet* 351:1133.

131. Bersoff-Matcha, S.J., W.C. Miller, J.A. Aberg, C. van Der Horst, H.J. Hamrick, Jr., W.G. Powderly, and L.M. Mundy. 2001. Sex differences in nevirapine rash. *Clin. Infect. Dis.* 32:124–129.

132. Bourezane, Y., D. Salard, B. Hoen, S. Vandel, C. Drobacheff, and R. Laurent. 1998. DRESS (drug rash with eosinophilia and systemic symptoms) syndrome associated with nevirapine therapy. *Clin. Infect. Dis.* 27:1321–1322.

133. D'Aquila, R.T., M.D. Hughes, V.A. Johnson, M.A. Fischl, J.P. Sommadossi, S.H. Liou, J. Timpone, M. Myers, N. Basgoz, M. Niu, and M.S. Hirsch. 1996. Nevirapine, zidovudine and didanosine compared with zidovudine and didanosine in patients with HIV-1 infection: A randomized, double-blind, placebo-controlled trial. National Institute of Allergy and Infectious Diseases AIDS Clinical Trials Group Protocol 241 Investigators. *Ann. Intern. Med.* 124:1019–1030.

134. Knobel, H., J.M. Miro, P. Domingo, A. Rivero, M. Marquez, L. Force, A. Gonzalez, V. De Miguel, J. Sanz, V. Boix, J.L. Blanco, and J. Locutura. 2001. Failure of short-term prednisone regimen to prevent nevirapine-associated rash: A double-blind placebo-controlled trial: the GESIDA 09/99 study. GESIDA 09/99 Study Group. *J. AIDS* 28:14–18.

135. Warren, K.J., D.E. Boxwell, N.Y. Kim, and B.A. Drolet. 1998. Nevirapine-associated Stevens-Johnson syndrome. *Lancet* 351:1133.

136. Metry, D.W., C.J. Lahart, K.L. Farmer, and A.A. Hebert. 2001. Stevens-Johnson syndrome caused by the antiretroviral drug nevirapine. *J. Am. Acad. Dermatol.* 44:354–357.

137. Barreiro, P., V. Soriano, E. Casas, V. Estrada, M.J. Tellez, R. Hoetelmans, D.G. de Requena, I. Jimenez-Nacher, and J. Gonzalez-Lahoz. 2000. Prevention of nevirapine-associated exanthema using slow dose escalation and/or corticosteroids. *AIDS* 14:2153–2157.

138. Havlir, D.V., and J.M.A. Lange. 1998. New antiretrovirals and new combinations. *AIDS* 12 (suppl A):S165–S174.

139. de Maat, M.M., R.M. Hoetelmans, R.A. Mathõt, E.C. van Gorp, P.L. Meenhorst, J.W. Mulder, and J.H. Beijnen. 2001. Drug interaction between St. John's wort and nevirapine. *AIDS* 15: 420–421.

140. Gangar, M., G. Arias, J.G. O'Brien, and C.A. Kemper. 2000. Frequency of cutaneous reactions on rechallenge with nevirapine and delavirdine. *Ann. Pharmacother.* 34:839–842.

141. Bellman, P.C. 1998. Clinical experience with adding delavirdine to combination therapy in patients in whom multiple antiretroviral treatment including protease inhibitors has failed. *AIDS* 12:1333–1340.

142. Harris, M., C. Alexander, M. O'Shaughnessy, and J.S. Montaner. 2002. Delavirdine increases drug exposure of ritonavir-boosted protease inhibitors. *AIDS* 16:798–799.

143. Bisseul, F., F. Bruneel, F. Habersetzer, et al. 1994. Fulminant hepatitis with severe lactate acidosis in HIV-infected patients on didanosine therapy. *J. Intern. Med.* 235:367–371.

144. Sulkowski, M.S., D.L. Thomas, and R.E. Chaisson. 2000. Hepatotoxicity associated with antiretroviral therapy in adults infected with human immunodeficiency virus and the role of hepaptitis C or B virus infection. *J.A.M.A.* 283:74–80.

145. Palmon, R., B.C.A. Koo, D.A. Shoultz, and D.T. Dieterich. 2002. Lack of hepatotoxicity associated with nonnucleoside reverse transcriptase inhibitors. *J. AIDS* 29:340–345.

146. Murphy, R. 1997. Non-nucleoside reverse transcriptase inhibitors. *AIDS Clin. Care* 9:75–79.

147. Castro, J.G., and L. Guitierrez. 2002. Rhabdomyolysis with actue renal failure probably related to the interaction of atorvastatin and delavirdine. Letter to the Editor. *Am. J. Med.* 112:505.

148. Scott, L.J., and C.M. Perry. 2000. Delavirdine: A review of its use in HIV infection. *Drugs* 60:1411–1444.

149. Murdaca, G., A. Campelli, M. Setti, F. Indiveri, and F. Puppo. 2002. Complete remission of AIDS/Kaposi's sarcoma after treatment with a combination of two nucleoside reverse transcriptase inhibitors and one non-nucleoside reverse transcriptase inhibitor. *AIDS* 16:304–305.

150. Hill, J.B., J.S. Sheffield, G.G. Zeeman, and G.D. Wendel, Jr. 2001. Hepatotoxicity with antiretroviral treatment of pregnant women. *Obstet. Gynecol.* 98:909–910.

151. Taylor, S., H. Reynolds, C.A. Sabin, S.M. Drake, D.J. White, D.J. Back, and D. Pillay. 2001. Penetration of efavirenz into the male genital tract: Drug concentrations and antiviral activity in semen and blood of HIV-1 infected men. *AIDS* 15:2051–2053.

152. Doser, N., P. Sudre, A. Telenti, V. Wietlisbach, P. Nicod, R. Darioli, and V. Mooser. 2001. Persistent dyslipidemia in HIV-infected individuals switched from a protease inhibitor-containing to an efavirenz-containing regimen. (Letter to the editor.) *J. AIDS* 26:389–395.

153. Peyriere, H., J.-M. Mauboussin, I. Rouanet, J. Fabre, J. Reynes, and D. Hillaire-Buys. 2001. Management of sudden psychiatric disorders related to efavirenz. *AIDS* 15:1323–1324.

154. Marzolini, C., A. Telenti, L. Decosterd, G. Greud, J. Biollaz, and T. Buclin. 2001. Efavirenz plasma levels can predict treatment failure and central nervous system side effects in HIV-1 infected patients. *AIDS* 15:71–75.

155. Nunez, M., D.G. de Requena, L. Gallego, I. Jimenez-Nacher, J. Gonzalez-Lahoz, and V. Soriano. 2001. Higher efavirenz plasma levels correlate with development of insomnia (Letter to the Editor). *J. AIDS* 28:399.

156. Blanch, J., B. Corbella, F. Garcia, E. Parellada, and J.-M. Gatell. 2001. Manic syndrome associated with efavirenz overdose. *Clin. Infect. Dis.* 33:270–271.

157. Bartlett, J.G., and J.E. Gallant. 2000. *Medical Management HIV Infection.* Baltimore, MD: Johns Hopkins University, Port City Press, 2000.

158. Yazaki, H., Y. Kikcuhi, and S. Oka. 2001. Skin eruption 8 days after a single dose of efavirenz-containing combination therapy. *Jpn. J. Infect. Dis.* 54:246–247.

159. Phillips, E.J., B. Kuriakose, and S.R. Knowles. 2002. Efavirenz-induced skin eruption and successful desensitization. *Ann. Pharmacother.* 36:430–432.

160. Domingo, P., and M. Barcelo. 2002. Efavirenz-induced leukocytoclastic vasculitis. *Arch. Int. Med.* 162:355–356.

161. Treudler, R., R. Husak, M. Raisova, C.E. Orfanos, and B. Tebbe. 2001. Efavirenz-induced photoallergic dermatitis in HIV (Correspondence). *AIDS* 15:1085–1087.

162. Behrens, G.M.N., M. Stoll, and R.E. Schmidt. 2001. Pulmonary hypersensitivity reaction induced by efavirenz. *Lancet* 357: 1503–1504.

163. Caso, J.A., J.dM. Prieto, E. Casas, and J. Sanz. 2001. Gynecomastia without lipodystrophy syndrome in HIV-infected men treated with efavirenz. *AIDS* 15:1447–1452.

164. Hughes, C.A., and G.D. Taylor. 2001. Metformin in an HIV-infected patient with protease inhibitor-induced diabetic ketoacidosis. *Ann. Pharmacother.* 35:877–880.

165. Centers for Disease Control and Prevention. 1998. USPHS task force recommendations for the use of antiretroviral drugs in pregnant women infected with HIV-1 for maternal health and for reducing perinatal HIV-1 transmission in the United States. *M.M.W.R.* 47:1–30. Updated February 2000. Available at http://www.hivatis.org.

166. Fundaro, C., O. Genovese, C. Rendeli, E. Tamburrini, and E. Salvaggio. 2002. Myelomeningocele in a child with intrauterine exposure to efavirenz. *AIDS* 16:299–300.

167. Moyle, G. 2003. Once-daily therapy: Less is more. *Int. J. STD AIDS* 14 (Suppl):1–5.

168. Wolf, K., H. Walter, N. Beerenwinkel, W. Keulen, R. Kaiser, D. Hoffmann, T. Lengauer, J. Selbig, A-M Vandamme, K. Korn, and R. Schmidt. 2003. Tenofovir resistance and resensitization. *Antimicrob. Agents Chemother.* 47:3478–3484.

169. Gallant, J.E., and S. Deresinski. 2003. Tenofovir disoproxil fumarate. *Clin. Infect. Dis.* 37:944–950.

170. Squires, K., A.L. Pozniak, G. Pierone, Jr. C.R. Steinhart, D. Berger, N.C. Bellos, S.L. Becker, M. Wulfsohn, M.D. Miller, J.J. Toole, D.F. Coakley, and A. Cheng. 2003. Tenofovir disoproxil fumarate in nucleoside-resistant HIV-1 infection: A randomized trial. Study 907 Team. *Ann. Intern. Med.* 139: 313–320.

171. Ristig, M., H. Drechsler, J. Crippin, M. Lisker-Melman, and P. Tebas. 2003. Management of chronic hepatitis B in an

HIV-positive patient with 3TC-resistant hepatitis B virus. *AIDS Patient Care STDS* 17:439–442.

172. Margot, N.A., E. Isaacson, I. McGowan, A. Cheng, and M.D. Miller, 2003. Extended treatment with tenofovir disoproxil fumarate in treatment-experienced HIV-1-infected patients: Genotypic, phenotypic, and rebound analyses. *J. AIDS* 33:15–21.

173. Aidsmed.com. reviewed by H. Grossman. 2003. Viread brand tenofovir disoproxil fumarate (tenofovir DF). Accessed December 23, 2003

174. Verheist, D., M. Monge, J.L. Meynard, et al. 2003. Fanconi syndrome and renal failure induced by tenofovir: A first case report. *Am. J. Kid. Dis.* 40:1331–1333.

175. Reynes, J., et al. 2003. Renal tubular injury and severe hypophosphoremia (Fanconi Syndrome) associated with tenofovir therapy. In: Tenth Conference on Retroviruses and Opportunistic Infections; Boston, February 10–14, 2003, Abstract 717.

176. Blick, G., et al. 2003. Tenofovir may cause severe hypophosphatemia in HIV-AIDS patients with prior adefovir-induced renal tubular acidosis. In: Tenth Conference on Retroviruses and Opportunistic Infections; Boston, February 10–14, 2003. Abstract 718.

177. Murphy, M.D., M. O'Hearn and S. Chou. 2003. Fatal lactic acidosis and acute renal failure after addition of tenofovir to an antiretroviral regimen containing didanosine. *Clin. Infect. Dis.* 36: (1082–1085). online (www.journals.uchicago.com)

178. Creput, C., et al. 2003. Renal lesions on HIV-1 positive patient treated with tenofovir. *AIDS* 17:935–937.

179. Moyle, G. 2003. Newer nucleoside analogues show fewer adverse effects. In: 43rd Interscience Conference on Antimicrobial Agents and Chemotherapy; Chicago, Illinois, September 14–17, 2003.

180. Birkus, G., M.J.M. Hitchcock, and T. Cihlar. 2003. Assessment of mitochondrial toxicity in human cells treated with tenofovir: Comparison with other nucleoside reverse transcriptase inhibitors. *Antimicrob. Agents Chemother.* 46:716–723.

181. Cihlar, T., G. Birkus, D.E. Greenwalt, and M.J.M. Hitchcock. 2002. Tenofovir exhibits low cytotoxicity in various human cell types: Comparison with other nucleoside reverse transcriptase inhibitors. *Antiviral Res.* 54:37–45.

182. Moyle, G. and M. Boffito. 2004. Unexpected drug interactions and adverse events with antiretroviral drugs. Lancet 364: 65–67.

183. Gulick, R.M., H.J. Ribaudo, C.M. Shikuma, et al. 2003. A comparative study of 3 protease inhibitor-sparing antiretroviral regimens for the initial treatment of HIV infection. In: 2nd IAS Conference on HIV pathogenesis and treatment; ACTG 5095. Paris, July 13–16, 2003, Abstract 41:2.

184. Grstoft, J., O. Kirk, N. Oabel, et al. 2003. Low efficacy and high frequency of adverse events in a randomized trial of the triple nucleoside regimen abacavir, stavudine, and didanosine. *AIDS* 17:2045–2052.

185. Farthing, D., H. Khanlou, V. Yeh, et al. 2003. Early virologic failure in a pilot study evaluating the efficacy of once daily abacavir (ABD), lamivudine (3TC), and tenofovir DF (TDF) in treatment naïve HIV-infected patients (oral presentation). Presented at the 2nd International AIDS Society meeting; Paris, France, July 13–16, 2003.

186. Gallant, J.E., A. Rodriguez, W. Weinberg, et al. 2003. Early nonresponse to tenfovir DF (TDF) + abacavir (ABC) and lamivudine (3TC) in a randomized trial compared to efavirenz (EFV) + ABC and 3TC: ESS 30009. Unplanned interim analysis (oral presentation #H-1722a) Presented at the 43rd Interscience Conference on Antimicrobial Agents and Chemotherapy, Chicago, IL, September 14–17, 2003.

187. Hoogewerf, M., R.M. Regez, W.E. Schouten, H.M. Weigel, P.H. Frissen, and K. Brinkman. 2003. Change to abacavir-lamivudine-tenofovir combination treatment in patients with HIV-1 who had complete virological suppression. *Lancet* 362: 1979–1980.

188. Grim, S.A., and F. Ramanelli. 2003. Tenofovir disoproxil fumarate. *Ann. Pharmacother.* 37:849–859.

189. Blanchard, J.N., M. Wohlfeiler, A. Canas, K. King, and J.T. Lonergan. 2003. Pancreatitis with didanosine and tenofovir disoproxil fumarate. *Clin. Infect. Dis.* 37:e57–62.

190. Robbins, B.L., C.K. Wilcox, A. Fridland, and J.H. Rodmann. 2003. Metabolism of tenofovir and didanosine in quiescent or stimulated human peripheral blood mononuclear cells. *Pharmacotherapy* 23:695–701.

191. Fulco, P.P., and M.A. Kirian. 2003. Effect of tenofovir on didanosine absorption in patients with HIV. *Ann. Pharmacother.* 37:1325–1328.

192. Deeks, S.G., M. Smith, M. Holodniy, and J.O. Kahn. 1997. HIV-1 protease inhibitors. A review for clinicians. *J.A.M.A.* 277: 145–153.

193. Debouck, C. 1992. The HIV-1 protease as a therapeutic target for AIDS. *AIDS Res. Hum. Retroviruses* 8:153–164.

194. McDonald, C.K., and D.R. Kurtzkes. 1997. Human immunodeficiency virus type 1 protease inhibitors. *Arch. Intern. Med.* 157:951–959.

195. Markowitz, M., M. Saag, W.G. Powderly, A.M. Hurley, A. Hsu, J.M. Valdes, D. Henry, F. Sattler, A. LaMarca, J.M. Leonard, and D.D. Ho. 1995. A preliminary study of ritonavir, an inhibitor of HIV-1 protease, to treat HIV-1 infection. *N. Engl. J. Med.* 333:1534–1539.

196. Condra, J.H., W.A. Schleif, O.M. Blahy, L.J. Gabryelski, D.J. Graham, J.C. Quintero, A. Rhodes, H.L. Robbins, E. Roth, M. Shivaprakash, et al. 1995. In vivo emergence of HIV-1 variants resistant to multiple protease inhibitors. *Nature* 374:569–571.

197. Graham, N.M. 2000. Metabolic disorders among HIV-infected patients treated with protease inhibitors: A review. *J. AIDS* 25 (Suppl)1:S4–11.

198. Hadigan, C., J.B. Meigs, C. Corcoran, P. Rietschel, S. Piecuch, N. Basgoz, B. Davis, P. Sax, T. Stanley, P.W. Wilson, R.B. D'Agostino, and S. Grinspoon. 2001. Metabolic abnormalities and cardiovascular disease risk factors in adults with human immunodeficiency virus infection and lipodystrophy. *Clin. Infect. Dis.* 32:130–139.

199. Tsiodras, S., C. Mantzoros, S. Hammer, and M. Samore. 2000. Effects of protease inhibitors on hyperglycemia, hyperlipidemia, and lipodystrophy cohort study. *Arch. Intern. Med.* 160:2050–2056.

200. Carr, A. 2000. HIV protease inhibitor-related lipodystrophy syndrome. *Clin. Infect. Dis.* 2:S135–142.

201. Paparizos, V.A., K.P. Kyriakis, C. Botsis, V. Papastamopoulos, M. Hadjivassiliou, and N.G. Stavrianeas. 2000. Protease inhibitor

therapy-associated lipodystrophy, hypertriglyceridaemia and diabetes mellitus. *AIDS* 14:903–905.

202. Domingo, P., A. Perez, O.H. Torres, J.A. Montiel, and G. Vazquez. 1999. Lipodystrophy in HIV-1-infected patients. *Lancet* 354: 868.

203. Mercie, P., S. Tchamgoue, F. Dabis, and J.L. Pellegrin. 1999. Lipodystrophy in HIV-1-infected patients. *Lancet* 354:867–868.

204. Buss, N., and F. Duff. 1999. Protease inhibitors in HIV infection. Lipodystrophy may be a consequence of prolonged survival. *B.M.J.* 318:122.

205. Buss, N. 1998. Saquinavir Soft Gel Capsule (Fortovase): Pharmacokinetics and Drug Interactions. In: Programme and abstracts from the 5th Conference on Retroviruses and Opportunistic Infections; Chicago, Illinois, February 1998 Abstract 354.

206. Mitsuyasu, R.T., P.R. Skolnik, S.R. Cohen, B. Conway, M.J. Gill, P.C. Jensen, J.J. Pulvirenti, L.N. Slater, R.T. Schooley, M.A. Thompson, R.A. Torres, and C.M. Tsoukas. 1998. Activity of the soft gelatin formulation of saquinavir in combination therapy in antiretroviral-naïve patients. NV15355 Study Team. *AIDS* 12:F103–109.

207. Dube, M.P., D.L. Johnson, J.S. Currier, and J.M. Leedom. 1997. Protease inhibitor-associated hyperglycemia. *Lancet* 350: 713–714.

208. Silva, M., P.R. Skolnik, S.L. Gorbach, D. Spiegelman, I.B. Wilson, M.G. Fernandez-DiFranco, and T.A. Knox. 1998. The effect of protease inhibitors on weight and body composition in HIV-infected patients. *AIDS* 12:1645–1651.

209. Carr, A., and D.A. Cooper. 1998. Images in clinical medicine. Lipodystrophy associated with an HIV-protease inhibitor. *N. Engl. J. Med.* 339:1296.

210. Aboulafia, D.M., and D. Bundaw. 1998. Images in clinical medicine. Buffalo hump in a patient with the acquired immundeficiency syndrome. *N. Engl. J. Med.* 339:1297.

211. Williamson, K., A.C. Reboli, and S.M. Manders. 1999. Protease inhibitor-induced lipodystrophy. *J. Am. Acad. Dermatol.* 40: 635–636.

212. Lo, J.C., K. Mulligan, V.W. Tai, H. Algren, and M. Schambelan. 1998. "Buffalo hump" in men with HIV-1 infection. *Lancet* 351:867–870.

213. van der Valk M., E.H. Gisolf, P. Reiss, F.W. Wit, A. Japour, G.J. Weverling, and S.A. Danner. 2001. Increased risk of lipodystrophy when nucleoside analogue reverse transcriptase inhibitors are included with protease inhibitors in the treatment of HIV-1 infection. *AIDS* 15:847–855.

214. Ho, T.T., K.C. Chan, K.H. Wong, and S.S. Lee. 1999. Indinavir-associated facial lipodystrophy in HIV-infected patients. *AIDS Patient Care STDS* 13:11–16.

215. Gun, S.K., K. Samaras, A. Carr, and D. Chisholm. 2001. Antiretroviral therapy, insulin resistance and lipodystrophy. *Diabetes Obes. Metab.* 3:67–71.

216. Goujard, C., F. Boufassa, C. Deveau, D. Laskri, and L. Meyer. 2001. Incidence of clinical lipodystrophy in HIV-infected patients treated during primary infection. *AIDS* 15:282–284.

217. Heath, K.V., R.S. Hogg, K.J. Chan, M. Harris, V. Montessori, M.V. O'Shaughnessy, and J.S. Montanera. 2001. Lipodystrophy-associated morphological, cholesterol and triglyceride abnormalities in a population-based HIV/AIDS treatment database. *AIDS* 15:231–239.

218. Krishnaswamy, G., D.S. Chi, J.L. Kelley, F. Sarubbi, J.K. Smith, and A. Peiris. 2000. The cardiovascular and metabolic complications of HIV infection. *Cardiol. Rev.* 8:260–268.

219. Garg, A. 2000. Lipodystrophies. *Am. J. Med.* 108:143–152.

220. Panse, I., E. Vasseur, M.L. Raffin-Sanson, F. Staroz, E. Rouveix, and P. Saiag. 2000. Lipodystrophy associated with protease inhibitors. *Br. J. Dermatol.* 142:496–500.

221. Padberg, J., D. Schurmann, M. Grobusch, and F. Bergman. 1999. Drug interaction of isotretinoin and protease inhibitors: Support for the cellular retinoic acid-binding protein-1 theory of lipodystrophy? *AIDS* 13:284–285.

222. Carr, H., K. Samaras, D.J. Chisholm, and D.A. Cooper. 1998. Pathogenesis of HIV-1-protease inhibitor-associated peripheral lipodystrophy, hyperlipidemia, and insulin resistance. *Lancet* 351:1881–1883.

223. Striker, R., D. Conlin, M. Marx, and L. Wiviott. 1998. Localized adipose tissue hypertrophy in patients receiving human immunodeficiency virus protease inhibitors. *Clin. Infect. Dis.* 27:218–220.

224. Hadigan, C., J.B. Meigs, J. Rabe, R.B. D'Agostino, P.W. Wilson, I. Lipinska, G.H. Tofler, and S.S. Grinspoon. 2001. Increased PAI-1 and tPA antigen levels are reduced with metformin therapy in HIV-infected patients with fat redistribution and insulin resistance. Framingham Heart Study. *J. Clin. Endocrinol. Metab.* 86:939–943.

225. Wolfort, F.G., C.L. Cetrulo, Jr., and D.R. Nevarre. 1999. Suction-assisted lipectomy for lipodystrophy syndromes attributed to HIV-protease inhibitor use. *Plast. Reconstr. Surg.* 104:1814–1820.

226. Ponce-de-Leon S., M. Iglesias, J. Ceballos, and L. Ostrosky-Zeichner. 1999. Liposuction for protease-inhibitor-associated lipodystrophy. *Lancet* 353:1244.

227. Ohta, Y., and I. Shinkai. 1997. Saquinavir. *Biorg. Med. Chem.* 5: 465–466.

228. Tian, R., N. Koyabu, H. Takanaga, H. Matsuo, H. Ohtani, and Y. Sawada. 2002. Effects of grapefruit juice and orange juice on the intestinal efflux of P-glycoprotein substrates. *Pharm. Res.* 19:802–809.

229. Hugen, P.W., D.M. Burger, P.P. Koopmans, J.W. Stuart, F.P. Kroon, R. van Leusen, and Y.A. Hekster. 2002. Saquinavir soft-gel capsules (Fortovase) give lower exposure than expected, even after a high-fat breakfast. *Pharm. World. Sci.* 24:83–86.

230. Cameron, D.W., M. Heath-Chiozzi, S. Danner, C. Cohen, S. Kravcik, C. Maurath, E. Sun, D. Henry, R. Rode, A. Potthoff, and J. Leonard. 1998. Randomised placebo-controlled trial of ritonavir in advanced HIV-1 disease. The Advanced HIV Disease Ritonavir Study Group. *Lancet* 351:543–549.

231. Sadler, B.M., P.J. Piliero, S.L. Preston, P.P. Loys, Y. Lou, and S.D. Stain. 2001. Pharmacokinetics and safety of amprenavir and ritonavir following multiple-dose, co-administration to healthy volunteers. *AIDS* 15:1009–1018.

232. Burger, D.M., P.W.H. Hugen, R.E. Aarnoutse, J.P. Dieleman, J.M. Prins, T. vander Poll, J.H. ten Veen, J.W. Mulder, P.L. Meenhorst, W.L. Blok, J.T.M. vander Meer, P. Reiss, and J.M.A.

Lange. 2001. A retrospective, cohort-based survey of patients using twice-daily indinavir + ritonavir combinations: Pharmacokinetics, safety, and efficacy. *J. AIDS* 26:218–224.

233. Mauss, S., G. Schmutz, and D. Kuschak. 2002. Unfavourable interaction of amprenavir and lopinavir in combination with ritonavir? *AIDS* 16:296–297.

234. Aceti, A., C. Pasquazzi, B. Zechini, and C. De Bac. 2002. Hepatotoxicity development during antiretroviral therapy containing protease inhibitors in patients with HIV: The role of hepatitis B and C virus infection. LIVERHAART Group. *J. AIDS* 29:41–48.

235. Nielsen, H. 1999. Hypermennorhoea associated with ritonavir [letter]. *Lancet* 353:811–812.

236. Routy, J.-P., G.H.R. Smith, D.W. Blank, and B.M. Gilfix. 2001. Plasmapheresis in the treatment of an acute pancreatitis due to protease inhibitor-induced hypertriglyceridemia. *J. Clin. Apheresis* 16:157–159.

237. Bachmeyer, C., L. Blum, F. Cordier, E. Launay, O. Danne, S. Aractingi, et al. 1997. Early ritonavir-induced maculopapular eruption. *Dermatology* 195:301–302.

238. James, C.W., K.C. McNelis, D.M. Cohen, S. Szabo, and A.K. Bincsik. 2001. Recurrent ingrown toenails secondary to indinavir/ritonavir combination therapy. *Ann Pharmacother.* 35:881–884.

239. Wang, M.W., S.L. Teitelbaum, P. Tebas, W.G. Powderly, and F.P. Ross. 2001. Indinavir inhibits bone formation while ritonavir inhibits osteoclast differentiation and function. In: 8th Conference on Retroviruses and Opportunistic Infections; Chicago, IL, 2001, Abstract 541.

240. Piliero, P.J., and A.G. Gianoukakis. 2002. Ritonavir-associated hyperparathyroidism, osteopenia and bone pain. *AIDS* 16:1565–1566.

241. Was, W., and P.B. DePetrillo. 2002. Ritonavir inhibition of calcium-activated neutral proteases. *Biochem. Pharm.* 63:1481–1484.

242. Nachman, S.A., J.C. Linsey, S. Pelton, L. Mofenson, K. McIntosh, A. Wiznia, K. Stanley, and R. Yogev. 2002. Growth in human immunodeficiency virus-infected children receiving ritonavir-containing antiretroviral therapy. *Arch. Pediatr. Adolesc. Med.* 156:497–503.

243. Mateu-de Antonio, J., S. Grau, J.-L. Gimeno-Bayon, and A. Carmona. 2001. Ritonavir-induced carbamazepine toxicity. *Ann. Pharmacother.* 35:125–126.

244. Moreno, S., D. Podzamczer, R. Blazquez, J.A. Iribarren, E. Ferrer, J. Reparaz, J.M. Pena, E. Cabrero, and L. Usan. 2001. Treatment of tuberculosis in HIV-infected patients: Safety and antiretrovirual efficacy of the concomitant use of ritonavir and rifampin. *AIDS* 15:1185–1187.

245. Sagir A, M. Wettstein, M. Oette, A. Erhardt, and D. Haussinger. 2002. Budesonide-induced acute hepatitis in an HIV-positive patient with ritonavir as a co-medication. *AIDS* 16:1191–1192.

246. Colson, A.E., M.J. Keller, P.E. Sax, P.T. Pettus, R. Platt, and P.W. Choo. 2002. Male sexual dysfunction associated with antiretroviral therapy. *J. AIDS* 30:27–32.

247. Rathrun, R.C., and D.R. Rossi. 2002. Low-dose ritonavir for protease inhibitor pharmacokinetic enhancement. *Ann. Pharmacother.* 36:702–702.

248. Martinez, L.J. 1996. Approval of new protease inhibitors. *Res. Init. Treat. Action* 2:1–3, 1996.

249. Bernasconi, E., J. Jost, B. Ledergerber, B. Hirschel, P. Francioli, and P. Sudre. 2001. Antiretroviral prophylaxis for community exposure to the human immunodeficiency virus in Switzerland, 1997–2000. *Swiss Med. Wkly.* 131:433–437.

250. Boubaker, K., P. Sudre, F. Bally, G. Vogel, J.Y. Meuwly, M.P. Glauser, and A. Telenti. 1998. Changes in renal function associated with indinavir. *AIDS* 12:F249–254.

251. Martinez, E., A. Mocroft, M.A. Garcia-Viejo, J.L. Blanco, J. Mallolas, L. Bianchi, I. Conget, J. Blanch, A. Phillips, and J. Gatell. 2001. Risk of lipodystrophy in HIV-1-infected patients treated with protease inhibitors: A prospective cohort study. *Lancet* 357:592–598.

252. Salahuddin, S., Y.S. Hsu, N.P. Ruchholz, J.P. Dieleman, I.C. Gyssens, and D.J. Kok. 2001. Is indinavir crystalluria an indicator for indinavir stone formation? *AIDS* 15:1079–1080.

253. Bernasconi, E., M. Uhr, L. Magenta, A. Ranno, and A. Telenti, 2001. Homocysteinaemia in HIV-infected patients treated with

highly active antiretroviral therapy. Swiss HIV Cohort Study. *AIDS* 15:1081–1082.

254. Food and Drug Administration. 1997. Protease inhibitors may increase blood glucose in HIV patients. *FDA Med. Bull.* 27:No. 2.

255. Lichtenstein, K.A., D.J. Ward, A.C. Moorman, K.M. Delaney, B. Young, F.J. Palella, Jr., P.H. Rhodes, K.C. Wood, and S.D. Holmberg, 2001. Clinical assessment of HIV-associated lipodystrophy in an ambulatory population. HIV Outpatients Study Investigators. *AIDS* 15:1389–1398.

256. Hanabusa, H., H. Tagami, and H. Hataya. 1999. Renal atrophy associated with long-term treatment with indinavir. *N. Eng. J. Med.* 340:392–393.

257. Hammer, A.M., K.E. Squires, M.D. Hughes, J.M. Grimes, L.M. Demeter, J.S. Currier, and J.J. Eron Jr. 1997. A controlled trial of two nucleoside analogues plus indinavir in persons with human immunodeficiency virus infection and CD4 counts of 200 per cubic millimeter or less. AIDS Clinical Trials Group 320 Study Team. *N. Engl. J. Med.* 337:725–733.

258. Kaul, D.R., S.K. Cinti, P.L. Carver, and P.H. Kazanjian. 1999. HIV protease inhibitors: Advanced in therapy and adverse reactions, including metabolic complications. *Pharmacotherapy* 19:281–298.

259. Zucker, S., X. Qin, S.D. Rouster, F. Yu, R.M. Green, P. Keshavan, J. Feinberg, and K.E. Sherman. 2001. Mechanism of indinavir-induced hyperbilirubinemia. *Proc. Natl. Acad. Sci. USA* 98: 12671–12676.

260. Jaeschke, H., K.D. Mullen, and D. Moradpour (eds.). Is "Gilbert's" the culprit in indinavir-induced hyperbilirubinemia? Hepatology Elsewhere. *Hepatology* 35:1269–1273.

261. Bouscarat, F., C. Bouchard, and D. Bouhour. 1998. Paronychia and pyogenic granuloma of the great toes in patients treated with indinavir. *N. Engl. J. Med.* 338:1776–1777.

262. Calista, D., and A. Boschini. 2000. Cutaneous side effects induced by indinavir. *Eur. J. Dermatol.* 10:292–296.

263. Teira, R., Z. Zubero, J. Munoz, J. Baraia-Etxaburu, and J.M. Santamaria. 1998. Stevens-Johnson syndrome caused by indinavir. *Scand. J. Infect. Dis.* 30:634–635.

264. Sollima, S., M. Osio, F. Muscia, P. Gambaro, A. Alciati, M. Zucconi, T. Maga, F. Adorni, T. Bini, and A. d'A. Monforte. 2001. Protease inhibitors and erectile dysfunction. *AIDS* 15:2331–2333.

265. Herman, J.S., N.J. Ives, M. Nelson, B.G. Gazzard, and P.J. Easterbroook. 2001. Incidence and risk factors for the development of indinavir-associated renal complications. *J. Antimicrobiol. Chemother.* 48:355–360.

266. Kosel, B.W., F.T. Aweeka, N.L. Benowitz, S.B. Shade, J.F. Hilton, P.S. Lizak, and D.I. Abrams. 2002. The effects of cannabinoids on the pharmacokinetics of indinavir and nelfinavir. *AIDS* 16:543–550.

267. Saag, M., M. Knowles, and Y. Chang. 1997. Durable effect of viracept (nelfinavir mesylate, NFV) in triple combination therapy. In: Programs and abstracts of the 37th International Conference on Antimicrobial Agents and Chemotherapy; Toronto, Canada, September 28–October 1, 1997, 1–101.

268. Manfredi, R., and F. Chiodo. 2001. Limits of deep salvage antiretroviral therapy with nelfinavir plus either efavirenz or nevirapine in highly pre-treated patients with HIV disease. *Int. J. Antimicrob. Agents* 17:511–516.

269. Saag, M.S., P. Tebas, M. Sension, M. Conant, R. Myers, S.K. Chapman, R. Anderson, and N. Clendeninn. 2001. Randomized, double-blind comparison of two nelfinavir doses plus nucleosides in HIV-infected patients (Agouron study 511). Viracept Collaborative Study Group. *AIDS* 15:1971–1978.

270. Nolan, D., R. Upton, E. McKinnon, M. John, I. James, B. Adler, G. Roff, S. Vasikaran, and S. Mallal. 2001. Stable or increasing bone mineral density in HIV-infected patients treated with nelfinavir or indinavir. *AIDS* 15:1275–1280.

271. Rudich, A., S. Vanounou, K. Riesenberg, M. Porat, A. Tirosh, I. Harman-Boehm, A.S. Greenberg, F. Schlaeffer, and N. Bashan. 2001. The HIV protease inhibitor nelfinavir induces insulin resistance and increases basal lipolysis in 3T3-L1 adipocytes. *Diabetes* 50:1425–1431.

272. Wensing, A.M.J., M. Reedjik, C. Richter, C.A.B. Boucher, and J.C.C. Borleffs. 2001. Replacing ritonavir by nelfinavir or nelfinavir/saquinavir as part of highly active antiretroviral

therapy leads to an improvement of triglyceride levels. *AIDS* 15:2191–2193.

273. Manfredi, R., L. Calza, and F. Chiodo. 2001. Gynecomastia associated with highly active antiretroviral therapy. *Ann. Pharmacother.* 35:438–439.

274. Huang, J.S., R.V. Mulkern, and S. Grinspoon. 2002. Reduced intravertebral bone marrow fat in HIV-infected men. *AIDS* 16: 1265–1269.

275. Cheseaux, J.-J., V. Jotterand, C. Aebi, H. Gnehm, C. Kind, D. Nadal, C. Rudin, C.-A.W. Lazarevitch, P. Nicod, and V. Mooser. 2002. Hyperlipidemia in HIV-infected children treated with protease inhibitors: Relevance for cardiovascular diseases. *J. AIDS* 30:288–293.

276. deWitte, S., F. Bonnet, M. Bonarek, P. Lamarque, P. Morlat, M.-C. Receveur, and J. Beylot. 2002. Adhesive capsulitis of the shoulder in an HIV patient treated with nelfinavir. *AIDS* 16:1307–1308.

277. Quiros-Roldan, E., S. Signorini, F. Castelli, C. Torti, A. Patroni, M. Airoldi, and G. Carosi. 2001. Analysis of HIV-1 mutation patterns in patients failing antiretroviral therapy. *J. Clin. Lab. Analysis.* 15:43–46.

278. Smith, W., N. Nassar, C. Gregg, and D. Skiest. 1999. Protease inhibitor-based therapy is associated with decreased HIV-related health care costs in men treated at a Veteran's Administration hospital. *J. Acquir. Immune Defic. Syndr. Hum. Retrovirol.* 20: 28–33.

279. Scott, T., C. Garris, M. Rogers, N. Graham, L. Garrett, L. Pedneault. 2001. Safety profile and "tolerability" of amprenavir in patients enrolled in an early access program. *Clin. Ther.* 23:252–259.

280. Package insert. 2000. Agenerase (amprenavir). Research Triangle Park, NC: Glaxo Wellcome, May, 2000.

281. James, C.W., K.C. McNelis, M.D. Matalia, D.M. Cohen, and S. Szabo. 2000. Central nervous system toxicity and amprenavir oral solution. *Ann. Pharmacother.* 35:174.

282. Demarles, D., C. Gillotin, S. Bonaventure-Paci, I. Vincent, S. Fosse, and A.M. Taburet. 2002. Single-dose pharmacokinetics of amprenavir coadministered with grapefruit juice. *Antimicrob. Agents Chemother.* 46:1589–1590.

283. Bankhead, C. 2003. Fosamprenavir a promising alternative in HIV infections. *Inpharma Weekly* 1378:9–11.

284. Gathe Jr., J.C., P. Ive, R. Wood, D. Schurmann, N.C. Bellos, E. DeJesus, A. Gladysz, C. Garris and J. Yeo. 2004. SOLO: 48-week efficacy and safety comparison of once-daily fosamprenavir/ritonavir versus twice-daily nelfinavir in native HIV-1 infected patients. AIDS 18: 1529–1537.

285. Sohma, Y., Y. Hayashi, T. Ito, H. Matsumoto, T. Kimura, and Y. Kiso. 2003. Develoment of water-soluble prodrugs of the HIV-1 protease inhibitor KNI-727: Importance of the conversion time for high gastrointestinal absorption of prodrugs based on spontaneous chemical cleavage. *J. Med. Chem.* 46: 4124–4235.

286. Horban, A. et al. 2003. Favourable increases in high-density lipoprotein cholesterol (HDL-C) concentrations in chronic HIV-infected therapy naïve subjects receiving 908/R QD in the SOLO Study. In: Program and Abstracts of the 9th European Conference on AIDS (9th EACS). October 29, 2003, Warsaw, Poland. Abstract F8/3.

287. Aids Alert. 2003. Atazanavir found to help improve lipid profile. IDSA study offers good news for HIV care.*Aids Alert* 18 (January): 7–8.

288. Sanne, I., P. Piliero, K. Squires, A. Thiry, and S. Schnittman. 2003. Results of a phase 2 clinical trial at 48 weeks (AI424-007): A dose-ranging, safety, and efficacy comparative trial of atazanavir at three doses in combination with didanosine and stavudine in antiretroviral-naïve subjects. AI424-007 Clinical Trial Group. *J. AIDS* 32:18–29.

289. Haas, D.W., C. Zala, S. Schrader, P. Piliero, H. Jaeger, D. Nunes, A. Thiry, and S. Schnittman, M. 2003. Therapy with atazanavir plus saquinavir in patients failing highly active antiretroviral therapy: A randomized comparative pilot trial. Session for the Protocol AI424-009 Study Group. *AIDS* 17:1339–1349.

290. Goldsmith, D.R., and C.M. Perry. 2003. Atazanavir. *Drugs* 63: 1679–93, 1694–1695.

291. Rollot, F., et al. 2003. Tenofovir-related Fanconi syndrome with nephrogenic diabetes insipidus in a patient with acquired immune deficiency syndrome: The role of lopinavir-ritonavir-didanosine. *Clin. Infect. Dis.* 37:174–176 online (www.jou.nok.urhing.edu).

292. Lim, M.L., et al. 2003. A two-way drug interaction between lopinavir/ritonavir and phenytoin. In: 10th Conference on Retroviruses and Opportunistic Infections; Boston, MA, February 10–14, 2003, Abstract 535(poster).

293. Viega, S., S. Henriques, N.C. Santos, and M. Castanho. 2004. Putative role of membranes in the HIV fusion inhibitor enfuvirtide mode of action at the molecular level. *Biochem. J.* 377:107–110.

294. Kilby, J.M., J.P. Lalezari, J.J. Eron, M. Carlson, C. Cohen, R.C. Arduino, J.C. Goodgame, J.E. Gallant, P. Volberding, R.L. Murphy, F. Valentine, M.S. Saag, E.L. Nelson, P.R. Sista, and A. Dusek. 2002. The safety, plasma pharmacokinetics, and antiviral activity of subcutaneous enfuvirtide (T-20), a peptide inhibitor of gp41-mediated virus fusion, in HIV infected adults. *AIDS Res. Hum. Retroviruses* 18:685–693.

295. Cervia, J.S., and M.A. Smith. 2003. Enfuvirtide (T-20): A novel human immunodeficiency virus type1 fusion inhibitor. *Clin. Infect. Dis.* 37:1102–1106.

296. Duffalo, M.L., and C.W. James. 2003. Enfuvirtide: A novel agent for the treatment of HIV-1 infection. *Ann. Pharmacother.* 37:1448–1456.

297. Koopmans, P.P. 2003. Enfuvirtide, the first representative of a new class of drugs for the treatment of HIV infection: HIV fusion inhibitors. *Ned. Tijdschr. Geneeskd.* 147:1726–1729.

298. Lalezari, J.P., J.J. Eron, M. Carlson, C. Cohen, E. DeJesus, R.D. Arduino, J.E. Gallant, P. Volberding, R.L. Murphy, F. Valentine, E.L. Nelson, P.I. Sista, A. Dusek, and J.M. Kilby. 2003. A phase II clinical study of the long-term safety and antiviral activity of enfuvirtide-based antiretroviral therapy. *AIDS* 17:691–698.

299. Barretina, J., J. Blanco, M. Armand-Ugon, A. Gutierrez, B. Clotet, and J.A. Este. 2003. Anti-HIV-1 activity of enfuvirtide (T-20) by inhibition of bystander cell death. *Antivir. Ther.* 8:155–161.

300. Gallant, J.E. 2003. The optimal use of enfuvirtide. *The Hopkins HIV Report* 15:1,2.

301. Lazzarin, A., B. Clotet, D. Cooper, J. Reynes, K. Arasteh, M. Nelson, C. Katlama, H.-J. Stellbrink, J.-F. Delfraissy, J. Lange, L. Huson, R. DeMasi, C. Wat, J. Delehanty, C. Drobnes, and M. Salgo. 2003. Efficacy of enfuvirtide in patients infected with

drug-resistant HIV-1 in Europe and Australia. TORO2 Study Group. *N. Engl. J. Med.* 348:2186–2195.

302. Lalezari, J.P., K. Henry, M. O'Hearn, J.S.G. Montaner, P.J. Piliero, B. Trottier, S. Walmsley, C. Cohen, D.R. Kuritzkes, J.J. Eron, J. Chung, R. DeMasi, L. Donatacci, C. Drobnes, J. Delahanty, and M. Salgo, 2003. Enfuvirtide, an HIV-1 fusion inhibitor, for drug-resistant HIV infection in North and South America. TORO1 Study Group. *N. Engl. J. Med.* 348:2175–2185. (Correction *N. Engl. J. Med.* 349:11, 2003).

303. Sista, P., T. Melby, U. Dhingra, et al. 2001. The fusion inhibitors T-20 and T-1249 demonstrate potential adtiviral activity against clade B HIV-1 isolates resistant to reverse transcriptase and protease inhibitors and non-B clades. In: 5th International Workshop on HIV Drug Resistance and Treatment Strategies; Scottsdale, AZ, June 4-8, 2001, Abstract 2.

304. Lalezari, J.P., I.H. Patel, X. Zhang, A. Dorr, N. Hawker, Z. Siddique, S. Kolis, and T. Kinchelow. 2003. Influence of subcutaneous injection site on the steady state pharmacokinetics of enfuvirtide (T-20) in HIV-1 infected patients. *J. Clin. Virol.* 28:217–222.

305. Chen, R.Y., J.M. Kilby, and M.S. Saag. 2002. Enfuvirtide. *Expert Opin. Investig. Drugs* 11:1837–1843.

306. Zhang, X., K. Nieforth, J.M. Lang, R. Rouzier-Panis, J. Reynes, A. Door, S. Kolis, M.R. Stiles, T. Kinchelow, and I.H. Patel. 2002. Pharmacokinetics of plasma enfuvirtide after subcutaneous administration to patients with human immunodeficiency virus: Inverse Gaussian density absorption and 2-compartmental deposition. *Clin. Pharmacol. Ther.* 72:10–19.

307. Ball, R.A., and T. Kinchelow. 2003. Injection site reactions with the HIV-1 fusion inhibitor enfuvirtide. ISR Substudy Group. *J. Am. Acad. Dermatol.* 49:826–831.

308. Tashima, K.T., and C.C.J. Carpenter. 2003. Fusion inhibition—a major but costly step forward in the treatment of HIV-1. *N. Engl. J. Med.* 348:2249–2250.

309. Vollmer, S. Patients, doctors cool to Fuzeon. The News and Observer. September 16, 2003. online (www.newsobserver.com.

310. Glutzer, E. 2003. Treatment with a new fusion inhibitor: Patient issues with enfuvirtide (T-20). A review of the presentation at the satellite symposium "New hope: Advancing the care

in HIV infection" at the 15th annual Association of Nurses in AIDS Care Conference, San Francisco, CA November 2002. *AIDS Read.* 13:S14–16.

311. Cohen, C., J. Hellinger, M. Johnson, S. Staszewski, N. Wintfeld, K. Patel, and J. Green. 2003. Patient acceptance of self-injected enfuvirtide at 8 and 24 weeks. *HIV Clin. Trials* 4:347–357.

312. Duckworth, M. 2003. First drug in a new class of HIV/AIDS treatments. ProCAARE, March 17, 2003, Centers for Disease Control and Prevention, South Africa. *Pharmacotherapy* 23: 695–701.

313. East, J.A., C. Cabrera, D. Schols, P. Cherepanov, A. Gutierrez, M. Witvrouw, C. Pannecouque, Z. Debyser, R.F. Rando, B. Clotet, J. Desmyter, and E. De Clercq. 1998. Human immuno-deficiency virus glycoprotein gp120 as the primary target for the antiviral action of AR177 (Zintevir). *Mol. Pharmacol.* 53:340–345.

Chapter 3

General (Non-antiretroviral) Antiviral Drugs

INTRODUCTION

Many clinical conditions are caused by viral infections and may range from encephalitis to gastroenteritis to rashes to mucous membrane lesions. In the past, the practitioner was limited to only treating symptoms as the virus ran its course. New developments in antiviral therapy are now progressing at an increasingly rapid pace and promise innovative treatment of viral infections.

The first portion of this chapter contains descriptions of viruses for which antivirals have been developed and approved. Viral infections are lumped by taxonomic group. In the latter part of this chapter, Food and Drug Administration (FDA)-approved and investigational non-HIV antiviral agents are discussed. (Table 3.1).

Well-known, established viruses continue to create morbidity and mortality worldwide, particularly in developing

Table 3.1 Current FDA-approved Antiviral Drugs (Excluding Antiretrovirals)

Herpes Simplex Virus (HSV)/ **Varicella Zoster Virus (VZV** Acyclovir (Zovirax) Valacyclovir (Valtrex) Famciclovir (Famvir) Foscarnet (Foscavir) Trifluridine (Viroptic) n-docosanol (Abreva)[a,b] Penciclovir (Denavir)[b]	**Hepatitis B Virus (HBV)** Interferon-alpha (Intron A) Lamivudine (Epivir-HBV) Adefovir (Hepsera) **Hepatitis C Virus (HCV)** Interferon-alpha (Intron A, Roferon-A) PEG-interferon-alpha (Peg- Intron, Pegasys)
Cytomegalovirus (CMV) Ganciclovir (Cytovene, Vitrasert) Valganciclovir (Valcyte) Foscarnet (Foscavir) Cidofovir (Vistide) Fomivirsen (Vitravene)	Interferon-alpha + Ribavirin (Rebetron) PEG-interferon-alpha and Ribavirin **Respiratory Syncytial Virus** Ribavirin (Virazole)
HHV-8 (Kaposi's Sarcoma) Interferon-alpha (Intron A, Roferon-A)	**Influenza Virus** Amantadine (Symmetrel) (Influenza A) Rimantadine (Flumadine)
Human Papillomaviruses **(HPV)** Interferon-alpha (Alferon N, Intron A) Imiquimod (Aldara)	(Influenza A) Zanamivir (Relenza) (Influenza A and B) Oseltamivir (Tamiflu) (Influenza A and B)

[a] Over the counter, has antiviral activity, but not specifically approved as an antiviral drug
[b] HSV only

countries (Fig. 3.1). Not only are the well-recognized viruses unchecked, but new viruses emerge each year—recently exposed to new host populations. Only a few of the newer diseases have antivirals or vaccines. Vaccines benefit the individual, but are only effective for the community if a significant number are vaccinated. Those who remain unvaccinated rely on post-exposure therapy, which may or may not be available.

The number of antiviral agents available to combat viral infection is expanding rapidly. Most of the approved drugs

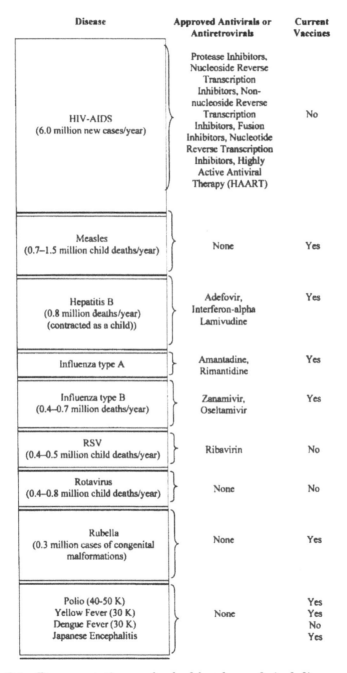

Fig. 3.1 Representative unchecked burdens of viral disease.

have been targeted for use for only a few viral infections, but many of these drugs may lead to new applications for other viral diseases or to the development of other agents that are more effective. New uses for these drugs are always under evaluation. This chapter provides an overview of viral infections that are targeted by these drugs and provides information on the wide range of efficacy of each antiviral agent. Antiviral drugs are introduced by chemical taxonomic grouping. Clinical studies and published reports of therapy provide valuable information to the reader. Molecular structure and the mechanism of action are also provided.

VIRAL INFECTIONS OTHER THAN HIV

Herpes Simplex Virus (HSV-1 and -2)

Herpes simplex virus occurs in both immunocompetent and immunocompromised populations. Herpes labialis, as characterized by orofacial herpes, fever blisters, and cold sores, is usually due to infection with HSV-1 (even though HSV-2 can also be a cause). Up to 30% of the American population may be affected by herpes labialis. Asymptomatic infection as detected by serum antibodies to HSV-1 is present in 60–80% of the general population and 95% of HIV positive patients. Genital herpes is usually caused by HSV-2, although the prevalence of HSV-1 in these infections is increasing. Other expressions of HSV-1 and HSV-2 are eczema herpeticum, herpetic encephalitis, neonatal herpes, herpes gladiatorum, herpetic whitlow, herpetic keratoconjuctivitis, and gingivostomatitis. Erythema multiforme is usually an indirect manifestation of HSV infection. Arguments for the initiation of antiviral drugs for the suppression of genital herpes are shown in Table 3.2. HSV-1 and -2 are unique in that these viruses may recur even though humoral immunity is present. These recurrences, called reactivation of latent infection, may affect the mucosal membranes or skin or may even result in encephalitis, keratoconjunctivitis, etc. Histopathological characteristics of primary and secondary occurrences focus on the inflammatory response from cell

Table 3.2　Reasons to Suggest Suppression of Genital Herpes with Acyclovir, Valacyclovir, or Famciclovir

1. **Number of outbreaks:** In the first two years after the first outbreak, the frequency is usually greatest.
2. **Severity of outbreaks:** Physical and/or emotional impact.
3. **Presence of a prodrome:** If the prodrome is not present, episodic therapy usually doesn't work well.
4. **Serostatus of the partner:** (The importance of this point is dependent on the fact that reducing asymptomatic shedding will reduce transmission).
   a. If the person at risk is female, the benefit may be greater than if the person at risk is male. (Rates for male-to-female transmission are up to 4 times that of female-to-male).
   b. If the person at risk is female and pregnant, the benefit may be greatest (i.e. three persons may benefit from one person taking a drug).
5. **Immuncompromised patient:** Immunocompromised patients usually suffer frequent and severe outbreaks.

death. Although asymptomatic infection is the most common, patients may present with oropharyngeal outbreaks, genital disease, central nervous system degeneration, and neonatal HSV caused by exposure of the infant to the mother's genital secretions during delivery.

HSV infection occurs when the virus comes in contact with mucosal surfaces or abraded skin. The infection causes cell ballooning and loss of plasma membranes. Pools of viral material collect between the dermis and epidermis, causing an inflammatory response. The vesicular fluid becomes pustular during healing with resultant scabbing. Shallow ulcers may occur.

Once viral replication occurs at the entry site, the virus moves to the dorsal root ganglia via retrograde transport of the virus (Fig. 3.2). After more replication, latency occurs and the severity and frequency of reactivation of the virus appears to be dependent upon the severity of the initial infection. Diagnosis of HSV-1 and 2 is by tissue culture, serology, and polymerase chain reaction (PCR). Currently, there is no approved vaccine for HSV-1 and -2. Prevention through education and

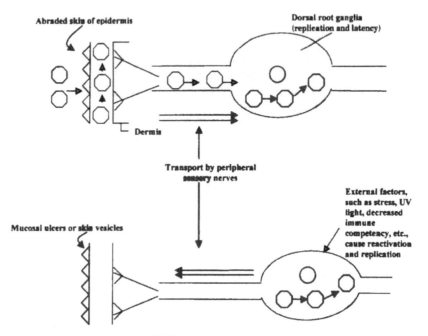

Fig. 3.2 Schematic of HSV infection, replication, latency, and reactivation.

use of condoms is warranted, especially for adolescents and adults who seem to be at the greatest risk. Neonatal infection is avoided through careful use of sterile instruments, caesarian section deliveries occurring within a few hours of an outbreak, care of maternal tissue which could be infective, and preventing exposure of the infant to any possible contaminant for HSV. Herpes-1 virus has been associated with Bell's palsy, treatable with acyclovir combined with prednisone (1).

HSV is treated with the nucleoside analogs (e.g., acyclovir) as well as foscarnet and trifluridine. Table 3.3 is an overview of how multiple manifestations of one virus (HSV) may be treated by a variety of therapies. As is often observed, drug resistance becomes a problem as new drugs with better efficacy become available, providing more options for treatment. HSV is an excellent model as it has been treated with numerous nucleoside analog antivirals.

Table 3.3 Treatment of Herpes Simplex Virus Infections

Symptom	Treatment
Herpes labialis	Topical application of 1% penciclovir cream every 2 hours while awake for 4 days. (Mucous membrane application is not recommended).
	Topical application of 10% docosanol cream 5 times daily.
	Acyclovir is often used off-label for oral treatment of herpes labialis, at 400 mg 3–5 times daily for 5 days.
	Famciclovir is often used off-label for oral treatment of herpes labialis, at 125 mg twice daily (b.i.d.) for 5 days, although a recent study showed that higher dosages are more optimal (500 mg 3 times a day (t.i.d.) for 5 days).
	Valacyclovir is often used off-label for oral treatment of herpes labialis, at 500 mg twice daily for 5 days, but FDA approval is for 2 g b.i.d. for 1 day.
	For chronic suppression, if needed (off-label): Acyclovir 400 mg twice daily, or famciclovir 250 mg twice daily or valacyclovir 500 mg once daily.
Herpes genitalis	Acyclovir 200 mg five times daily (or 400 mg t.i.d.) for 10 days (initial infection) or 5 days (recurrent attacks). Intravenous acyclovir may be given for severe primary infections, at 5 mg/kg over 1 hour every 8 hours for 7 days, followed by oral therapy. Daily suppressive therapy may be given to prevent frequent attacks, at 400 mg twice daily.
	Valacyclovir 1 gram twice daily for 10 days for initial episodes, and 500 mg twice daily for three-five days for recurrent attacks. For chronic suppressive therapy, 1 gram daily is given for patients with 10 or more recurrences per year, and 500 mg once daily is given for those with less frequent outbreaks.
	Famciclovir 250 mg t.i.d. for 10 days for initial episodes, and 125 mg twice daily for 5 days for recurrent outbreaks. For continuous suppressive therapy, 250 mg twice daily is given.
Other cutaneous HSV infections (i.e., herpetic whitlow)	No controlled studies have evaluated acyclovir, valacyclovir, or famciclovir for therapy of HSV infections in other cutaneous areas. If disease is severe and recurrent, prescribe oral acyclovir (or valacyclovir or famciclovir) initially at dosages

(continued)

Table 3.3 (*Continued*)

Symptom	Treatment
	utilized to treat primary genital HSV infections. If suppressive therapy is planned, those dosages utilized for frequently recurrent genital HSV infection are appropriate.
Mucocutaneous HSV infections in immunocompromised patients	Intravenous acyclovir infusion at 5 mg/kg over 1 hour, given every 8 hours for 7 days. For children less than 12 years of age, the dosage is 250 mg/m² at the same schedule.
	For limited disease, topical application of acyclovir 5% ointment every 3 hours (6 times daily) for 7 days.
Recurrent orolabial or genital HSV infections in HIV-infected patients	Famciclovir 500 mg twice daily for 7 days. This same dosage is also used on a daily basis for chronic suppression of recurrent episodes in HIV-infected persons.
	Valacyclovir 500 mg to 1000 mg b.i.d. can also be used for episodic therapy (e.g., 7 days) or on a daily basis for chronic suppression in these patients.
Herpes simplex keratoconjunctivitis	Trifluridine 1% ophthalmic solution for primary keratoconjunctivitis and recurrent epithelial keratitis due to HSV, given as one drop in the affected eye(s) every 2 hours while awake (maximum of 9 drops per day). This is continued until re-epithelialization of the corneal ulcer occurs, followed by one drop every 4 hours while awake for 7 more days.
	Topical acyclovir for HSV ocular infections is effective, but probably not superior to trifluridine, and is no longer recommended.
Herpes simplex encephalitis	Intravenous acyclovir infusion at 10 mg/kg over 1 hour, given every 8 hours for 14 days. For children 6 months to 12 years of age, the dosage is adjusted to 500 mg/m².
Neonatal herpes simplex infection	Intravenous acyclovir infusion at 10 mg/kg over 1 hour, given every 8 hours for 14 days (SEM[a] disease) to 21 days (encephalitis or multiorgan disease).
Acyclovir-resistant HSV infections	Intravenous foscarnet infusion at 40 mg/kg over 1 hour either every 8 or 12 hours, for 2–3 weeks or until all lesions are healed.
	Cidofovir 1% cream or gel may be compounded as an alternative therapy.

[a] SEM = Skin, eyes, mucous membranes

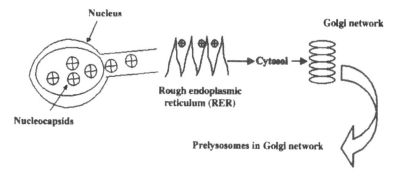

Fig. 3.3   Infection and replication of varicella zoster virus (VZV).

Varicella Zoster Virus (VZV)

VZV is spread in the air or via direct contact and then (Fig. 3.3) replicates in the nuclei of cells (2). Nucleocapsids of VZV are produced in the nuclei of infected host cells. Capsids receive a primary viral envelope from the inner nuclear membrane. Eventually these attach to rough endoplasmic reticulum (RER). Nucleocapsids move through the cytosol to the Golgi apparatus (trans-Golgi network) where they obtain a final envelope. The distribution of VZV is worldwide, but is less prevalent in tropical climates than those that are more temperate. Varicella zoster virus infection occurs as chickenpox in the young and manifests itself as shingles (herpes zoster) when reactivated in adults. More than 90% of the adult population has serological evidence of prior infection with VZV, although they may not have had an active, recordable case. Primary VZV infection in adults, adolescents, and immunocompromised patients may be more severe and require extended treatment. Shingles, the recurrence of VZV, is associated with painful lesions that heal but may leave the patient with post-herpetic neuralgia (PHN) for months or even years. Painful PHN has been associated with high suicide rates among the elderly. Antiviral therapies are first line treatment options although higher doses are utilized for the slower growing, more fastidious VZV than for HSV infection. Varicella in children manifests itself as a rash that requires two weeks to heal and fever that lasts approximately 5 days. Prior to the development of vaccines for infants and children to prevent "chickenpox," most children were exposed to chickenpox as an aerosol by close contact with classmates who were incubating VZV prior to their development of a rash. Complications include external bacterial infections in the skin and internal infections in the lungs. Reye's syndrome is not seen as frequently as physicians now instruct parents not to give aspirin for the symptomatic treatment of the fever associated with chickenpox outbreaks. Varicella may cause neutropenia and thrombocytopenia, renal complications, arthritis, joint, or ocular complications. In the immunocompromised, varicella, combined with other secondary infections, may be fatal. Zoster has become the greater health hazard when compared with varicella. The localized skin eruptions occur with reactivation of the virus often at an advanced age. Zoster eruptions in older patients may cause painful, long-lasting inflammation of the nerves (i.e., PHN). Symptomatic treatment for pain associated with PHN has been lacking although initiation of gabapentin concomitant with a nucleoside analog within the first 72 hours of vesicle eruption shows promise for decreasing the incidence, severity, and duration of PHN (3). Acyclovir is indicated for the treatment of varicella (chickenpox) but valacyclovir and famciclovir are also used in adolescents and adults; all three nucleoside analogs can be used to treat zoster (shingles).

Epstein-Barr Virus (EBV)

Epstein-Barr virus (EBV) is found in human mucosal epithelial cells and B lymphocytes. Other cell types may also be infected. Burkitt's lymphoma, originally identified in Africa, was found to be due to Epstein-Barr virus, named after its two discoverers (4). Epstein-Barr virus later became associated with not only African Burkitt's lymphoma, but Hodgkin's disease and nasopharyngeal carcinoma (5,6). Infectious mononucleosis is the most common manifestation of EBV. Infectious mononucleosis has a large public health impact on young college students and military recruits. Both are populations living in close quarters, exposed to many new people, and where mucosal contact via oral secretions may occur. Symptoms present in >50% of patients include fever, pharyngitis and sore throat, lymphadenopathy, malaise, headache, and splenomegaly. Complications involve the neurological, respiratory, cardiac, hematological, hepatic and renal systems. There is a rash in 10% of the cases (7). EBV-associated lymphoproliferative diseases and malignancies occur as solid tumors (nasopharyngeal carcinoma and cervical lymphadenopathy), B-cell lymphoproliferative disorders (Hodgkin's lymphoma, Burkitt's lymphoma, and lymphoproliferative disease in the immunocompromised), and T-cell lymphoproliferative disorders (oral lymphoma in HIV-infected patients, angiocentric cutaneous lymphoma including papules, nodules, bullae, panniculitis, histiocytoid cutaneous lymphoma, and vesiculopapular lesions of the face) (8). In HIV-positive persons, oral hairy leukopenia (OHL) is a benign focus of hyperplasia. EBV is sometimes identified in breast tumors (9–11). EBV has a latent circular genome and a linear genome. OHL develops when the linear genome replicates via a viral polymerase. Antiviral agents which inhibit this enzyme are an effective therapy for OHL. These include: 1) high doses of acyclovir (800 mg five times/day); 2) valacyclovir and famciclovir (with better bioavailability); and 3) ganciclovir, foscarnet or cidofovir for HIV-infected patients with CMV (OHL seems to improve at the same time).

Cytomegalovirus (CMV)

A variety of cutaneous manifestations may occur with CMV mononucleosis syndrome, congenital CMV infection, and coinfection of HIV with CMV. In vitro, CMV infection shows sensitivity to many of the antiviral agents used to treat HSV and VZV. CMV infection can be life-threatening to neonates, transplant recipients, and HIV-positive patients. CMV retinitis requires particular attention to prevent blindness. CMV replicates by rolling-circle replication. For CMV to replicate requires eleven genetically determined proteins to be in place. These proteins are contained within a variety of related molecules: DNA polymerase, a polymerase-associated protein, single-stranded DNA binding protein, helicase primase, transactivators, and two unknown functions (12). This specificity provides a number of molecular targets for potential antiviral drug development and intervention. As with many viruses, transmission is relatively simple and may occur through intrauterine infection from primary-infected mothers, perinatal infection from breast milk, postnatal infection primarily from saliva and/or sexual contact, blood transfusions, and organ transplantation. Laboratory diagnoses of active CMV infection include PCR, histopathology, isolation of the virus, antigen detection, and serological assays. CMV can be prevented by utilizing seronegative blood for transfusions, especially for pregnant women and immunocompromised patients. Day care centers may be the reservoir for transmission of CMV among a variety of individuals. CMV is asymptomatic in most cases, but saliva, a saliva-coated toy, or eating utensils (fomites) may spread the disease among teethers, droolers, and toddlers. Children may then infect siblings, pregnant mothers or day care workers. Infected workers risk transmittal to the children. Since this mode of transmission occurs within the realm of daycare centers, daycare workers must be careful to utilize appropriate hand washing and other good hygiene practices.

Exposure to CMV appears to be a life-long event. The percentage of women with IgG antibodies against CMV increases as their ages increase. Approximately 40% of women under the age of 16 have IgG antibodies against CMV compared with nearly 80% of those women over 41 years of age (13). CMV in the immunosuppressed can also have serious consequences. Studies indicate that seronegative CMV transplant recipients can acquire CMV from organs of seropositive donors (14). CMV has been associated with thrombotic microangiopathy in HIV-infected patients (15,16). Vaccines for better protection are needed and are being developed and tested. The antivirals, ganciclovir, valganciclovir, foscarnet, cidofovir, and fomivirsen, are FDA approved for treatment of CMV. These currently available drugs have issues of toxicity, modest efficacy and poor oral bioavailability. New compounds being tested include novel inhibitors of protein kinase and viral proteins of DNA origin. Certain non-nucleosides also can inhibit the viral process (17).

Human Herpesvirus 8 (HHV-8)

Kaposi's sarcoma (KS) occurs as four main types. Classic Kaposi's sarcoma occurs in elderly Mediterranean men or those of Ashkenazi Jewish descent. An endemic form affects persons of all ages in tropical Africa. The two most common forms seen in the medical profession are an immunosuppressive form in organ transplant recipients and the AIDS-associated form. Mediterranean, Jewish, Arabic, or African ancestry is often associated with KS in organ transplant recipients. In Africa, where endemic KS is the cause of up to 10% of all histologically proven malignancies, sexual transmission is believed to be the most common mode of transmission. Perinatal transmission from mother to child is also suspected (18). Kaposi's sarcoma, prior to the introduction of highly active antiretroviral therapy (HAART), affected nearly 20% of patients with AIDS (19–21), and was primarily treated with destructive therapies similar to those used with HPV. Radiation therapy and chemotherapy were also used. The development of alitretinoin, a gene expression regulator, has shown promise in treating Kaposi's sarcoma with a topical, at-home therapy. However, alitretinoin is not as effective for the large fungating lesions, but it could be combined with chemotherapy for treatment of large tumors. Antiherpes drugs seem to be more effective as a preventive drug for KS in HHV-8 infected immunosuppressed persons than as a therapy for active KS. KS is composed of large latently infected spindle cells. These antiviral drugs seem to block the lytic phase of viral replication which occurs when HHV-8 is establishing itself in the dermis (22–25). Interferon-alpha is currently FDA-approved for treatment of Kaposi's sarcoma (26).

Human Papillomavirus (HPV)

HPV is the most commonly sexually transmitted disease in the United States. HPV expresses itself as genital warts or lesions on the cervix and the virus has been directly connected to the development of cervical cancer (27). There are over 100 genotypes of HPV with genotypes 16 and 18 most commonly associated with the development of cervical cancer (Fig. 3.4).

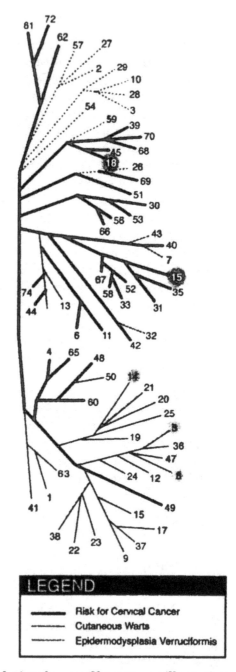

Fig. 3.4 Relational map of human papillomaviruses by genotypes.

The prevalence of genotypes worldwide demonstrates isolation by distance with additional pockets of introduced genotypes or mutations occurring overtime. Sexual behavior and possibly fomite contamination are leading causes of transmission. Electrocautery and laser therapy present a risk to the surgeon and other medical staff as HPV DNA is contained in the smoke caused by the procedure (28).

The genetic make-up of the infected person may affect development of cervical dysplasia or neoplasia. There appears to be genetic propensity to develop either long-term infection leading to cervical cancer (if left untreated) or automatic clearing of the infection (experienced by the majority of women). Other lesions indicate HPV infection, including, but not limited to, plantar warts, common warts, flat or planar warts (29,30), epidermodysplasia verruciformis, other anogenital diseases, respiratory papillomatosis (especially in children), and other mucosal papillomas (Fig. 3.4).

While treatment with antiviral drugs is needed to help those already infected, vaccine development is also needed as a preventive method. Most treatments for HPV have been ablative— trichloroacetic acid, podophyllotoxin, cryotherapy, laser ablation, surgical excision, and electrosurgery/cautery. Not only can genital warts be treated with antiviral drugs, but some of the therapies may prove effective in treating common warts. Imiquimod users have a 56% complete response rate with a 13% relapse rate for the treatment of anogenital warts (31,32). Interferon-alpha is also FDA approved for the treatment of HPV (i.e., condyloma acuminatum).

Molluscum Contagiosum Virus (MCV) and other Poxviruses

Currently, no antiviral agents are FDA-approved for treatment of MCV lesions. Most lesions are treated with cytodestructive methods. There are reports of various antiviral agents having some efficacy in treating MCV, but more thorough investigations and clinical studies are needed. In HIV-positive patients, antiretroviral agents, such as highly active antiretroviral therapy (HAART), improve the immune system and contribute to the success of additional antiviral drugs (33,34).

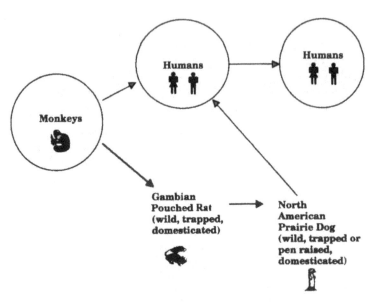

Fig. 3.5   Recent epidemiology of monkey pox.

Two other poxviruses have gained recent attention: small-pox as a bioterrorism threat and monkeypox as a hitchhiker to the United States on the Gambian pouched rat with subsequent infection of U.S.-endemic prairie dogs being sold as pets. The handlers of the pet prairie dogs then developed monkeypox. Monkeypox was initially identified as a poxvirus in laboratory primates before it was linked to an orthopoxvirus from central and western Africa. It is a rare zoonosis and isolation of most cases makes vaccine development unlikely. However, the potential for animal to animal and human to human transmission (Fig. 3.5) may stimulate development of new vaccines or additional antiviral therapy. Prior to this event in the summer of 2003, monkeypox transmission was only by monkeys and squirrels to humans and human to humans subsequently. Skinning or handling wild animals and consumption of incompletely cooked wild monkey meat was thought to be the primary route of transmission. Smallpox vaccination reduces susceptibility to monkeypox and lessens the severity of the disease (33).

Initially variolation with pustule fluid or scab material was used to protect against smallpox. Refinements in vaccine development led to the eradication of epidemic smallpox.

Recent advances in smallpox vaccine development and administration are discussed in chapter 4 (Vaccines). A possible treatment
for complications from vaccination is vaccinia immune globulin.
Cidofovir has antipoxvirus effects and the potential to treat vaccinia and smallpox (34). Ribavirin displays modest antiviral activity against cowpox. Trifluridine is used to treat ocular keratitis.

Hepatitis B Virus (HBV)/Hepatitis C Virus (HCV)

HBV and HCV have similar treatments and are sensitive to similar drugs. Both hepatitis B and C have the potential to develop
fatal sequellae, such as cirrhosis of the liver and hepatocellular
carcinoma. Injection drug use accounts for 21% of the known
cases in the United States and Western Europe (35). The primary
means for HBV transmission is through blood or blood products,
sexual contact or perinatal exposure. Fomites, such as contaminated dental instruments, acupuncture needles, tattoo needles,
and other invasive medical instruments, may also transmit hepatitis B. Travelers are subject to infection, particularly those in
third-world countries. Transfusion and dialysis are other modes
of transmission. Seven genotypes, encompassing 12 subtypes,
have been described. Nearly 5% of the world's population has
chronic HBV infection (36). The incubation period for HBV
ranges from 60 to 180 days. Patients may experience jaundice
and, perhaps, liver failure (37,38). Unfortunately, patients may
not know they have HBV until they present with ascites, bleeding esophageal variances, or encephaly (39). Biochemically,
serum bilirubin and aminotransferase levels are used for initial
diagnosis but serological and virological confirmation is
required. Necrotizing vasculitis and polyarteritis nodosa are
associated with HBV infections, and are linked to cryoglobuline-
mia (35,40,41). Chronic infection may occur in hemodialysis, diabetic, and elderly stroke or head injury patients with very high
rates (43–59%) of chronic infection after an acute exposure. HIV
positive patients are also at greater risk. Treatment of symptoms
without knowledge of the presence of HBV can be problematic as
many drugs are potentially hepatotoxic.

With better diagnostics for HCV infection, it is estimated
that 3.9 million Americans (1.8% of the population) are
infected with HCV (42) with over 170 million infected worldwide.

The genome displays genetic heterogeneity which makes it less likely to activate the human immune system. Appropriate animal models for HCV are lacking and mechanistic molecular studies of replication have been limited. Humans may be multiply infected overtime and there may be a failure to develop a high rate of immunity after the initial infection occurs (43,44). As with other hepatitis infections, clinical manifestations do not occur until the disease has become chronic. The presence of fibrosis is the end stage of hepatitis C over time and is predictive of progression to cirrhosis. HCV progresses over a period of 10–30 years from infection to liver cirrhosis. There are six definite genotypes with subtypes of each genotype. Leukocytoclastic vasculitis, lichen planus, poryphyria cutanea tarda, and polyarteritis nodosa have been linked to chronic HBV and/or HCV infections (39,45,46). Prevention via modification of risky behaviors, passive immunoprophylaxis, and immunization (i.e., HBV) are the best strategy. Education and information campaigns to reduce the transmission of hepatitis B and vaccines have been effective in reducing the numbers of cases of hepatitis B in the United States (35). Currently approved treatments for hepatitis B include interferon-alpha, adefovir, and lamivudine. Lamivudine is discussed in chapter 2 **Page 48**. Hepatitis C treatments are pegylated (PEG) interferon-alpha, and PEG-interferon-alpha + ribavirin. Currently available drugs have issues of toxicity, modest efficacy, and poor oral bioavailability. New compounds being tested include novel inhibitors of protein kinase, viral protease, and viral proteins of DNA origin. Certain non-nucleosides also can inhibit the viral process (17).

Influenza Virus

Influenza is responsible for pandemic or worldwide outbreaks of new strains of flu that originate in localized geographic areas. The advent of world travel has opened every country's door to a sudden invasion of new influenza strains at a moment's notice. Fortunately, faster and better communications about the disease—prevention, clinical manifestations, treatment, etc.—assist with harnessing resources to prevent further spread. Animals, particularly those domesticated for agricultural use, are often the culprit, such as the swine influenza virus that was responsible for the 1918 pandemic with 40 million deaths worldwide. There are three influenza viruses: A, B, and C. Only A is subdivided and only five of those subtypes are known to affect humans. A and B have eight different RNA segments; C has only seven.

Rapid detection of influenza in pediatric patients is important for early therapy. The use of an enzyme-linked immunosorbent assay can detect influenza A. The end result is that this rapid detection system decreases the use of ancillary tests and indiscriminate use of antibiotics (47). On the other hand, for adults, clinical modeling indicates that testing strategies for influenza before prescribing antivirals is more expensive than just prescribing the antiviral. Running tests for influenza are more costly and less effective when the probability of influenza exceeds 30% (48).

Human influenza virus may co-infect with an animal strain to produce new pandemic strains, much as hybridization occurs among higher level organisms. In this case, however, replication occurs and the new viral strain has few, if any, enemies. Each strain requires a new set of antibodies to be produced for future resistance.

Pandemic influenza viruses are characterized by rapid onset and easy dissemination of infection. The short (only days) incubation periods accompanied by high levels of virus in respiratory secretions at the onset of illness create multiple waves of infection. Hands or fomites may also spread influenza (49).

Factors which contribute to the spread of an influenza virus are travelers, seasonally by geographic area, and initiation of school in the fall. Mortality rates are highest in the elderly and the very young, particularly those with respiratory or cardiovascular disease. Nursing home outbreaks require special care and a number of recommendations have been made to avoid major outbreak catastrophes (49–51). Nosocomal infections occur where there are high concentrations of people.

Influenza outbreaks vary by the proportional activity of the three subtypes. Dramatic changes occur in those proportions annually. Thus, this year's vaccine combination may not be effective for the following years. The ancestral genetic origin of pandemic strains is often avian. A limitation on vaccinations for influenza is the "drift" (proportional reassortment) of wild virus strains each year (52). For example, the composition of the 2002–2003 vaccine was A/Moscow/10/99 (H3N3)-like, A/Ner Caledonia/20/99 (H1N1)-like, and B/Hong Kong/330/2001-like strains (53).

Treatment of influenza is symptomatic and antiviral. Ventilation may be necessary. Antivirals such as amantadine, ramantadine, oseltamivir and zanamivir are effective. Ribavirin is under investigation as is interferon-alpha (54–56).

Respiratory Syncytial Virus (RSV)

Respiratory syncytial virus (RSV) is the most common cause of inflammation in the small airways in the lung and pneumonia in infants and small children. Most children have had RSV by the age of 3 (57). RSV is seasonal and peaks in February. Native Americans and Alaskan natives seem to be more susceptible (58).

RSV is a labile paramyxovirus that causes human cell fusion-the syncytial effect. Two strains, A and B, cause either asymptomatic illness (Type B) or more clinical illness (Type A).

Babies who are born premature and are less than 6 weeks of age, with congenital problems, such as heart disease, chronic lung disease, and immunodeficiency, are at high risk. Other contributing factors are lower socioeconomic states, crowded living conditions, presence of secondary cigarette smoke, older siblings in the home, and daycare attendance. Breast-fed infants seem to be at less risk than their bottle-fed counterparts.

Children with runny noses (rhinorrhea), wheezing and coughing, low-grade (102°F) or higher (104°F) fever (if coinfected), and nasal flaring may have RSV. RSV can be positively identified by using direct antigen tests that provide a positive response in little over an hour. RSV has been indicated as a risk factor for asthma development. An antiviral, such as ribavirin, inhibits replication during the viral replication stage (54–57).

Rhinovirus

Rhinovirus infection has been responsible for years for the common cold, which was treated symptomatically. Rhinovirus has also been associated with complications, such as acute sinusitis, otitis media, acute bronchitis, and pneumonia. Rhinovirus is also associated with the development of asthma and cystic fibrosis exacerbations in children.

Rhinosinusitis involves the nasal passages, paranasal sinuses, naso- and oropharynx, Eustachian tubes, middle ear, larynx, and large airways. Systemic involvement is usually mild in adults. Rhinovirus infections in immunocompromised patients, as with other infections, are more serious when combined with multiple infections.

Adults who are taught the characteristics of allergic rhinitis and cold are able to distinguish between the two (59).

Symptomatic and anti-inflammatory treatment includes decongestants, fever relief, cough cessation, etc., but does not cure the infection. Antivirals identified for their potential usefulness include interferon α to reduce viral replication. Capsid binding agents and 3 C protease inhibitors are being evaluated. Pleconaril and AG7088 are under investigation in clinical trials.

NUCLEOSIDE ANALOGS

The (non-antiretroviral) nucleoside analogs include acyclovir, valacyclovir, famciclovir, penciclovir, ganciclovir, and valganciclovir as well as ribavirin. Nucleoside analogs are important antivirals in the therapy of HIV and herpesvirus infections.

Most nucleoside analogue antivirals have the capacity to induce chromosomal aberrations, but these aberrations are not evident in gene arrays. Genotoxicity is being investigated in this group but, thus far, there is no conclusive evidence that nucleoside analogs cause tumors in humans. Antiviral nucleosides for HIV therapy, in addition to being highly effective, may also cause side effects that become serious enough to consider alternative therapies (60).

Acyclovir

Introduction

Acyclovir, an analog of 2′-deoxyguanosine, has become the most widely prescribed antiviral in the world since its introduction in 1983 (Fig. 3.6). Acyclovir does not appear to alter

Generic Name Acyclovir	Structure	Viral Diseases Treated (FDA Approved)
Brand Name(s) Zovirax **Other Name(s)**	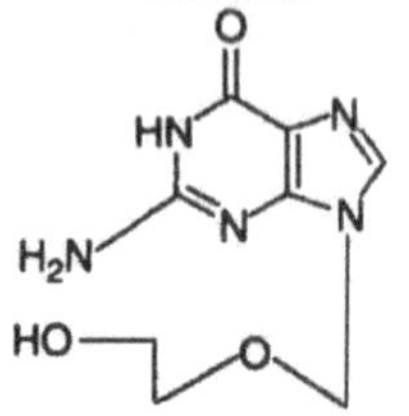	Herpes simplex virus 1 (HSV-1) Herpes simplex virus 2 (HSV-2) Varicella zoster virus (VZV)

Fig. 3.6 Associated names, structure, and applicability of acyclovir.

the development of long-term immunity to varicella zoster virus when administered for the treatment of chickenpox in otherwise healthy patients. A limiting factor is considered to be its poor bioavailability. Viral resistance to acyclovir is not a major concern in normal clinical practice, but has occurred in a few patients with immunosuppression. There are conflicting studies as to whether acyclovir treatment in AIDS patients is associated with prolonged survival. Use of highly active anti-retroviral therapy (HAART) has virtually eliminated further studies of acyclovir as an agent for prolonged survival in AIDS patients.

Mechanisms of Action

Acyclovir is first phosphorylated to acyclovir monophosphate by the virus-specific enzyme, thymidine kinase (Fig. 3.7). Host cellular enzymes further phosphorylate the compound to convert it to its active triphosphate form (61). The final product inactivates viral DNA polymerase which leads to irreversible inhibition of further viral DNA synthesis (62–65). Acyclovir potency against HSV-1 replication can vary among cell lines. It has been suggested that the effect of acyclovir is due to proficient phosphorylation of acyclovir and/or a favorable dGTP/acyclovir triphosphate level in macrophage cells (66).

Studies to Support Use of Acyclovir

Acyclovir has been extensively studied for treatment of many viral diseases. Studies of interest are shown in Table 3.4 (64, 65,67–120).

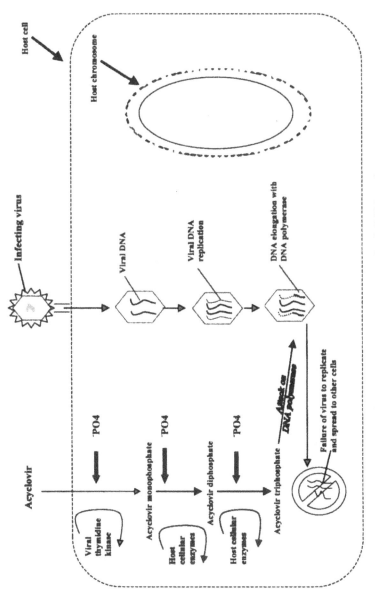

Fig. 3.7 Phosphorylation of acyclovir to inactivate viral DNA polymerase.

Table 3.4 Clinical Studies and Reported Observations to Support Use of Acyclovir as an Antiviral Agent

Topic	Findings	References
Use within acute herpes infection	Acyclovir, valacyclovir, or famciclovir is the choice of treatment.	64,65
Treatment of recurrent herpes episodes	Acyclovir, valacyclovir, or famciclovir is the choice of treatment.	64,67
Reduction of viral shedding	Acyclovir, valacyclovir, or famciclovir is the choice of treatment.	68
Topical acyclovir to treat herpes labialis in otherwise healthy patients	Little therapeutic effect of topical acyclovir; better with oral valacyclovir or famciclovir.	69–73
Varicella zoster virus (VZV) infections (chickenpox and herpes zoster)	In immunocompetent children and adults, oral acyclovir that is begun within 24 hours after the onset (20 mg/kg 4 times daily for 5 days) decreases the severity of the disease.	74–76
Cutaneous healing of herpes zoster	Oral acyclovir (800 mgPO) given 5 times daily for 7–10 days causes faster healing and less severity of acute pain.	77–82
Reanalysis of placebo-controlled trial	Median duration of zoster-associated pain in acyclovir recipients was 20 days, compared with 62 days for the placebo counterparts.	83
Early trials for reducing duration of post-herpetic neuralgia in herpes zoster	Little benefit of acyclovir.	77,78,84
Meta-analysis of data from immunocompetent patients involved in 5 clinical trials of herpes zoster	Oral acyclovir treatment initiated within 72 hours of rash onset may reduce the incidence of residual pain at 6 months by 46% in immunocompetent adults.	85
Epstein-Barr dacryoadenitis (Sjögren's syndrome)	Treatment with systemic acyclovir, followed by cyclosporin A and prednisone to suppress the inflammatory response (i.e., off-label use).	86

(continued)

Table 3.4 *(Continued)*

Topic	Findings	References
Acyclovir, alone or combined with prednisolone, for 21 days vs 7 days of acyclovir alone	A 7-day regimen of acyclovir monotherapy is effective, but there is no added benefit to using the acyclovir for 21 days, either combined with prednisolone or given as monotherapy.	87
Prednisone + acyclovir for treatment of herpes zoster	Patients with acyclovir + prednisone returned to usual daily activities, had better sleep patterns, experienced less pain, and, in general faster cessation of acute neuritis, but no difference in the resolution of PHN during the 6 months following outbreak onset.	88
Maternal transfer of acyclovir to breast milk	The mother's dosage of acyclovir ranged from 200-800 mg 5 times daily and the level of acyclovir in babies ranged from .2 mg to 0.732 mg/kg/day. This is much less than the dosage prescribed for an infant with herpes encephalitis (30 mg/kg/day).	89–91
Viral resistance as a result of repeated dosage	Not a significant problem in clinical practice; majority of cases occur in patients with immunosuppression, particularly AIDS.	92–97
Viral resistance rates to acyclovir therapy	Rates of resistance in immunocompromised patients varied from 2% to 10.9%.	98–100
Treatment of acute infectious mononucleosis	Oral or intravenous acyclovir has little or no clinical benefit on the treatment of acute infectious mononucleosis.	101–103
Treatment of oral hairy leukoplakia (OHL)	Acyclovir is somewhat effective for treatment (off-label). Recurrence of OHL lesions after discontinuation of acyclovir is frequent and almost inevitable.	104–106

(continued)

Table 3.4   *(Continued)*

Topic	Findings	References
Herpes simplex encephalitis	Acyclovir is treatment of choice, but morbidity is very high (28%).	107,108
UV radiation-induced herpes labialis in the immuncompromised	Acyclovir (5%) and hydrocortisone (1%) (ME609) provides benefits by reducing lesion incidence, healing time, lesion size, and lesion tenderness.	109
Penciclovir vs acyclovir for HSV-1 infection (animal study)	Penciclovir efficacy in lesion number reduction, lesion area, and virus titer was significantly higher than that of acyclovir in guinea pigs.	110
Post-herpetic neuralgia	56 days of intravenous and oral acyclovir therapy had little or no effect on the clinical course of post-herpetic neuralgia.	111
Ramsay-Hunt syndrome (VZV)	Treatment with acyclovir (800 mg 5 times daily) combined with oral prednisone (60 mg. daily for 3–5 days) within 7 days of onset; also effective for Bell's palsy.	112
HSV esophagitis in immunocompetent host	Therapy may shorten duration of illness	113
HSV-1	Trichosanthin, combined with acyclovir and interferon, enhances the anti-herpetic effect.	114
Neonatal herpes	High doses of acyclovir reduce mortality rates.	115
Retinal vasculitis from chickenpox (VZV)	10 days of treatment with acyclovir resolved vasculitis and speeded a return of normal visual acuity.	116
Herpetic whitlow (HSV)	Intravenous acyclovir (5 mg/kg twice daily) cleared herpetic lip lesions and herpetic whitlow of the fingers.	117

(continued)

Table 3.4   (*Continued*)

Topic	Findings	References
Oral valacyclovir vs intravenous acyclovir	Oral valacyclovir is convenient and possibly safer than intravenous acyclovir. It also has a comparable systemic exposure with reduced peak levels.	118
Acyclovir-resistance in neonatal HSV	New mutation in the TK gene developed within 7 days of treatment.	119
Eczema herpeticum	Recurrences less extensive after treatment.	120

Treatment

Acyclovir can be administered topically, orally or intravenously with few adverse events (Table 3.5). Acyclovir is considered to be safe and well-tolerated with a 20 year history of usage, although its bioavailability (15–20%) is a limiting factor. Acyclovir is effective in decreasing severity in chickenpox (121,122). Acyclovir 5% ointment is used to treat initial herpes genitalis and limited mucocutaneous herpes simplex virus infections in immunocompromised patients. Acyclovir in ointment form is used cutaneously and should not be applied to the eye. Acyclovir is noncarcinogenic and nonteratogenic (i.e., class B) (123).

Intravenous acyclovir is more readily assimilated and can be used for serious or disseminated infections. Immunocompromised patients with HSV or VZV infections who develop chickenpox, disseminated herpes zoster, severe cases of trigeminal zoster (particularly ophthalmic zoster), eczema herpeticum (Kaposi's varicelliform eruption), herpes encephalitis, and neonatal herpes may be treated with intravenous acyclovir. During administration of intravenous acyclovir, adequate fluid intake by patients is important and renal insufficiency may require dosage adjustments.

Acyclovir and its related analogs are ideal for treating and suppressing genital herpes and related HSV episodes.

Table 3.5 Treatment Modalities Using Acyclovir

Symptom	Treatment
Initial herpes genitalis	Acyclovir 5% ointment to be applied to all lesions every 3 hours (6 times daily) for 7 days. Oral acyclovir 200 mg 5 times daily or 400 mg 3 times daily for 10 days.
Mucocutaneous herpes simplex virus infections in immunocompromised patients	Acyclovir 5% ointment to be applied to all lesions every 3 hours (6 times daily) for 7 days. For limited disease, topical application of acyclovir 5% ointment every 3 hours (6 times daily) for 7 days.
Intermittent treatment of episodes of herpes genitalis	Begin acyclovir at the earliest symptoms of recurrence with 200 mg 5 times daily for 5 days or 400 mg 3 times daily for 5 days
Chronic suppressive therapy of herpes genitalis	400 mg of acyclovir given twice daily, then reevaluate the patient's frequency of recurrences after 2–3 years. Indicators for initiation of suppressive therapy are shown in Table 3.2.
Severe mucocutaneous herpes simplex infection in the immunocompromised	Intravenous acyclovir is administered at a rate of 5 mg/kg over 1 hour, given every 8 hours for 7 days. Children under 12 should be given 250 mg/M^2 over 1 hour, every 8 hours.
Severe initial genital herpes in the immunocompetent	Intravenous regimen of 5 mg/kg over 1 hour, given every 8 hours, for 5 days, followed by oral acyclovir 400 mg b.i.d. (indefinitely for suppression). Children between 6 mo and 12 years are treated with 500 mg/m^2 over at least 1 hour, given every 8 hours for a total of 10 days.
Recurrent eczema herpeticum	200 mg 5 times a day (or 400 mg t.i.d.) for 5 days has given good responses; recurrences become less extensive over time.
Herpes labialis	Acyclovir is often used at 400 mg t.i.d. for 5 days.
Other cutaneous HSV infections	Although these are very rare in controlled studies using acyclovir to treat HSV in other cutaneous areas, it would seem prudent to prescribe oral acyclovir initially at doses utilized to treat primary HSV infections.

(continued)

Table 3.5 (*Continued*)

Symptom	Treatment
HSV ocular infections	Topical acyclovir is not superior to trifluridine and is not commonly recommended.
HSV encephalitis	Intravenous acyclovir infusions at 10 mg/kg over 1 hour, given every 8 hours for 14 days. For children from 6 mo to 12 yrs of age, the dosage is adjusted to 500 mg/m².
Neonatal herpes simplex infection	Intravenous acyclovir infusion at 10 mg/kg over 1 hour, given every 8 hours for 14 days (SEM disease) to 21 days (encephalitis or multi-organ disease).
Chickenpox in immunocompetent children and adults	Oral acyclovir 20 gm/kg 4 times daily for five days to decrease severity in children and adults if begun within 24–72 hours of the onset of the varicella rash (76–78,123,124). Acyclovir is approved for the treatment of chickenpox in adults and children over 40 kg at a dosage of 800 mg 4 times daily for 5 days. (Many physicians treat chickenpox in adolescents and adults with the herpes zoster regimen, which is 800 mg 5 times daily for 7 days.)
Herpes zoster in immunocompetent patients	Oral acyclovir (800 Mg) is administered 5 times daily for 7–10 days to reduce severity of pain.

Treatment should be initiated for a variety of reasons. These are summarized in Table 3.5. The argument is that the therapy is based on reducing the available time of exposure to others, thus preventing transmission, and the suppression of painful lesions.

Once therapy is needed to control HSV infection, there are a number of therapies available, depending upon the age and immune status of the patient.

Adverse Events

In general, acyclovir is well tolerated by most patients, whether administered topically, orally, or intraveneously. There are few rare adverse events present, if they occur at all. These are:

Nausea.

Vomiting.

Diarrhea.

Headache.

Central nervous system. If patients have a preexisting renal impairment, treatment with acyclovir may induce nephrotoxicity or neurotoxicity. One patient, treated for suspected viral meningoencephalitis with acyclovir, began to improve until right arm myoclonia developed followed by a progressive comatose state. Acyclovir neurotoxicity should be suspected if continuing treatment with acyclovir is accompanied by worsening neurological status. High plasma and CSF acyclovir levels can confirm the toxicity. Hemodialysis may be effective in reducing levels of acyclovir. Measuring blood creatinine permits prompt dosage adjustment (124).

Crystalluria. Adverse reactions of crystalluria include urinary insufficiency, elevated serum creatinine, and altered renal function that may lead to acute tubular necrosis. Risks that promote crystal development are dehydration, high dose of acyclovir and rapid induction rate (125). Crystalluria may occur in patients if the infusion rate for the administration of intravenous acyclovir occurs too rapidly. Therefore it is important that each dose of acyclovir be administered evenly during a one-hour period. Crystalline formation may cause renal impairment which is usually reversible. In at least one incidence, discontinuation of acyclovir resulted in resolution of crystalluria with 24 hours with no evidence of renal toxicity (126).

Phlebitis and infusion-site inflammation. Both phlebitis and inflammation at the infusion site may be caused by the intravenous administration of acyclovir.

Other Considerations

Acyclovir-resistant herpes simplex virus. Laboratory isolates and clinical specimens reveal that the frequency of acyclovir resistance ranges from 7.5 × 10^{-4} to 15 × 10^{-4} and are not significantly different (127,128).

Acyclovir-resistent varicella-zoster infection in HIV-positive patients. Acyclovir resistance has been reported in HIV-positive patients who are coinfected with VZV (129–132).

Pregnant women and breast-fed infants. Data from the treatment of 1000 pregnant women who received acyclovir before or during early pregnancy indicates that there was no increase in rates of miscarriage or in birth defects of the offspring. However, it is recommended that acyclovir be given to pregnant women only if the benefit outweighs the risk to the fetus. Acyclovir may concentrate in breast milk as it has been shown that breast milk acyclovir concentrations may be 0.6 to 4.1 times greater than the drug concentration in the corresponding maternal plasma (89). The amount of acyclovir exposure to breast-fed infants depends upon the maternal dose of acyclovir and quantity of milk ingested. In mothers who received acyclovir in dosages ranging from 200–800 mg five times daily, the level of acyclovir in the infants equated to a dosage of 0.2 mg/kg/day to 0.731 mg/kg/day (89–91). This quantity is less than the dosage indicated for infants with herpes encephalitis (30 mg/kg/day) that is given intravenously.

Transfer of antiviral agents to breast milk may provide therapeutic benefits in reducing the vertical transmission of viruses and clinical sequelae in the breast-feeding infant (133).

Probenicid coadministration. If probenicid is coadministered with intravenous acyclovir, there may be an increased half-life and systemic exposure of acyclovir, requiring dose adjustments.

Coadministration with antiretrovirals. Acyclovir, famciclovir, and valacyclovir are all safe and effective in HIV seropositive patients and have no negative interactions with HAART (134,135).

Generic Name Valacyclovir	Structure	Viral Diseases Treated (FDA Approved)
Brand Name(s) Valtrex Zelitrex **Other Name(s)**	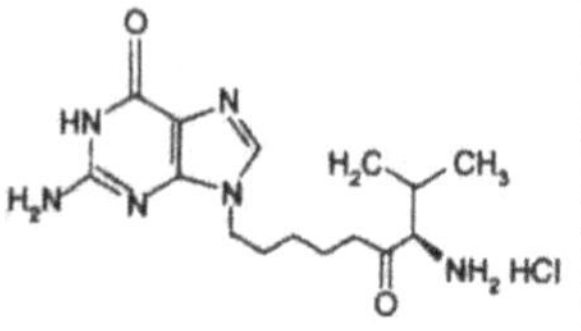	Herpes simplex virus 1 (HSV-1) Herpes simplex virus 2 (HSV-2) Varicella zoster virus (VZV)

Fig. 3.8 Associated names, structure, and applicability of valacyclovir.

Valacyclovir

Introduction

Valacyclovir is a prodrug of acyclovir with significantly improved bioavailability (136) (Fig. 3.8). Once absorbed, over 99% of the dosage is hydrolyzed by valacyclovir hydrolase to acyclovir. The oral bioavailability of valacyclovir is 3–5 times that of acyclovir, but the bioavailability of valacyclovir remains lower than that of famiciclovir. The increased bioavailability provides valacyclovir with the benefit of less frequent dosing, a boon for those who tend to forget to take medications. Valacyclovir was approved by the FDA in 1995 for use in the treatment of herpes simplex viruses and varicella zoster virus infections. A variety of off-label uses is also known. It is likely that valacyclovir will eventually replace acyclovir for treatment of HSV or VZV infections in HIV-positive or other immunocompromised persons (137).

Mechanism of Action

Valacyclovir is the L-valyl ester and prodrug of acyclovir. The conversion of valacyclovir to acyclovir by valacyclovir hydrolase translates into higher blood levels of acyclovir (Fig. 3.9). The metabolism and mechanism of action are identical to that of acyclovir. The greater affinity (100 times greater than that of penciclovir triphosphate) of acyclovir triphosphate for viral DNA polymerase is such that viral DNA chain termination

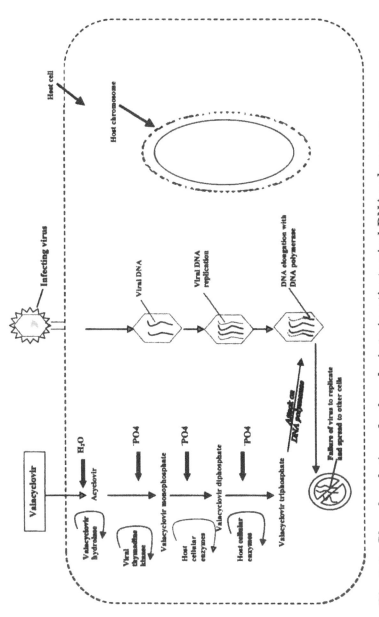

Fig. 3.9 Phosphorylation of valacyclovir to inactivate viral DNA polymerase.

requires less concentrations of acyclovir. Acyclovir and valacyclovir are obligate viral DNA terminators. It is unknown if there is any importance to the relationship between the greater viral DNA polymerase affinity and obligate/conditional viral DNA chain termination.

Clinical Studies to Support the Use of Valacyclovir

Valacyclovir is used to treat HSV, VZV, and (occasionally) CMV (136,138–150) (Table 3.6). Valacyclovir is considered to be as effective as acyclovir and famciclovir, with more convenient dosing than with acyclovir.

Treatment

Valacyclovir is administered orally with limited adverse events, similar to acyclovir and famciclovir. In addition, the increased bioavailability of valacyclovir means that patients only take medications 2–3 times per day rather than 5 times (with acyclovir). Table 3.7 highlights treatment options for HSV-1 and -2 and VZV.

Adverse Effects

Like acyclovir, side effects do not differ significantly from those of the placebo. There are a few rare adverse effects such as:

Nausea.

Headaches.

Thrombotic microangiopathy (TMA). Thrombotic microangiopathy, similar to thromboic thrombocytopenic purpura/hemolytic uremic syndrome (TTP/HUS), may occur in immunosuppressed patients who have received high dosages of valacyclovir (8 g/day) for extended periods of time when used for suppression of CMV. Valacyclovir has not been shown to be the cause of the TMA as rates seen in this study were similar to those of all patients with advanced HIV disease. Of 18 patients, eight developed TMA during treatment with the study drug, whereas 10 patients developed TMA after it had been discontinued for a median of 8 weeks.

Table 3.6 Clinical Studies and Reports of the Effectiveness of Valacyclovir in the Treatment of HSV, VZV, and CMV

Topic	Findings	References
Oral bioavailability	Oral bioavailability of valacyclovir is 3 to 5 times greater than acyclovir, but less than famciclovir.	136
Treatment of herpes zoster for cutaneous healing with acyclovir vs valacyclovir in immunocompetent adults aged 50+	For cutaneous healing, 7 days of acyclovir is just as effective for treatment of herpes zoster as 7 or 14 days of valacyclovir, but valacyclovir is more convenient; 14 days of valacyclovir are no more effective than 7 days.	138
Treatment of herpes zoster for reduction of duration of postherpetic neuralgia with acyclovir vs valacyclovir in immunocompetent adults aged 50+	Both regimens of valacyclovir (7 and 14 days) were associated with a greater reduction in the duration of postherpetic neuralgia than acyclovir.	138
Treatment of herpes zoster for duration of persistent pain with acyclovir vs valacyclovir in immunocompetent adults aged 50+	Both regimens of valacyclovir (7 and 14 days) were associated with a greater reduction in the duration of pain than acyclovir.	138
Treatment of first episode of genital herpes	Valacyclovir and acyclovir had comparable efficacy related to duration of viral shedding, time to healing, duration of pain, time of loss of all symptoms, and adverse effects, but valacyclovir is more convenient.	139
Length of time of administration of valacyclovir for episodic therapy of recurrent genital herpes	There is no difference in the effects of valacyclovir when 500 mg of valacyclovir is administrated 2 times daily	140

(continued)

Table 3.6   (*Continued*)

Topic	Findings	References
	for 3 or 5 days. FDA now recommends the 3-day course of valacyclovir.	
Suppression of genital herpes	Well tolerated and often preferred because of fewer doses needed (i.e., once daily).	141
Transmission of genital herpes	Valacyclovir (once daily) reduces risk of transmission of genital herpes	142
Herpes labialis	2 g b.i.d. for only one day, starting with the first symptom of recurrence, is effective therapy.	
HSV outbreaks after laser resurfacing	Valacyclovir is effective, as is famiciclovir and acyclovir.	143,144
Oral valacyclovir vs. intravenous acyclovir	Oral valacyclovir is as safe, much less expensive, and more convenient than intravenous acyclovir. Valacyclovir has reduced peak loads and a comparable systemic exposure.	145
Treatment of CMV viremia, viruria, and herpes simplex in CMV seropositive and seronegative renal transplant patients	Valacyclovir decreased the CMV viremia, viruria, and herpes simplex disease, although it is not FDA approved for this indication.	146
Pain cessation after herpes zoster outbreak	Valacyclovir more effective for pain suppression after 30 days than acyclovir.	147
Renal failure	Bioavailability improvements mean dosage should be lowered to prevent renal problems.	148
Bell's palsy	Treatment with prednisone and valacyclovir.	149,150

Table 3.7 Treatment Regimen for Valacyclovir

Symptom	Treatment
Episodic treatment of recurrent genital herpes	500 mg of valacyclovir twice daily for 3 days.
Herpes labialis	2 g b.i.d. for only one day, starting with the first symptom of recurrence.
Initial episodes of genital herpes	1 g valacyclovir twice daily for 10 days.
Chronic suppressive daily therapy (for persons with 10 or greater outbreaks in previous year)	1 g of valacyclovir administered once daily.
Chronic suppressive therapy for individuals with less than 10 recurrences each year	500 mg of valacyclovir administered once daily.
Herpes zoster	Valacyclovir is most effective if started within 72 hours of onset of rash, but is probably beneficial after 72 hours. Dose is 1 gram orally 3 times daily for 7 days.
Chickenpox in adolescents and adults (off-label)	1 gram orally 3 times daily for 7 days

This syndrome has not been observed in healthy patients who received doses of 3 g/day nor has it been seen in HIV-positive patients receiving valacyclovir for suppression of genital herpes.

Probenecid and cimetidine coadministration. Coadministration of valacyclovir with probenecid causes reduced renal clearance of acyclovir. Dosage adjustments are not necessary unless renal impairment exists and is not clinically significant in patients with normal renal function.

Neurologic toxicity. Valacyclovir very rarely may cause neurotoxicity as its bioavailability is 54% compared with 20% for acyclovir. Valacyclovir hydrolyzes to acyclovir following systemic exposure and may cause unexpected overdoses, but clinical manifestations are rare (148).

Treating Bell's Palsy

Antivirals bind to viral enzymes so the viruses do not replicate. Adverse effects of valacyclovir are rare but can include headache, nausea, diarrhea, constipation, and dizziness (149, 150) (see Table 3.6). When treatment begins within 3 days of onset of paralysis caused by Bell's palsy, patients treated with acyclovir have less neural degeneration and more favorable recoveries (150). Therefore, valacyclovir is being studied for this indication.

Famciclovir

Introduction

Famciclovir, an oral prodrug of penciclovir expresses the highest bioavailability (77%) of the nucleoside analogues. Like acyclovir, famciclovir, a diacetyl-6-deoxy analog, is effective against HSV-1, HSV-2, and VZV (Fig. 3.10). It is approved for the treatment of herpes zoster and for the episodic treatment and suppression of recurrent genital herpes in otherwise healthy adults. Originally FDA-approved in 1995, famciclovir has been found to significantly reduce the pain, burning, tenderness, and tingling of recurrent genital herpes and its metabolite, penciclovir, is used for therapy of herpes labialis (151). For the immunocompromised, famciclovir is an effective treatment for herpes zoster although famciclovir,

Generic Name Famciclovir	Structure	Viral Diseases Treated (FDA Approved)
Brand Name(s) Famvir **Other Name(s)**	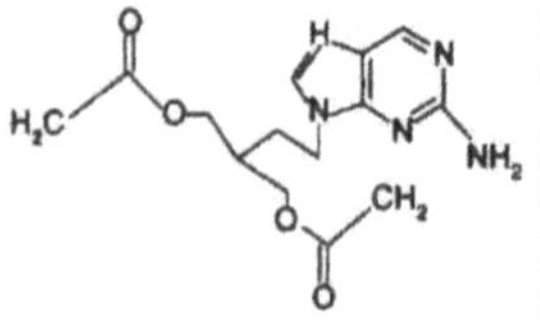	Herpes simplex virus 1 (HSV-1) Herpes simplex virus 2 (HSV-2) Varicella zoster virus (VZV)

Fig. 3.10 Associated names, structure, and applicability of famciclovir.

like valacyclovir, is not currently approved for the treatment of herpes zoster in this population (152). Famciclovir can be used to treat ophthalmic zoster (153) as well as shorten zoster-associated pain (154).

Mechanisms of Action

Famciclovir is a guanine analog that is also classified as a purine analog, a modified cyclic or acyclic sugar. Famciclovir is metabolized to the active agent, penciclovir triphosphate. In hepatitis B guanine analogs inhibit priming by binding to tyrosine at the priming site of the polymerase. They also inhibit DNA elongation of both strands of DNA of the virus. Although elongation is initiated, it is terminated only two or three nucleotides later. Famciclovir is a prodrug, and its deacytylation and oxidation form, penciclovir, is the active antiviral form (Fig. 3.11). D-famciclovir is more potent than l-famciclovir (155). Once it is rapidly metabolized to penciclovir by the gastrointestinal tract, blood, and liver, the remaining metabolism is identical to that of acyclovir (156).

Clinical Studies and Published Reports to Support the Use of Famciclovir

Famciclovir studies often compare the efficacy of famciclovir with acyclovir (153,157–170) (Table 3.8). For herpes zoster, famciclovir generally is as effective or more effective than acyclovir. Famciclovir is also useful in both immunosuppressed and immunocompetent patients. Aoki, in a review, cites the use of famciclovir in the treatment of both HIV-negative and HIV-positive patients for the management of recurring genital herpes (HSV) (171). In the treatment of VZV adult patients, famciclovir is usually prescribed at 500 mg orally three times a day in the USA and 250 mg three times daily in most other countries. Famciclovir and valacyclovir are preferred over oral acyclovir for the treatment of zoster in otherwise healthy adults (172). In a comparison study to treat Chinese patients with hepatitis B, lamivudine was significantly more effective than famciclovir (173).

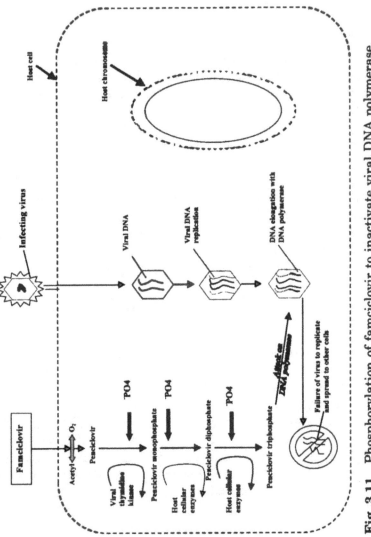

Fig. 3.11 Phosphorylation of famciclovir to inactivate viral DNA polymerase.

Table 3.8 Clinical Studies and Published Reports that Support the Use of Famciclovir

Topic	Findings	Reference
Dosage for off-label treatment for herpes labialis	Genital herpes regimen dosing is not sufficient for treatment of herpes labialis. Use of higher doses may be necessary to reduce lesion healing time (e.g., 500 mg TID for 5 days).	157
Efficacy in reducing number of recurrences of genital herpes	Famciclovir delays the time of the first recurrence of genital herpes. The number of patients remaining lesion free was 3 times higher in famciclovir than in placebo recipients.	158,159
Comparison of famciclovir with acyclovir for treatment of HSV in HIV-positive patients	Both acyclovir and famciclovir are well tolerated, generally safe to use, and effective	160
Symptomatic and asymptomatic viral shedding in women	For those women with a history of recurrent genital herpes, famciclovir reduces the frequency and delays the onset of viral shedding.	161
Genital herpes recurrences	Famciclovir is effective in increasing the time to first recurrence of genital herpes and increasing the number of recurrence-free patients.	159,160
Suppression of HSV reactivation in HIV-positive patients	Famciclovir treatment of 500 mg twice daily for 8 weeks significantly reduces symptoms and viral shedding.	161
Herpes zoster in immunocompetent patients; reduction of postherpetic neuralgia	Famciclovir is effective at reducing PHN when used 500 mg t.i.d. for 7 days, especially among persons 50 years of age and older.	162,163

(*continued*)

Table 3.8 *(Continued)*

Topic	Findings	Reference
Rapid resolution of zoster-associated pain	Famciclovir is as effective and more convenient than acyclovir for rapid resolution of zoster-associated pain.	163,164
Ophthalmic zoster	Famciclovir 500 mg 3 times daily was well tolerated and demonstrated efficacy similar to acyclovir 800 mg 5 times daily	153
Ramsey Hunt syndrome	A 7–10 day course of famciclovir (500 mg 3 times daily) combined with 3–5 days of oral prednisone (60 mg/day) is effective against VZV-mediated Ramsey Hunt syndrome.	112,165
Treatment of herpes zoster in immunosuppressed patients	Famciclovir is safe and effective.	166
Hepatitis B virus (HBV)	Only limited in vivo effect on HBV.	167–169
HBV disease in liver transplant recipients and recurrent HBV disease	Famciclovir administered independently seems to be of limited efficacy in the treatment of HBV after liver transplantation.	170

Treatment

Dosages for treatment vary according to the disease treated, the severity of an outbreak, and the recurrence rate of outbreaks as shown in Table 3.9.

Adverse Events

Headache.

Nausea.

Diarrhea.

Increased serum concentrations of penciclovir. Serum concentrations of penciclovir may occur if famciclovir is

Table 3.9 Treatment Table for Famciclovir

Symptom	Treatment
Herpes zoster initiation	Famciclovir 500 mg every 8 hours for 7 days, begun at the earliest signs of the disease.
Chickenpox in adolescents and adults	Famciclovir 500 mg every 8 hours for 7 days.
Episodic treatment of genital herpes	Famciclovir 125 mg twice daily for 5 days.
Chronic suppressive treatment of recurrent genital herpes	Famciclovir 250 mg twice daily for 1–2 years, followed by a reevaluation of patient's recurrences.
Recurrent orolabial or genital herpes in HIV-positive patients.	Famciclovir 500 mg twice daily for 7 days.
Initial outbreak of HSV in HIV-positive patients	250–750 mg t.i.d. for 5–10 days
Recurrent anogenital herpes in HIV-positive patients with CD4+ counts of <200 × 10^6 cells/ml	500 mg twice daily for 7 days is as effective as acyclovir 400 mg 5 times daily for 7 days.

used concurrently with probenecid (or other drugs significantly eliminated by active renal tubular secretion).

Special Considerations

Renal impairment. For patients with renal impairment, all regimens in Table 3.9 will require dosage adjustments.

Coadministration with probenecid or other related drugs. Administration of drugs eliminated by active renal tubular secretion with famciclovir may cause increased serum concentrations of penciclovir.

Drug resistance. For hepatitis B, five domains (labeled A–E) have been identified. Domains B and E may affect primary and template positioning. Structural changes in these domains may affect oral resistance to nucleoside analogues. Famciclovir promotes mutations in the B domain. A mutation at position 528 (Leu replaced by

Table 3.10   Nucleotide changes that induce resistance
to famciclovir in genotype A hepatitis B virus

V521L
P525L
L528M
L528V
T532S

Met or Val) also occurs during lamivudine therapy and
may cause cross-resistance. A summary of susceptible
positions for the B-domain resistance for famciclovir is
shown in Table 3.10.

Approval. Famciclovir has been approved for the episodic
therapy and for chronic suppression of recurring HSV
as well as treatment of herpes zoster in North America
and in some, but not all, European countries (137).

Penciclovir

Introduction

Penciclovir is acyclic nucleoside analogue which has *in vitro*
activity against HSV-1, HSV-2, and VZV (175) (Fig. 3.12). FDA
approval is only for topical treatment of recurrent herpes labialis as the oral bioavailability is extremely low. Intravenous
penciclovir shows promise for the treatment of mucocutaneous
herpes simplex infections in those with immunosuppression.

Generic Name Penciclovir	Structure	Viral Diseases Treated (FDA Approved)
Brand Name(s) Denavir Vectavir **Other Name(s)**	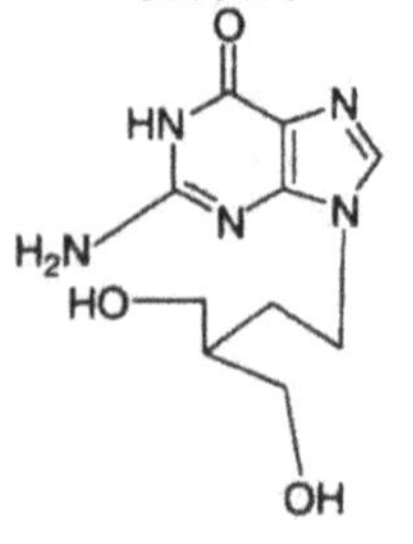	Herpes simplex virus 1 (HSV-1)

Fig. 3.12   Associated names, structure, and applicability of
penciclovir.

The active form of penciclovir is significantly more stable in HSV-infected cells (in vitro half-life of 10–20 hours) when compared to acyclovir (0.7 to 1 hour) (174).

Mechanisms of Action

Like acyclovir, penciclovir must be phosphorylated by viral thymidine kinase and cellular kinases prior to its competitive inhibition of viral DNA polymerase (Fig 3.13). However, penciclovir is not an obligate DNA-chain terminator like acyclovir (175,176).

Clinical Studies to Support the Use of Penciclovir

There is only one major study involving immunocompetent patients that demonstrates that penciclovir treatment results in improvement in a variety of facets. These improvements were observed at all stages of a herpes labialis outbreak: prodrome, erythema, papule, and vesicle. Table 3.11 (151) highlights the parameters measured and analyzed.

Treatment

Herpes labialis lesions may be treated with topical cream (Table 3.12). Treatment should be initiated as early as possible during the course of an outbreak. The systemic uptake of penciclovir is negligible.

Adverse Events

Adverse events are similar to those of acyclovir and valacyclovir.

Table 3.11 Efficacy of Penciclovir in Treating Herpes Labialis

Topic	Findings	Reference
In immunocompetent patients:	Topical 1% penciclovir decreases:	151
a. Healing time	Average healing time by 0.7 days	
b. Pain duration	Average duration of pain by 0.6 days	
c. Viral shedding	Significantly shortened.	

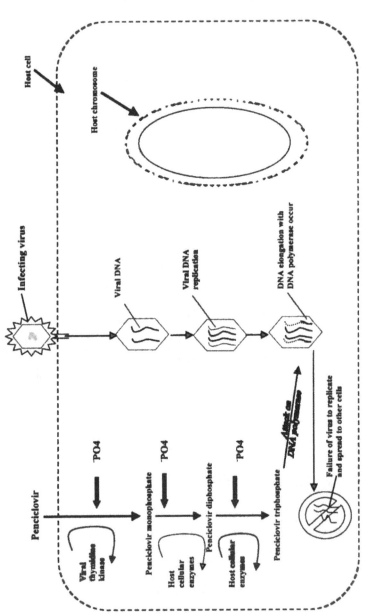

Fig. 3.13   Phosphorylation of penciclovir to inactivate viral DNA polymerase.

Table 3.12   Treatment of Viral Diseases with Penciclovir

Symptom	Treatment
Herpes labialis lesions (immunocompetent patients)	Apply topical 1% penciclovir cream to herpes labialis lesions every 2 hours while awake for 4 days to reduce healing time, pain duration, and viral shedding.

Ganciclovir

Introduction

Ganciclovir, a nucleoside analogue, is used to prevent and treat the manifestations of CMV in immunocompromised patients (177–179). This is important as CMV infection in immunocompetent individuals tends to be brief and self-limited. However, CMV can be severe and life-threatening in neonates, transplant recipients, and HIV-positive patients. Oral ganciclovir is available for CMV prophylaxis, but it is not considered to be as effective as other means. Valganciclovir a prodrug of ganciclovir, has improved bioavailability. Ganciclovir may also have in vitro efficacy against EBV (HHV-4) replication (Fig. 3.14).

Generic Name Ganciclovir Brand Name(s) Cytovene Cymvene Other Name(s) DHPG	Structure ![structure]	Viral Diseases Treated (FDA Approved) Cytomegalovirus (CMV) retinitis Human cytomegalovirus (HCMV)

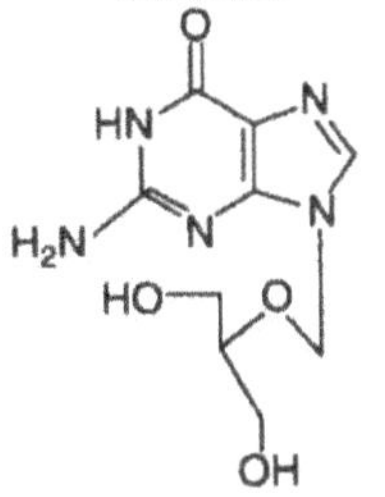

Fig. 3.14   Associated names, structure, and applicability of ganciclovir.

Mechanism of Action

The viral-encoded phosphotransferase (thymidine kinase) monophosphorylates ganciclovir, a nucleoside analogue, to the active triphosphate form. This triphosphate form becomes part of a newly synthesized DNA chain. This inhibits further

DNA synthesis by inhibiting DNA polymerase and by inducing premature chain termination (180–183) (Fig. 3.15). The thymidine kinase (TK) encoded by HSV or VZV has a broad substrate specificity that permits interaction by acyclovir or ganciclovir. Phosphorylation of ganciclovir in CMV-infected cells is dependent upon a protein kinase. The role of the kinase is not completely understood and is under study. In HHV-6, a similar mechanism activates ganciclovir. Mutations for drug resistance most often occur in the UL97 gene that affects the monophosphorylation process or the UL54 gene that codes for DNA polymerase in human CMV (184). Graft-versus-host-disease can be prevented when donor T cells are transfected to express herpes simplex virus thymine kinase. Cells that express this enzyme are susceptible to ganciclovir, which opens a new avenue for addressing drug resistance.

Clinical Studies and Reports that Support the Use of Ganciclovir

Oral ganciclovir is available for CMV prophylaxis, but is not as effective as intravenous treatment. Valganciclovir has better availability (177,178,183,185–193) (Table 3.13).

Treatment

Intravenous ganciclovir is the drug of choice for treatment of CMV in transplant recipients or AIDS patients (194) (Table 3.14). The ocular implant of ganciclovir for treatment of CMV retinitis provides a better clinical outcome for disease regression and the convenience of ambulatory therapy. This, however, must be balanced against the potential of intra-ocular side effects or contralateral eye infection by CMV (185). Late-onset cytomegalovirus disease among organ transplant recipients is common and the current thought is that antiviral prophylaxis, such as with ganciclovir, be used preemptively. Allograft rejection is often associated with CMV risk. Those patients on ganciclovir may benefit from extended and/or enhanced antiviral prophylaxis (195). Stem cell transplantation (SCT) has similar challenges in that SCTs are at increased risk of developing CMV pneumonia where the best available therapy has a mortality

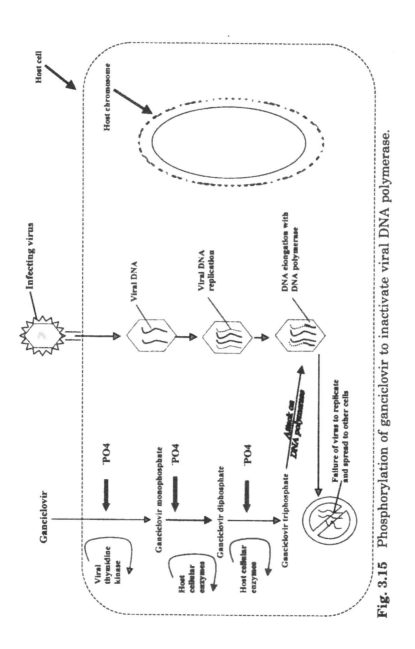

Fig. 3.15 Phosphorylation of ganciclovir to inactivate viral DNA polymerase.

Table 3.13   Clinical Studies and Reports of Ganciclovir Usage

Topic	Findings	Reference
Bioavailability	Oral bioavailability is 8–9%. Needs to be administered by daily intravenous infection.	183
Treatment and prevention of CMV in immunocompromised patients	Ganciclovir is usually administered intravenously because of poor oral bioavailability.	177,178, 183
CMV retinitis	The ocular implant may be used to treat CMV, although it requires surgical insertion every six months.	185
Foscarnet vs ganciclovir	Ganciclovir is preferred due to less severe side effects.	186
Ganciclovir vs valganciclovir	Valganciclovir has better oral bioavailability and fewer severe side effects.	
EBV-positive tumor in the positive immunocompetent (Phase I/II trial)	Induce latent viral TK gene and enzyme in tumor cells using arginine butyrate, followed by ganciclovir treatment in standard treatment doses.	187
HHV-6	HHV-6 reactivation in transplant patients is controlled with ganciclovir.	188
CMV with acute lymphoblastic leukemia	Ganciclovir can be used to manage CMV infection.	189
Cytotoxicity in retinas (in vitro)	Ganciclovir shows no toxicity in micromolar concentration.	190
CMV after solid organ transplantation	Ganciclovir is effective for kidney, liver, heart, and lung transplant recipients as preemptive therapy.	191
Globulin plus ganciclovir to treat CMV in a solid organ transplant patient	Oral ganciclovir given preemptively reduces invasion of tissue by CMV-associated disease.	192
CMV retinitis intravitreal vs intravenous therapy	Induction therapy should be prolonged until complete inactivation of CMV retinitis is obtained before beginning maintenance therapy.	193

Table 3.14 Treatment with Ganciclovir

Symptom	Treatment
Failed monotherapy for CMV retinitis	Combine foscarnet and ganciclovir.
CMV retinitis	Ocular implants.

rate of 45–78%; therefore, post-operative prevention of CMV is critical (196).

Adverse Effects

Dosage of ganciclovir must often be limited due to:

Bone marrow suppression. Bone marrow suppression may also be accompanied by thrombocytopenia, neutropenia, anemia, and granulocytopenia.

Retinal toxicity. High doses of intravitreal ganciclovir may cause retinal damage (197).
Also involved may be:

Renal insufficiently.

Neutropenia.

Fever.

Rash.

Headache.

Irritation and phlebitis. Irritation and phlebitis may occur at the infusion site.

Nausea. May occur with arginine butyrate combined with ganciclovir to treat Epstein-Barr tumors.

Ganciclovir resistance. A recent study demonstrated that 26 of 210 patients with CMV retinitis expressed phenotypic or genotypic ganciclovir-resistance (198).

Special Considerations

Animal studies. Ganciclovir was found to be teratogenic, carcinogenic, and mutagenic in animal studies. It also caused aspermatogenesis.

Combination therapy with foscarnet. In cases of failure of monotherapy, ganciclovir can be combined with foscarnet for treatment.

Monitoring of CMV infection in immunocompromised transplant patients. The results of quantitative antigenemia, which uses buffy coat cell preparations, may differ significantly from quantitative PCR, which uses plasma for the analysis of ganciclovir resistance. Once ganciclovir is initially introduced for treatment of CMV, quantitative PCR levels drop. A subsequent use of both quantitative PCR and antigenemia may be indicative of the emergence of ganciclovir-resistant CMV. Once foscarnet is administered, both the PCR and antigenemia levels drop. The results of the quantitative PCR can often be used to provide pre-emptive treatment before traditional clinical indicators appear (199). PCR with plasma performed best in a comparison with seven other laboratory assays. This permitted pre-emptive treatment with ganciclovir (200).

Arginine butyrate/ganciclovir treatment of EB tumors. Arginine butyrate/ganciclovir treatment does not appear to activate HIV transcription rates (187).

Pregnant women. Only limited studies have been done, but no large-scale safety data exists (201).

Neonates and pediatric patients. Ganciclovir has been used effectively in pediatric transplant patients, but safety of use in neonates with CMV infection has not been established (202).

Effect of corticosteroids on efficacy. In transplant patients, corticosteriod use may promote early pp65 antigenemia rather than emergence of a ganciclovir-resistant virus. Therefore, an immediate switch from ganciclovir to foscarnet (with more severe side effects) may not be warranted. Instead, dose intensification with ganciclovir should continue to be the medication of choice (203,204).

Valganciclovir

Introduction

Valganciclovir is used to treat CMV retinitis, an infection in eyes of immunocompromised patients. Valganciclovir does not cure CMV, but it can keep symptoms from becoming worse or

Generic Name Valganciclovir Brand Name(s) Valcyte Other Name(s)	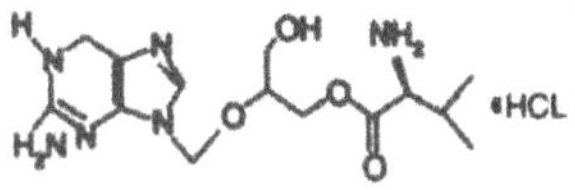 Structure 	Viral Diseases Treated (FDA Approved) Cytomegalovirus (CMV) retinitis

Fig. 3.16 Associated names, structure, and applicability of valganciclovir.

cause some improvement. Oral valganciclovir has increased availability when compared with oral ganciclovir. As with all other antivirals, valganciclovir-resistant strains are emerging (205) (Fig. 3.16).

Mechanism of Action

Valganciclovir is a valylester prodrug of ganciclovir with approximately 10 times the bioavailability of oral ganciclovir (Fig. 3.17).

Clinical Findings and Reports That Support the Use of Valganciclovir

Valganciclovir has been used to treat CMV retinitis (205) (Table 3.15).

Treatment

Oral tablets are available in the United States. Adults should take 900 mg two times a day with food (Table 3.16).

Adverse Effects

Anemia and other blood problems. Valganciclovir can suppress the numbers of white blood cells, increasing the opportunity for infection. Valganciclovir also lowers blood platelet number which may increase blood clotting time.

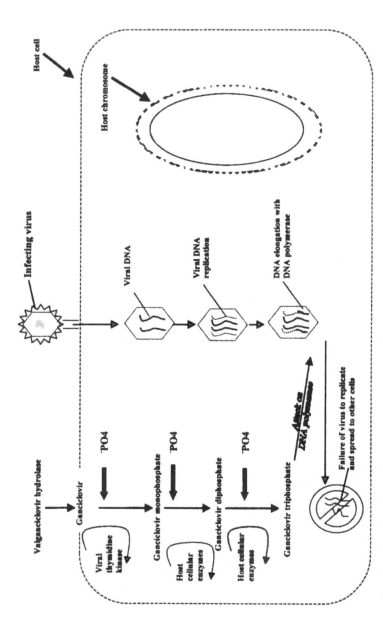

Fig. 3.17 Phosphorylation of valganciclovir to inactivate viral DNA polymerase.

Table 3.15 Published Reports of Valganciclovir Usage

Topic	Findings	Reference
CMV retinitis	Mutations increased with drug exposure over time.	205
Effect of valganciclovir or ganciclovir resistance on CMV retinitis	Retinitis progression, however, could not be linked to UL97 genotype mutation.	

Gastrointestinal. Presence of blood in urine or stools, with stools possibly appearing black or tarry, and painful or difficult urination are common side effects of valganciclovir. Abdominal pain, diarrhea, nausea, and vomiting are normally less serious side effects.

Respiratory distress or infection. Cough, hoarseness, troubled breathing, nasal congestion, sore throat, chills, fever, lower back or side pain, unusual bleeding, bruising, or fatigue could be seen if a patient is taking valganciclovir.

Mucocutaneous. Ulcers, sores or white spots may appear in the mouth, paler than usual appearance of the skin, pinpoint red macules on skin, or allergic (hive-like) swelling or itching are indicators of adverse effects of valganciclovir.

Ophthalmological. Seeing flashes of light, floating spots before the eyes, or a "veiled curtain" appearing across the field of vision can be indicators of side effects of valganciclovir.

Neurological. Rare but serious side effects may be confusion, illogical thinking, seizures, or false sensations. Agitation may also occur.

Table 3.16 Treatment with Valganciclovir

Symptom	Treatment
CMV prophylaxis	900 mg b.i.d. with food.

Special Considerations

Concomitant therapy. Taking valganciclovir with didanosine, mycophenolate, or probenecid may increase the chance of side effects.

Pregnant and breast-feeding women. Valganciclovir has not been studied in pregnant women but animal studies indicate that valganciclovir causes birth defects and other problems. Men who are taking valganciclovir should use a condom to avoid impregnating their spouse, not only during the course of treatment but for at least 90 days following treatment. Use of valganciclovir during pregnancy should be avoided whenever possible.

Studies to determine the transfer of valganciclovir from nursing mothers to their infants have not been completed. Valganciclovir is not recommended during breast-feeding because it may cause unwanted effects in nursing babies.

Pediatric use. No studies have been done on pediatric patients.

Elderly. No studies have been done on elderly patients and it is not known if valganciclovir causes different side effects or problems in older people.

Kidney disease. Valganciclovir increases the chances of side effects as it accumulates in the blood in patients with kidney disease.

Blood diseases. Low platelet count, low red blood cell count, or low white blood cell count may be exacerbated by valganciclovir.

Ribavirin

Introduction

Severe viral pneumonia—respiratory syncytial virus RSV—in children can be effectively treated by ribavirin. Ribavirin is a broad-spectrum antiviral nucleoside. In addition to being used to treat RSV pneumonia, it is also used to treat strains of influenza A and B and Lassa fever, off-label. It is emerging as a

Generic Name Ribavirin	Structure	Viral Diseases Treated (FDA Approved)
Brand Name(s) Virazole Virazid Virazide Rebetol Copegus **Other Name(s)** Tribavirin	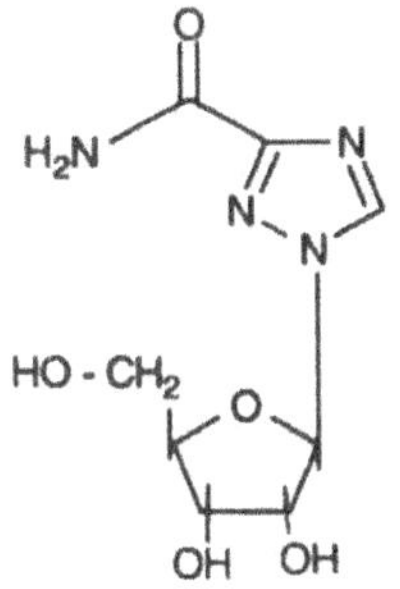	Respiratory syncytial virus (RSV) Hepatitis C virus

Fig. 3.18 Associated names, structure, and applicability of ribavirin.

possible treatment for adenovirus (206). As summarized by Gavin and Katz, adenovirus sites are found throughout the body as cystitis, pneumonia, enteritis, colitis, hepatitis, nephritis, etc., and survival-rate improvements are high enough to consider IV ribavirin a feasible treatment modality (206). Many other viruses respond to ribavirin, including hepatitis A, B, and C, particularly when combined with pegylated interferon-alpha (for more information, refer to ribavirin-PEG-interferon, **page 213**). Ribavirin is a white crystalline powder with high solubility in water and limited solubility in anhydrous alcohol. Figure 3.18 shows the structure of ribivarin.

Mechanisms of Action

Ribavirin, a broad-spectrum antiviral nucleoside (guanosine) analog, phosphorylates easily. Although the mechanisms of ribavirin remain unclear (207), ribavirin appears to be a non-specific antiviral with most of its efficacy due to incorporation of the ribavirin into the viral genome. Ribavirin undergoes dehydration synthesis to form new products (Fig. 3.19). When cells are exposed to ribavirin, there is a reduction in intracellular guanosine triphosphate—a requirement for translation, transcription, and replication in viruses and a reason for the broad-spectrum attributes of ribavirin (208). Ribavirin significantly increases the mutation rate of RNA in poliovirus and

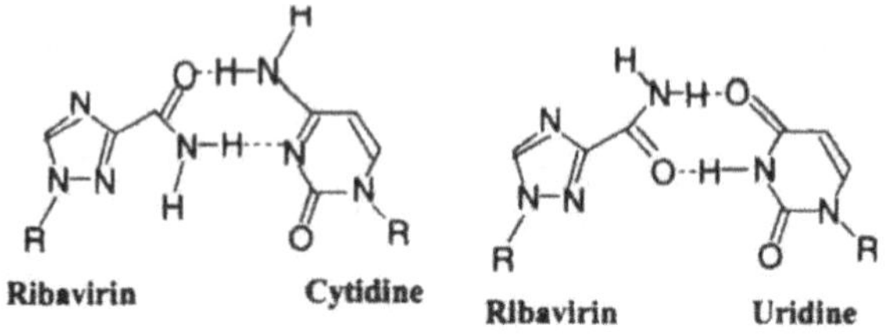

Fig. 3.19   Ribavirin bonding to cytosine and uracil.

reduces viral fitness (Fig. 3.20). Thus, an understanding of the in-depth mechanisms of ribavirin activity could contribute to the development of lethal mutagenesis as an effective antiviral strategy.

Studies that Support Treatment with Ribavirin

Ribavirin may help treat orthopoxviruses, influenza and chronic hepatitis A and B (206,209,210) (Table 3.17).

Treatment

Ribavirin is usually prescribed as an inhalant for infants and small children. Elderly patients, teenagers, and adults are usually not prescribed ribavirin. Ribavirin is readily absorbed with oral administration and there is a linear relationship between the time of last administration and the dosage. Although the tablets are taken with food, there is insufficient data to determine the effect of different types of diets (high fat, high protein, vegetarian, etc.) on ribavirin absorption. Dosages and types of administration are shown in Table 3.18.

Adverse Effects

Unusual tiredness and weakness. May occur in patients taking ribavirin by mouth or injection for Lassa fever.

Headache. Occurs rarely.

Itching, redness, and swelling of the eyes. Occurs rarely.

Skin rashes. Occurs rarely.

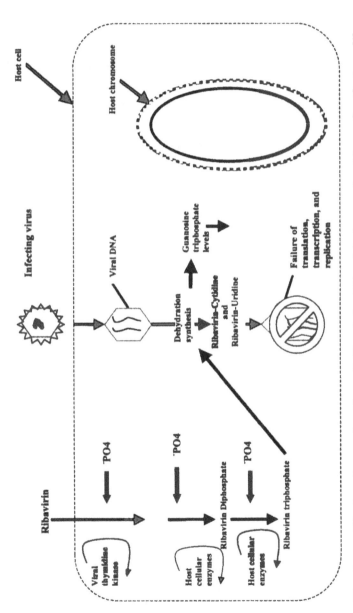

Fig. 3.20 Mechanisms of action of ribavirin. Ribavirin is a nucleoside analog that readily phosphorylates to ribavirin triphosphate. Ribavirin is incorporated into the viral genome by binding to cytosine and uracil.

Table 3.17   Studies that Support the Use of Ribavirin

Topic	Finding	Reference
Severe adenovirus disease in immunocompromised children	Two of five children recovered, whereas non-treatment would have resulted in five non-recoveries. Early intervention (diagnosis via PCR) with ribavirin may make earlier, more effective treatment possible	206
Orthopoxviruses (in vivo)	Ribavirin has an inhibitory activity against orthopox viruses.	209
Lassa fever	Ribavirin given orally or by injection.	210
Influenza A and B	Ribavirin given by aerosol inhalation.	210

Table 3.18   Treatment Modalities for Ribavirin

Symptoms	Treatment
Chronic hepatitis C	Capsules: Must be combined with Interferon –alpha therapy to be effective. (See Table 3.28.)
Respiratory syncytial virus (RSV)	Inhalation therapy: Dosage for treating infants must be determined by physicians. Dosage has not been determined for adults and teenagers. Usually not prescribed for the elderly.
Influenza A and B	Given by aerosol inhalation as a fine mist by using a nebulizer attached to an oxygen hood, tent, or facemask.
Lassa fever	Given either orally or by injection.
Adenoviruses	Intravenous ribavirin can be used as a compassionate-use medicine in severely immunocompromised patients with adenovirus.

Combination Therapy with Interferon-alpha. The adverse events of this combination therapy are significant and include severe depression with suicidal tendencies, hemolytic anemia, suppression of bone marrow function, pulmonary dysfunction, pancreatitis, and diabetes.

Special Considerations

Combination with Interferon-alpha. Combination therapy of ribavirin with interferon alpha has been shown to be effective in the treatment of hepatitis C. Ribavirin monotherapy is not effective. However, there may be severe adverse effects (see the preceding section). For example, patients with autoimmune hepatitis become worse when treated with this therapy.

Allergies. Some patients are allergic to ribavirin. The possibility exists that children who are allergic to food, preservatives, dyes, or other substances may also be allergic to ribavirin.

Pregnancy. Ribavirin for inhalation therapy for very young children may cause exposure to women who are pregnant (or may become pregnant) if they spend time at the bedside when the inhalation therapy is being administered. The effect of ribavirin on prenatal development *has not* been tested in humans, but breast milk containing ribavirin has been shown to cause birth defects and other problems in certain animal studies.

Hepatic dysfunction. In patients with decreased hepatic function, the pharmacokinetics of ribavirin cannot be accurately predicted. Therefore, the dosage may need to be increased for efficacy, but monitored carefully to reduce adverse effects.

Breast milk. In animal studies, ribavirin passes to the offspring through breast milk and can cause problems in nursing animals and the young. There have been no tests on humans.

NUCLEOTIDE ANALOGS

The derivatives of nucleosides that are monophosphorylated belong to the nucleotide analogs. Those with antiviral properties include cidofovir, adefovir, and tenofovir. Tenofovir is used to treat HIV infection and is discussed in Chapter 2, **page 62**.

Phosphorylation of nucleosides occurs within the cytoplasm of cells that are beginning mitotic division. The synthesis of bases that contribute to DNA chain elongation is limited by the inclusion of nucleotide analogs. Mitochondrial DNA-polymerase may also be affected.

Cidofovir

Introduction

Cidofovir has received much attention as a therapy for many viral diseases (Fig. 3.21). Although preemptive antiviral therapy for CMV infection following allogenic stem cell transplantation is recommended as an effective strategy for preventing CMV disease, some studies do not support this hypothesis (211). Cidofovir is considered an option for the treatment of acyclovir-resistant HSV although it has not been FDA-approved for this purpose. However, there is an increasing need for additional therapies as more herpes viral strains

Generic Name Cidofovir	Structure	Viral Diseases Treated (FDA Approved)
Brand Name(s) Vistide (i.v.) **Other Name(s)**	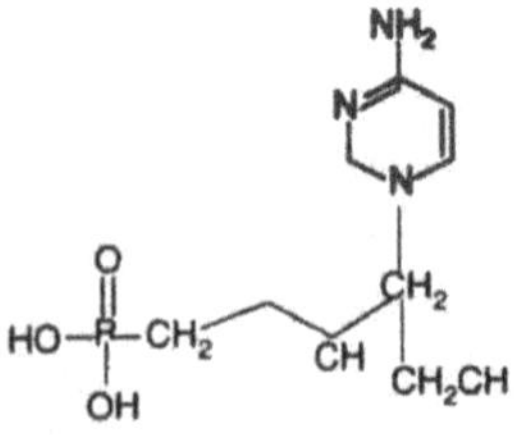	Cytomegalovirus (CMV) retinitis

Fig. 3.21 Associated names, structure, and applicability of cidofovir.

become acyclovir-resistant. Cidofovir shows promise as a therapy against TK-deficient strains of HSV. As the first acyclic phosphonate nucleotide approved for use in the United States, cidofovir can be used to treat CMV retinitis inpatients with AIDS. AIDS patients treated with cidofovir for CMV retinitis often report an improvement in AIDS-related Kaposi's sarcoma.

Cidofovir is the most effective anti-orthopoxvirus agent currently under preclinical investigation (212). Other diseases for which cidofovir is used include VZV, CMV, HPV, polyoma viruses, adenoviruses, and other poxviruses (213). Cidofovir shows efficiency against JC virus in vitro (214). Cidofovir is considered to be the second-line therapy for CMV disease after the first antiviral failed (215). Anogenital warts respond to cidofovir topical gel (216).

Mechanism of Action

Cidofovir is considered to be an acyclic phosphonate nucleotide. Cidofovir is similar to foscarnet in that it does not require thymidine kinase for phophorylation (Fig. 3.22). To become activated, the drug is phosphorylated by cellular kinase to cidofovir diphosphate (217–219), which makes it effective against TK-deficient strains of HSV. HHV-8 replication is sensitive to cidofovir. Although cidofovir is poorly absorbed by mouth, aerosolized cidofovir may help create a barrier against aerosolized virus infections. Cidofovir acts as a chain terminator for viral DNA polymerase. After intracellular phosphorylation to a diphosphate form, activity occurs at the 3' end of the viral DNA with termination at the end of two sequences.

Clinical Studies and Reports that Support the Use of Cidofovir

Several studies document the treatment of acyclovir-resistant and normal strains of HSV with topical cidofovir. Representative studies are highlighted in Table 3.19 (213,215,220–251). The FDA did not approve the use of cidofovir gel for acyclovir-resistant herpesvirus infection due to a lack of sufficient phase-three data (229). However, the manufacturer has reported successful treatment of HSV with compounded cidofovir cream (230). Cidofovir delays the progression of CMV retinitis in

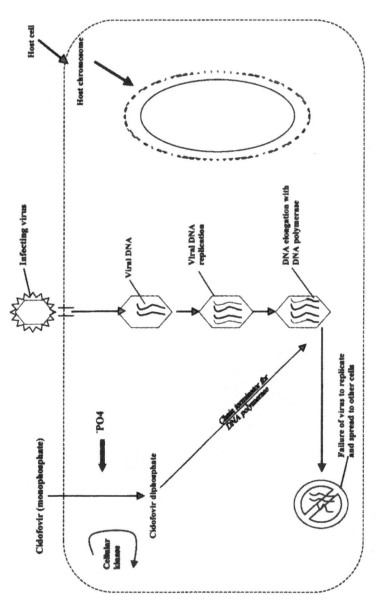

Fig. 3.22 Phosphorylation of cidofovir to inactivate viral DNA polymerase.

Table 3.19 Studies and Reports of Cidofovir Usage

Topic	Findings	Reference
CMV retinitis in AIDS patients	Intravenous cidofovir, given once weekly for 2 weeks, followed by maintenance therapy once every 2 weeks, delays the progression of CMV retinitis in AIDS patients.	220–224
HHV-8	Kaposi's sarcoma in an HIV-negative patient was unresponsive to intralesional cidofovir.	225–227
Kaposi's sarcoma	Cidofovir used to treat CMV retinitis may also improve Kaposi's sarcoma.	
HSV	Cidofovir is effective in treating acyclovir-resistant HSV.	228–230
HPV	Treatment of CIN-III (cervical intraepithelial neoplasia, grade III), laryngeal, and cutaneous papilloma lesions	213
Poxviruses	Use for molluscum contagiosum lesions and orf lesions.	231–233
Perianal condylomata in HIV-positive patient (HPV)	Topical cidofovir (1% gel) was used once daily for 2 weeks for complete clearance of HPV lesions.	234–236
Use of cidofovir for CMV, preemptive therapy and secondary preemptive therapy	In allogenic stem cell transplant patients, 50% of those with CMV responded to therapy, 66% of preemptive therapy cases, and 62% of those categorized as secondary preemptive therapy also responded.	215
Use of alkoxyalkyl or alkoxyglycerol to improve oral bioavailability for CMV therapy (in vitro)	Alkyl ethers of propanediol or ethonediol provide multilog increases in antiviral activity against laboratory wild strains, clinical isolates, and ganciclovir-resistant strains of human CMV.	237

(continued)

Table 3.19 (*Continued*)

Topic	Findings	Reference
Laryngeal papillomatosis	Treatment with cidofovir (combined with IV hydration and probenecid) resulted in pharyngeal and bronchial lesions disappearing. Laryngeal papillomas disappeared after 9 mos. Treated lesions were significantly reduced and no new lesions were formed.	238
Adenovirus in allogenic hematopoietic stem cell transplantation or bone marrow transplantation	Cidofovir is effective, particularly if administered before the disease develops. Effective against hemorrhagic cystitis and simultaneous CMV reactivation.	239–241
Aerosolized cowpox virus infection (mouse)	Aerosolized cidofovir may be an effective prophylaxis or early postexposure therapy of human smallpox or monkeypox virus infection.	242
Intranasal administration to combat cowpox (mouse)	Mice, exposed to cowpox virus and treated with 3 different compounds, responded best overall to cidofovir.	243,244
Lung transplant	Patient suffered acute renal failure with cidofovir therapy with no viral load reduction (actually an increase).	245
Orf in a renal-transplant patient	Cidofovir was successful in treating an immunocompromised patient with orf (ecthyma contagiosum, a poxvirus). Topical application did not alter renal function.	246
HPV-induced skin lesions	Cidofovir cream 1% or injection treatment for relapsing HPV-associated lesions.	247,248

patients with AIDS (220–224). The use of cidofovir alone may not change the course of progressive multifocal leukoencephalopathy in non-HIV-positive patients (249).

Cidofovir has shown to be effective against HHV-8 (in vitro). HAART therapy usually benefits KS lesions, but a case report indicates cidofovir treatment may be considered for the control of KS lesions and to reduce HHV-8 replication (250).

Treatment

Genital warts and common warts can be effectively treated with cidofovir, although it is not currently FDA-approved for this purpose. Table 3.20 highlights other treatments. Dosages may vary with little effect on toxicity. For patients receiving 3 mg/kg vs 5 mg/kg of cidofovir, the only toxic condition deemed significant ($p < 0.04$) was an increase in baseline creatinine. Other conditions included nausea and vomiting. Cidofovir must be used with caution if combined with other known nephrotoxic drugs or used concomitant with cyclosporin (215).

Adverse Effects

A number of side effects have been reported with the use of cidofovir (211–251).

Table 3.20   Treatment with Cidofovir

Symptom	Treatment
CMV retinitis in AIDS patients	Intravenous application given once weekly for 2 weeks, followed by maintenance therapy once every 2 weeks to delay progression in AIDS patients.
Genital or common warts	1% or 3% cidofovir gel or cream, applied once daily for 5 or 10 days.
Intravenous administration	5 mg/kg/week for 2 weeks, then 5 mg/kg every other week with hydration and probenecid to prevent nephrotoxicity.

With HSV:

Pain.

Pruritus.

Skin changes. May cause localized fibrosis if cidofovir is injected.

Ulcerations.

Erythema. Some HPV (condylomata acuminata) HIV-positive patients experience transient erythema from cidofovir use with no long-term side effects (248).

Neutropenia.

Nephrotoxicity. Occurs as serum creatinine levels rise to 1.5–2 times normal. Some patients develop tubular toxicity. Pretreatment with intravenous normal saline and probenecid is mandatory to decrease the risk of nephotoxicity.

Metabolic acidosis.

Ocular hypotony.

Uveitis. (250).

Special Considerations

Probenecid. Probenecid can be used with intravenous normal saline to reduct the risk of nephrotoxicity (213).

Other nephrotoxic agents. Concomitant use is contraindicated.

Cidofovir gel availability. Compounding of the drug is expensive.

Smallpox vaccination study. Currently, smallpox vaccinations are being tested. Should volunteers develop complications of vaccinia, cidofovir will be the drug of choice for antiviral therapy.

Adefovir

Introduction

Adefovir dipivoxil is a diester prodrug of adefovir with specific activity against the human hepatitis B virus (HBV). Adefovir was approved in September 2002. Those who take the oral drug have experienced improved liver histology and have a

Generic Name	Structure	Viral Diseases Treated
Adefovir dipivoxil		(FDA Approved)
Brand Name(s)	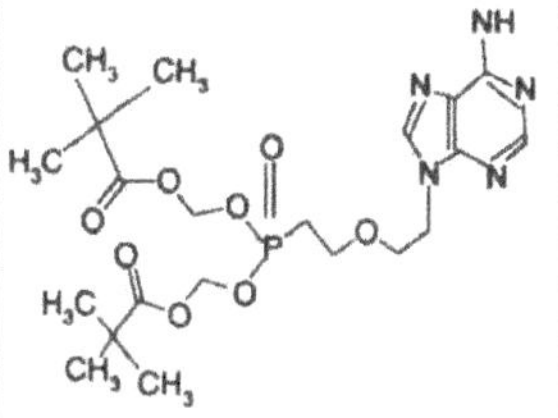	Hepatitis B virus (HBV)
Hepsera		
Other Name(s)		

Fig. 3.23 Associated names, structure, and applicability of adefovir dipivoxil.

reduced serum HBV DNA concentration if they were infected with the precore mutant strain of the virus (252). With precore mutant HBV, the virus' ability to produce "e" antigen is destroyed by the viral genome. Precore mutant virus is associated with more severe liver disease and is more commonly found in Asian and Mediterranean countries. The wild type also responds favorably to adefovir. Brand name, chemical structure, and antiviral uses of adefovir are shown in Fig. 3.23.

Mechanisms of Action

Adefovir is a nucleotide analog of adenosine monophosphate that is acyclic. Nucleotide analogs block HBV DNA polymerease, the enzyme involved in correct replication of the virus in cells. Adefovir is actually adefovir dipivoxil, a diester prodrug of adefovir. Adefovir is phosphorylated to the active metabolite, adefovir diphosphate, by host cellular kinases. The diphosphate form inhibits the reverse transcriptase of the DNA polymerase by competing with the normal DNA substrate, deoxyadenosine triphosphate. Once the adefovir compound is incorporated into the viral DNA, the DNA chain ceases to elongate. This mechanism is shown in Fig. 3.24.

Studies to Support the use of Adefovir

A variety of studies were performed on adefovir before the FDA gave approval, and are shown in Table 3.21 (252–255).

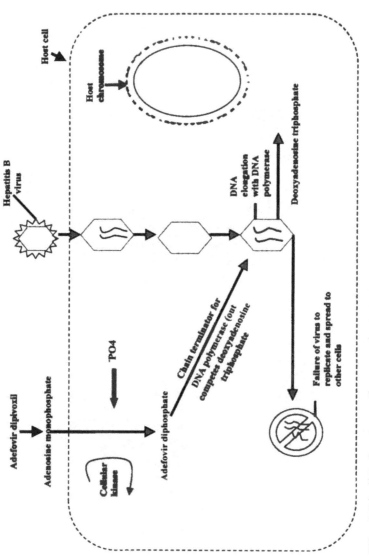

Fig. 3.24 Mechanism of action of adefovir.

Table 3.21 Reports that Support Use of Adefovir

Topic	Findings	Reference
Chronic hepatitis B	Loss of serum HBV DNA and HBcAg after 12 weeks therapy with adefovir.	252
Evaluation of safety, antiviral activity and viral resistance	Long-term treatment not associated with toxicity levels that would limit patient use of adefovir.	253
Changes in liver histology after treatment with adefovir	Levels of HBV DNA and alanine aminotransferase (ALT) were more normal after treating chronic hepatitis B with adefovir. Histological improvement of the liver was noted.	254
Safety and efficacy of adefovir in HIV-positive (advanced) patients	Adefovir can cause considerable nephrotoxicity. Adefovir added to normal background antiretroviral therapy has no added benefit in advanced HIV disease.	255

Treatment

Adefovir is administered as an oral tablet. Each table contains 10 mg of adefovir dipivoxil and a number of inactive ingredients. In laboratory studies, 0.2–0.25 µM of adefovir achieved a 50% reduction in viral DNA synthesis. Adefovir is excreted by glomular filtration and active tubular secretion by the kidneys. The potential for CYP 450 interactions with adefovir as a inhibitor or substrates with other medicinal products is negligible given the renal elimination of adefovir. Adefovir may be taken without regard to food.

Adverse Events

In initial clinical trials, a number of adverse events were reported, such as asthenia, headache, abdominal pain, nausea, flatulence, diarrhea, and dyspepsia. However the reports between those receiving adefovir and the placebo were not significantly different. Pre- and post-liver transplant patients reported some additional concerns that may be important on a case-by-case basis: changes in serum creatinine and serum phosphorus, pruritus and rash, abnormal liver functions, and some respiratory complications.

Discontinuation of adefovir treatment. Once patients who have been on adefovir or other anti-HBV therapy discontinue therapy, severe acute exacerbation of hepatitis has occurred. Monitoring of hepatic function of patients who discontinue anti-HBV therapy should continue over time. Resumption of anti-HBV therapy may be needed if alanine aminotransferase (ALT) levels rise significantly. Patients with poor liver function (hepatitis or cirrhosis) may be at higher risk. Deaths have occurred, so patients should be closely monitored.

Nephrotoxicity. Patients with normal renal function have a low risk of nephrotoxicity. However, for patients with or at risk of renal dysfunction, chronic administration of the standard dosage of adefovir may cause nephrotoxicity.

Coadministration with nephrotoxic agents. Coadministration of cyclosporine, tacrolimus, aminoglycosides, vancomycin, and non-steroidal anti-inflammatory drugs with adefovir may increase the chances that nephrotoxicity may occur.

Coadministration with ibuprofen. Ibuprofen at a dosage of 800 mg three times/day increased adefovir exposure by 23% although the significance of this observation is unknown.

Pregnancy. No adequate or well-controlled studies on pregnant women have been conducted. Fetal malformations occurred in pregnant rats when administered doses 38 times human systemic exposure, although there is no indication that this would be predictive of human response. Adefovir should be administered to pregnant women only after careful consideration of the risks and benefits and only if clearly needed.

Pediatric and geriatric use. Insufficient studies have been done to establish safety and effectiveness.

Overdosage. Doses of adefovir of 500 mg daily for 2 weeks and 250 mg daily for 12 weeks have been associated with gastrointestinal side effects. In case of overdose, the patient should be monitored for evidence of toxicity and standard supportive treatment used, as necessary.

HIV. For those with HIV, adefovir may interfere with the efficacy of usual HIV medications. Patients should have an HIV test prior to administration of adefovir.

Lactic acidosis. Nucleoside analog medications, such as adefovir, may cause a build-up of acid in the blood called lactic acidosis, which should be treated as a medical emergency. Symptoms of lactic acidosis are weakness or tiredness, unusual muscle pain, trouble breathing, stomach pain with nausea and vomiting, cold extremities, dizziness or light-headedness, or a fast or irregular heartbeat.

Special Considerations

Renal impairment. Patients with moderately or severely impaired renal function or undergoing dialysis for end-stage renal disease may experience decreased half-life and clearance rates for adefovir. The dosing interval of adefovir may need to be adjusted for these patients.

Hepatic impairment. In non-chronic HBV patients, the pharmacokinetics remains the same in patients with moderate and severe hepatic impairment compared with unimpaired patients. No change in dosage is anticipated for these patients.

ANTISENSE DRUGS

Antisense oligonucleotides containing locked (poorly binding) nucleic acids are a new class of therapeutic agents for viral infections, cancer, inflammatory, and cardiovascular diseases. Some drawbacks of antisense drugs include low-binding to active sites and toxic side effects (256). Oligonucleotides may be inhibitors of HIV (257). It still remains a challenge for oligonucleotides to provide efficient and specific antisense activity with reduced toxicity. Fomivirsen is an example of an antisense drug.

Generic Name Fomivirsen Brand Name(s) Vitravene Other Name(s)	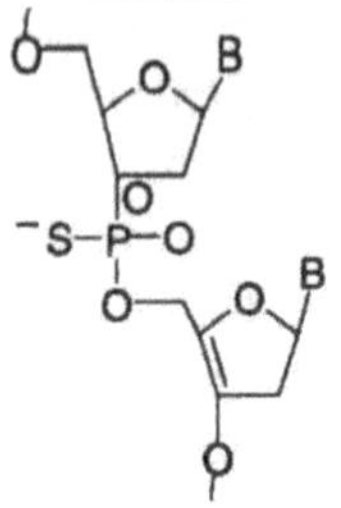 Structure	Viral Diseases Treated (FDA Approved) Human cytomegalovirus (HCMV) retinitis

Fig. 3.25 Associated names, structure, and applicability of fomivirsen.

Fomivirsen

Introduction

Fomivirsen, an antisense drug, is the first in this group to be FDA-approved. Patients who have CMV retinitis as a result of their AIDS infection may be treated with fomivirsen, particularly if they have a contraindication to, or an intolerance for, other CMV retinitis treatments (Fig. 3.25). Fomivirsen is effective when certain CMV strains are known to be ganciclovir, foscarnet, and cidofovir resistant.

Mechanism of Action

Fomivirsen is a DNA analogue that complements a unique sequence of nucleotides with the mRNA of CMV. Formivirsen is a single-stranded antisense oligonucleotide (Fig. 3.26). This region of mRNA is responsible for the regulation of viral gene expression that is necessary to produce infectious CMV. As the CMV genetic material begins to reproduce, messenger RNA is used to encode a specific protein. Fomivirsen is a complementary (antisense) sequence that binds to the messenger RNA sequences and prohibits the development of new CMV proteins. Because it is more specific to CMV, fomivirsen produces few side effects. Because fomivirsen interferes with CMV replication, CMV may not be able to develop resistance as it has to ganciclovir and other antivirals.

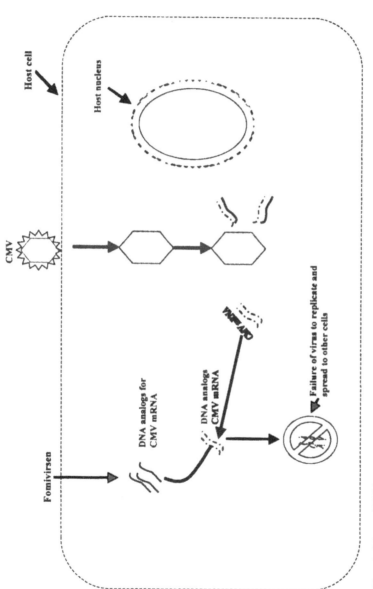

Fig. 3.26 mRNA suppression in cytomegalovirus by fomivirsen.

Table 3.22   Clinical Studies and Reports of Fomivirsen Usage

Topic	Findings	References
CMV retinitis in an AIDS patient (2 case studies)	Bull's-eye maculopathy developed after intravitreal injection of fomivirsen. Resolution occurs after discontinuation of fomivirsen.	258,259
Drug induced immune recovery uveitis (IRU)	Fomivirsen may cause drug-induced IRU.	260

Clinical Studies and Reports of Fomivirsen Usage

Most clinical studies have involved the use of fomivirsen in the treatment of CMV retinitis (258–260) (Table 3.22).

Treatment

Treatment for CMV-retinitis is shown in Table 3.23.

Adverse Effects

In AIDS patients, pigmentary retinopathy, alterations in the electro-retinogram, rings of over-or under-pigmented retinal epithelium around the cornea (bull's-eye maculopathy), and cataracts have been reported. Other common adverse effects are:

> **Ocular inflammation.** Vitreitis and/or iritis may occur.
> **Intraocular pressure.** Elevation of intraocular pressure occurs in 10–20% of cases.

Special Considerations

Fomivirsen has a narrow therapeutic index. It can cause toxic effects in some patients when the same dose is safe for others. Widespread retinal epithelial charge can occur, causing severe peripheral loss (261,262).

Table 3.23   Treatment with Fomivirsen

Symptom	Treatment
CMV-retinitis in AIDS patients	Intravitreal

Generic Name Imiquimod	Structure	Viral Diseases Treated (FDA Approved)
Brand Name(s) Aldara Other Name(s)	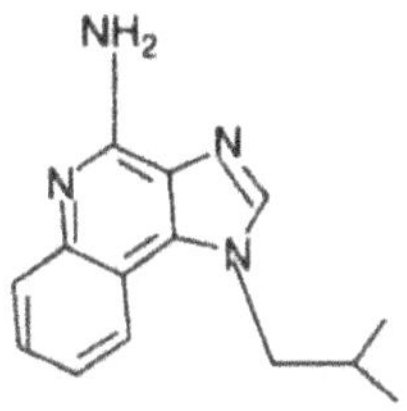	Anogenital warts

Fig. 3.27 Associated names, structure, and applicability of imiquimod.

TOPICAL IMMUNE MODULATORS

Imiquimod

Introduction

Imiquimod has no direct antiviral activity, but it induces numerous cytokines in human peripheral mononuclear blood cells (Fig. 3.27). As an immune response modifier, it stimulates interleukin-1 (IL-1), IL-6, IL-8, tumor necrosis factor (TNF), and interferon-alpha. Imiquimod has been shown to be highly effective in the treatment of common and/or genital warts caused by the human papillomavirus. Imiquimod should be considered the first line of therapy for most genital warts as it has a high rate of efficacy, it is easy to use, and recurrence rates of genital warts are low (263). It is FDA approved for therapy of actinic keratoses and superficial basal cell carcinomas. Other conditions in which successful use of imiquimod has been reported include squamous cell carcinoma in situ and lentigo maligna (264).

Mechanism of Action

The regression of warts is strongly associated with a decrease in HPV DNA and mRNA expression of both early and late viral proteins. Tyring et al. (265) indicates that the clearance of genital warts and the reduction in baseline wart area result from the induction of interferon-alpha, -beta, -gamma, and TNF-alpha (Fig. 3.28). Imiquimod acts as an immune response modifier by affecting the innate and acquired immune response.

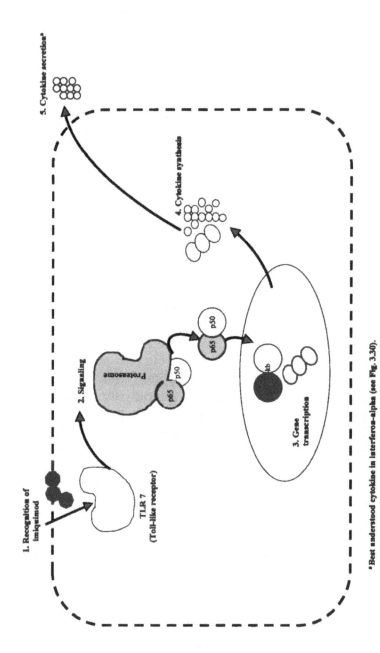

Fig. 3.28 Mechanisms of action of imiquimod.

It stimulates natural-killer cell activity, contributes to the maturation of Langerhans cells, and augments the effectiveness of T cells (266).

Clinical Studies and Reports of Imiquimod Usage

Most antiviral studies of imiquimod involve its usage with human papilloma virus infections (See Table 3.24) (264–272,275–282).

Treatment

Imiquimod is applied as a cream (Table 3.25). Most patients tolerate imiquimod, and the medication can be applied at home. Imiquimod cream applied to the skin does not enhance phototoxicity or UV-damage to cells or DNA (274). Generally, imiquimod is effective for self-treatment of genital warts at home with some minor, local adverse effects. These inflammatory reactions stop when treatment is stopped temporarily. Localized skin reactions can often be controlled by fewer applications per week or by leaving medication on for a shorter period of time. For those patients who have recurring warts, a second treatment regimen with imiquimod is often effective. Imiquimod is considered to be a cost-effective treatment for condylomata accuminata when compared with surgical excision, loop electrosurgical excision, electrodessication, CO_2 laser, podofilox, and pulsed-dye lasers. The ease of use of imiquimod and other factors, such as fewer office visits and the low recurrence rate following imiquimod use, contribute to the choice of this treatment modality (283).

Adverse Effects

The main side effects of imiquimod are at the site of application. Skin reactions are common and treatment may be temporarily discontinued for a few days. These reactions include:

Erythema. This is the most common local skin reaction (270).
Itching.
Burning.
Pain. Usually mild pain in patients with daily treatments over time.

Table 3.24   Clinical Studies and Reports of Imiquimod Usage

Topic	Findings	Reference
Clearance of genital warts	Imiquimod 5% cream cleared 56% of warts with a recurrence rate varying from 13–19%. Reduction of baseline wart area of 80% or more in 62% of patients.	267,268
Treatment of common warts and molluscum contagiosum	Imiquimod 5% cream, self-applied, once daily for 5 days/week for overnight is effective.	269
Anogenital warts in female patients	Imiquimod 5% cream 3 times per week for 16 weeks is effective in 75% of patients if those with partial clearance continued treatment longer than 16 weeks. Recurrence was 15% with 75% of these accomplishing clearance later.	270
Topical imiquimod and valacyclovir for HIV patients with acyclovir-resistant HSV (off label).	Lesions were treated with imiquimod. As soon as healing of ulcers occurred, 1g of valacyclovir hydrochloride (twice daily) was begun. All lesions healed and patients (3) continued to take 500 mg valacyclovir hydrochloride daily.	271,272
Treatment of infantile hemangioma (off label)	Infants (2) with emerging infantile hemangiomas treated with 5% imiquimod 3 times per week had complete resolution of lesions after 3–5 months of therapy initiation with no scarring and a normal neurological examination.	264
Recurrent HSV lesions treated with imiquimod and glycoprotein vaccine (guinea pigs)	Imiquimod and vaccine combination extended the duration and extent of protection for recurrences when compared with imiquimod treatment alone.	265

(continued)

Table 3.24 *(Continued)*

Topic	Findings	Reference
Effect of imiquimod on UV-exposed skin	Imiquimod had no detectable potential to induce photocontact allergy or phototoxicity. Imiquimod cream (5%) does not enhance UVR-induced damage to epidermal cells or DNA.	266
High-grade vaginal intraepithelial neoplasia	Reduced grade of neoplasia after treatment with 5% imiquimod cream vaginally. Treatment was 3 times per week for 8 weeks.	275
External anogenital warts in HAART-treated HIV patients.	Persistent anogenital warts on males (4) responded to treatment with imiquimod, possibly due to the immune restoration by HAART.	276
High grade cervical intraepithelial neoplasia	Significant benefit with 5% imiquimod cream with low recurrence rate.	277
Penile genital warts	Imiquimod is better utilized with treatment of 3 times per week rather than 1 times daily due to local skin reactions. Total clearance was 62% in 3 times weekly application group.	278
Bowenoid papulosis on labia majora	Imiquimod 5% cream applied on alternate days for 10 days and then for 2 hours daily for the next 10 days gave complete clinical resolution. Histology also became more normal.	279
Condyloma acuminata in inguinal area and thigh	Imiquimod may be useful as a primary or adjunct therapy in treatment of non-genital lesions caused by HPV.	280
Patients with HIV and anal warts	Application of 5% imiquimod cream 3 times per week for 8 weeks was effective in clearing warts.	281

(continued)

Table 3.24   (*Continued*)

Topic	Findings	Reference
Anogenital warts in children	Both podofilox and imiquimod 5% cream are safe and effective to use on children with anogenital warts, but imiquimod is associated with a lower recurrence rate.	282

INTERFERON-ALPHA AND COMBINATIONS

Introduction

Interferon is an antiviral protein that may be formulated from purified, natural, human interferon -alpha proteins or produced as a glycoprotein using recombinant DNA techniques. One drawback to interferon has been its sustainable bioavailability and short "time in residence" in the body. The advent of pegylated interferon (PEG-interferon)—a combination of equal amounts of polyethylene glycol and interferon -alpha to form a 40 kDa branched structure—provided a longer-lasting interferon with fewer injections required to administer a sustained virological response rate. By coadministering ribavirin with PEG-interferon alpha -2a, sustained virological responses of 56% are recorded. A comparison with PEG-interferon alone or standard alpha interferon -2b with ribavirin yields responses of

Table 3.25   Treatment with Imiquimod

Symptom	Treatment
Clearance of genital warts	Imiquimod cream (5%) applied to wart area without occlusion, 3 times per week prior to bedtime. After 6–10 hours, the area should be washed with soap and water to remove the medication. Continue for 16 weeks or until there is a complete clearance of warts.

30% and 45% respectively (284). These early reports have led to the testing of other treatments being combined with PEG-interferon for a variety of diseases. A histamine dehydrochloride is currently being tested. Another study focuses on a new molecule that is interferon-alpha fused to albumin. Therapies that provide longer-acting therapy and improved side-effect profiles are the future.

Interferon-Alpha

Introduction

Interferon-alpha has FDA approval for the treatment of hairy-cell leukemia, Kaposi's sarcoma, condyloma acuminata, chronic HBV or HCV infection, and melanoma (after local excision). Natural and recombinant interferon-alpha can be used to treat condyloma acuminata (285,286). The most important application of interferon-alpha is as antiviral therapy for hepatitis B and C as there is a potentially fatal sequelae of these infections, such as cirrhosis and hepatocellular carcinoma. Interferon-alpha as an intralesional injection can be used for refractory or recurring external condylomata acuminata. Interferon is also FDA-approved for treatment for AIDS-related Kaposi's sarcoma and melanoma after excision (Fig. 3.29). Interferon alpha-2b is effective in early control of HCV infection to prevent chronic HCV infection (287).

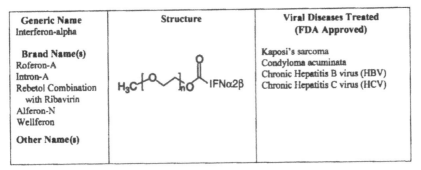

Generic Name Interferon-alpha	Structure	Viral Diseases Treated (FDA Approved)
Brand Name(s) Roferon-A Intron-A Rebetol Combination with Ribavirin Alferon-N Wellferon **Other Name(s)**	H₃C—O—...—O—IFNα2β	Kaposi's sarcoma Condyloma acuminata Chronic Hepatitis B virus (HBV) Chronic Hepatitis C virus (HCV)

Fig. 3.29 Associated names, structure, and applicability of interferon-alpha.

Mechanism of Action

Alpha interferons filter through the glomeruli of the kidneys, degrade to smaller proteins, and enter the circulatory system. Interferons bind to specific membrane receptors on a cell's surface. There is high species specificity for binding to these receptors. The binding begins a cascade of events that induce protein synthesis and a variety of cellular responses, including the inhibition of viral replication and cell proliferation. Macrophages stimulate phagocytosis, lymphocyte cytotoxicity is boosted, and human leucocyte antigen expression occurs when interferons are introduced. It is not clear which one or more of these events enhance the therapeutic effect of interferons (Fig. 3.30).

Clinical Studies and Reports that Support the Use of Interferon Alpha

Interferon-alpha has been shown to have positive benefits as well as side effects (19,20,35–40,286–300) (Table 3.26).

Treatment

Use of interferon-alpha for therapy is shown in Table 3.27. When treating molluscum contagiosum virus (MCV) with interferon-alpha, those patients without systemic symptoms, and with a relatively intact immune system and limited lymphadenopathy experience the best results. For AIDS-related Kaposi's sarcoma, treatment should be continued until there is no further evidence of the tumor unless adverse effects preclude further therapy. PEG-interferon has recently been approved and appears to be more effective than standard interferon therapy for HCV infection.

Adverse Effects

> **Injections.** Intralesional injections are painful and time-consuming.
> Systemic adverse effects include:
> **Neutropenia.**
> Constitutional symptoms include:

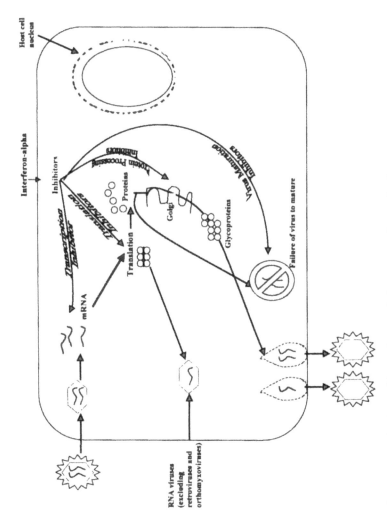

Fig. 3.30 Action of interferon-alpha on various viral structures.

Table 3.26 Clinical Studies and Reports that Support the Use of Interferon-Alpha

Topic	Findings	Reference
Kaposi's sarcoma	Partial improvement.	19–20
Chronic HBV	Interferon-alpha has long-term effectiveness in 30–40% of patients with chronic HBV.	35–40,287
Chronic HCV	Interferon-alpha has long-term effectiveness in 25% of patients with chronic HCV. HCV genotype 1 (most prevalent in the United States) has the lowest response rate.	287–294
Subcutaneous application of interferon-alpha	May cause exacerbation of asthma in those previously predisposed to asthma.	294,295
Condylomata acuminata	Partial improvement.	286
Psoriasis	May worsen with interferon-alpha treatment.	295
Lichen planus	May improve or worsen with interferon-alpha treatments	286
Molluscum contagiosum virus (MCV)	Overall response rates to systemic interferon-alpha range from 30–46%, the majority of which are partial responses.	296–300

Fatigue.

Fever.

Myalgias.

Lethargy.

Headaches (influenza-like syndrome).

Central nervous system dysfunction, including depression.

Gastrointestinal disturbances.

Bone marrow suppression. Bone marrow suppression often occurs when this medication is combined with other medications.

Table 3.27   Treatment with Interferon-Alpha

Symptom	Treatment
Chronic HBV	Intron A (children): 3.0 million IU 3 times a week for first week. Escalate dose to 6 million (max 10 million), 3 times a week for 16–24 weeks. Intron A (adults): 30–35 million IU/ week (5 million IU daily or 10 million 3 times a week for 16 weeks).
Chronic HCV	Intron A: 3.0 million IU 3 times a week. Continue treatment to 18–24 months if ALT is normal at 16 weeks of therapy.
HPV treated with Intron A	Intron A: Inject 1.0 million IU into each lesion 3 times a week for 3 weeks, with a maximum of 5 lesions per session.
HPV treated with Alferon N	Alferon N: Inject 0.05 ml (250,000 IU) into each lesion twice each week for up to 8 weeks. The maximum dose allowed per treatment session is 0.5 ml (2.5 million IU).
Disseminated AIDS-related Kaposi's sarcoma	Interferon alpha-2b (Intron A) administered subcutaneously or intramuscularly at a dosage of 30 million IU/M^2 three times a week.[a] Interferon alpha-2a (Roferon A) given subcutaneously or intramuscularly at 36 million IU daily for 10–12 weeks for induction therapy. Follow up with 36 million IU 3 times a week until there is no further evidence of tumor for maintenance therapy.[a]

[a] If a severe reaction occurs during treatment, dosage reduction by 50% or temporary discontinuation is indicated. An escalation dosage regimen may alternatively be used to decrease the risk of acute toxicity.

Possible autoimmune phenomena include:

Psoriasis. May worsen with treatment (295).

Asthma. May be exacerbated with treatment (294,295).

Special Considerations

Failure of other therapies. Interferon-alpha should be reserved for cases where other therapies have failed or for which no other effective therapy is available.

Combination therapy with cytodestructive or surgical treatment. Treatment of condyloma acuminatum with Interferon-alpha is most effective when combined with additional cytodestructive/surgical treatments.

PEG-Interferon

Introduction

Pegylated interferon-alpha is a combination of interferon-alpha with polyethylene glycol (PEG). Polyethylene glycol is commonly used in the food and cosmetic industries. Pegylating interferon enhances the pharmacological activity of the protein—better efficacy, fewer and less serious adverse events, and better patient satisfaction. PEG-interferon combined with ribavirin is most effective in treating hepatitis C (see "PEG-Interferon and Ribavirin", **page 214**) (Fig. 3.31).

Generic Name PEG-Interferon-alpha	Structure	Viral Diseases Treated (FDA Approved)
Brand Name(s) Pegasys Peg-Intron **Other Name(s)**	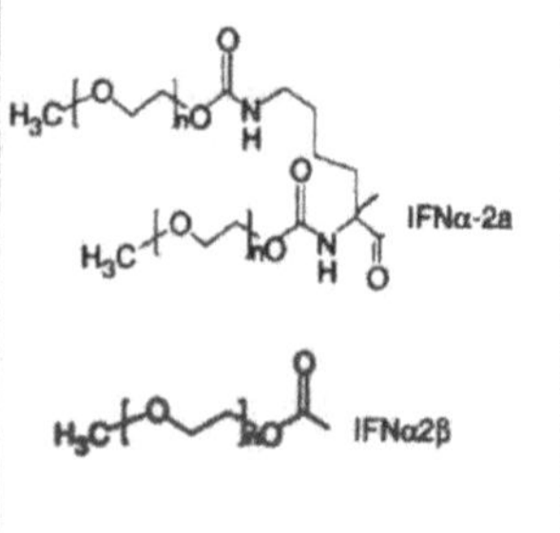	Hepatitis C virus (HCV)

Fig. 3.31 Associated names, structure, and applicability of PEG-interferon alpha-2a and alpha-2b.

Mechanism of Action

To retard renal and cellular clearance of interferon and other protein molecules, a minimum mass of 40–60 kDa is required. Smaller molecules will continue to pass through the glomerulus (301,302). Branched chains are less susceptible to proteolysis than are linear chains. The polyethylene glycol chains may attach at a single site or multiple sites, with multiple sites being less preferred. Native interferon has a half-life of 2.1 hrs with a 1.0 hr residence time. Two linear 20 kDa pegylated interferon chains linked by lysine have a half-life of 23 hours and a residence time of 32 hours. Branched monopegylated chains (2 × 20 kDa) have a half-life of 15 hours and a 20 hr plasma residence time. These peglyated chains are combined with others to improve absorption, distribution, and elimination characteristics of interferon alpha-2a. The primary differences between interferons and pegylated interferons is size. Larger-sized (pegylated) interferons have better distribution and absorption, and less elimination (Fig. 3.32).

Clinical Findings and Reports That Support the Use of PEG-Interferon

While pegylated interferon-alpha suppresses viral acitivity, other studies indicate that coadministration of pegylated interferon-alpha with another antiviral or immunomodulator enhances the performance of the antiviral or other therapy. More recent clinical studies are focusing on dual or three-way therapy; these are discussed later in this section.

Treatment

When treating chronic hepatitis C, the results of the first few weeks of therapy are often a better predictor of long-term results than extensive "predictive" testing by genotyping, viral load analyses, and extent of cirrhosis damage. Antiviral therapy is recommended for persons whose alanine aminotransferase levels are abnormal, and who have HCV RNA in serum and evidence of cirrhosis (presence of fibriosis, inflammation, and necrosis) (303). The primary measures of efficacy

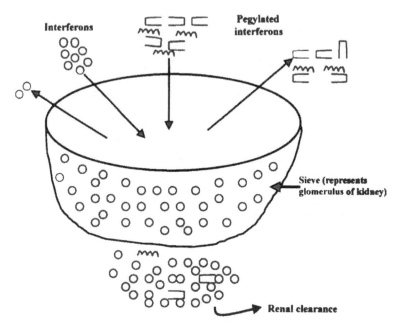

Fig. 3.32   Comparison of interferon and pegylated interferon.
Pegylated interferons are larger in structure and are more difficult
to remove from the kidneys. Therefore, unpegylated interferons
experience renal clearance much faster.

are a reduction in viral load and normalization of liver function. Virus loads should drop below the detection limit for a
validated PCR-RNA technique with a normal blood level of
the liver enzyme AGT. Interferon alpha-2b is administered
frequently (usually 3 times a/week for chronic hepatitis C or
daily for melanoma) because of rapid clearance via the glomerulus. By pegylating interferon-alpha, delayed clearance
occurs and administration of pegylated interferon-alpha can
often be reduced to once a week (304).

Adverse Effects

Pegylated interferon-alpha has an adverse event frequency
profile similar to that of standard interferon alpha-2a. Side
effects usually decrease in severity as treatment continues.

Depression.

Pyrexia.

Rigors.

Nausea and vomiting.

Impaired concentration.

Alopecia.

Psychiatric events. May include severe depression, psychosis, and personality disorders.

Special Considerations

Hepatitis C patients. Hepatitis C patients with cirrhosis of the liver often have other issues pertaining to safety and tolerability, such as neutropenia and thrombocytopenia. Myalgia, arthralgia, and injection-site inflammation are commonly reported by chronic hepatitis C patients. Other adverse events occur as often as with standard interferon-alpha.

There may be contraindications to taking pegylated interferon in patients with a history of heart disease, kidney disease, seizures, or depression.

Ribavirin and Interferon-Alpha/PEG-Interferon Alpha

Introduction

Ribavirin is approved to treat respiratory syncytial virus (RSV). It is also approved for synergistic use with interferon-alpha in the treatment of chronic hepatitis C when interferon-alpha monotherapy has failed (305–308). The combination is well tolerated, but more adverse effects are to be expected with the combined treatment. Hepatitis C is prevalent in HIV-positive persons and treatment of HCV in this population can be challenging.

Mechanism of Action

The mechanisms of the enhanced efficacy of ribavirin therapy combined with interferon therapy are unknown. What is known, however, is that the two combined with each other are more effective than either taken alone.

Clinical Studies and Reports to Support Ribavirin and Interferon Alpha Usage

The most effective therapy for treating chronic hepatitis C is the ribavirin–PEG-interferon-alpha combination therapy (309–316) (Table 3.28).

Treatment

Interferon-alpha and ribavirin is used to treat chronic hepatitis C viral infection (Table 3.29).

Adverse Effects

Ribavirin can cause :

> **Hemolytic anemia.** Usually compensated for by reducing the ribavirin dosage (317).

Interferon can cause:

> **Neutropenia.**
> Constitutional symptoms include:
> **Fatigue.**
> **Fever.**
> **Myalgias.**
> **Lethargy.**
> **Headaches (influenza-like syndrome).**
> **Central nervous system dysfunction**, including depression.
> **Gastrointestinal disturbances.**
> **Bone marrow suppression.** Bone marrow suppression often occurs when interferon-alpha is combined with other medications.
> Possible autoimmune phenomena include:
> **Psoriasis.** May worsen with treatment.
> **Asthma.** May be exacerbated with treatment.
> **Myasthenia gravis** (318).

Table 3.28 Clinical Studies and Reports of Ribavirin and Interferon-Alpha Usage

Topic	Findings	Reference
Hepatitis C (recurrent/ severe after liver transplantation)	Early virological response did not change progressive course of hepatitis C disease.	309
Chronic hepatitis C	interferon and ribavirin increases response rates over 24–48 weeks of therapy.	310
Side effects	Two drug-combination has greater side-effects.	310
Early intervention of therapy to treat hepatitis C	Early intervention is more effective rather than waiting until infection becomes chronic.	311
Interferon levels in chronic hepatitis C treated with interferon-alpha and ribavirin	Combining interferon-alpha and ribavirin enhances type-1 T helper cell activity.	312
Review of viral hepatitis therapy	Most effective therapy is pegylated interferon-alpha and oral ribavirin.	313
Cost effectiveness of ribavirin and interferon alpha-2b	Combination therapy increases quality adjusted life expectancy and is cost-effective.	314
Combination therapy in dialysis patients with chronic hepatitis C infection	Ribavirin can be used with interferon-alpha as long as dosage of ribavirin is reduced and close monitoring of plasma and hemoglobin levels occurs.	315
Virological and histological responses to combination therapy for hepatitis C	Combination therapy is appropriate for hepatitis C relapsers and non-responders.	316

Table 3.29   Treatment with Ribavirin and Interferon-Alpha

Symptom	Treatment
Chronic HCV	Oral ribavirin tablets taken 2 times daily for 6 months and interferon alpha-2b injections 3 times per week during the same time period.

Special Considerations

Ribavirin is teratogenic. As a precaution against pregnancy and birth defects, female patients on ribavirin must practice effective contraception during the treatment period and for 6 months thereafter.

PEG-interferon and ribavirin. Clinical studies have demonstrated that this combination therapy is currently the most effective treatment for hepatitis C infections.

Concomitant use of ribavirin and zidovudine. This usage combination should be avoided as in vitro studies indicate that ribavirin interferes with the activity of zidovudine against HIV.

Triple therapy. Other combinations may provide enhanced therapy with fewer side effects, such as triple therapy of interferon-alpha, ribavirin, and ursodeoxycholate to improve liver chemistry (319). Other combinations will surely follow.

ION CHANNEL FUNCTION INHIBITORS OF M2 PROTEINS AND NEURAMINIDASE INHIBITORS

(Amantadine, Rimantadine, Zanamivir, and Oseltamivir)

Although amantadine and rimantadine have been in use for some time, their effectiveness is limited to the treatment of influenza A. Both interfere with the ion channel function of the M2 protein and act indirectly on hemagglutinin. Influenza B does not have an M2 protein. Both amantadine and rimantadine can cause gastrointestinal (GI) and central nervous system (CNS) symptoms that are especially troubling in the elderly. Viral resistance occurs in up to 30% of the population and mutant viruses have been isolated from patients who have never been treated (320–322).

The influenza virus has two glycoprotein areas that facilitate virus attachment and help distribute newly formed virons. These glycoprotein areas are called hemagglutinin (HA) and neuraminidase (NA). HA initiates viral adsorption and penetration. The NA allows for the release of the virions from the infected cell and from each other. NA may also play a role in the movement of the virus into the respiratory tract mucin layer. Zanamivir, a neuraminidase inhibitor, was designed based on the interaction of the influenza virus NA and cell-surface receptors. The active site is conserved in all known influenza A and B strains, making zanamivir a broad-spectrum treatment for influenza. By delivering high concentrations of zanamivir via oral inhalation, viral replication in the respiratory tract is hindered.

Oseltamivir was later developed as an orally active inhibitor based on the antiviral properties of zanamivir. By replacing the sugar ring with one of cyclohexene, placing an amino group in the 4' position on the ring, and replacing the glycerol side chain with a hydrophobic pentyl ether group, oseltamivir phosphate can be administered as a solid capsule or oral suspension medication.

An additional inhibitor, known as biocryst, is being developed and tested. In vitro and in vivo studies with mice indicate that efficacy is comparable to zanamivir and oseltamivir (323). Biocryst is a hybrid, in that it has a guanidine group, as in zanamivir, and the hydrophobic group, as in oseltamivir. This structure may cause biocryst to facilitate reduced development of drug resistance by the influenza virus as mutations are less likely to occur (324). Both zanamivir and oseltamivir have very few side effects.

Amantadine

Introduction

Amantadine was first introduced as an antiviral in the 1960s. It was incidentally found to be a drug for the treatment of Parkinson's disease because it has the ability to release

Generic Name	Structure	Viral Diseases
Amantadine		Treated
		(FDA Approved)
Brand Name(s)		
Symmetrel		Influenza A virus
Other Name(s)		

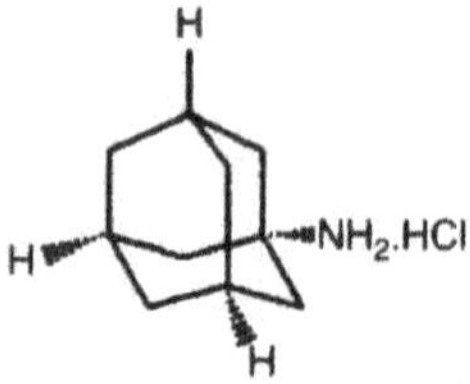

Fig. 3.33 Associated names, structure, and applicability of amantadine.

dopamine. Amantadine has been extensively tested as a possible treatment for drug dependence with limited success (325–330). However, more recently amantadine has been restudied as an antiviral agent, particularly in patients with chronic hepatitis C infection, with greater efficacy and less cost than interferon-alpha. Amantadine has activity against influenza and some of the Flaviviridae (Fig. 3.33). It is identified as a potential blockade to new cell infections (331). With the success of combining interferon treatment with ribavarin, testing is being expanded to include amantadine and interferon combination treatment to address the expanding concern over drug resistance of hepatitis C (332). The advent of pegylated interferons may result in better treatment options for combination therapy with amantadine—a better pharmaco-dynamic profile and antiviral efficacy (333).

Mechanisms of Action

How amantadine causes antiviral activity is not understood. Amantadine may be a major blocker of new cell infections rather than a cure, per se, for viral infections, such as influenza. Figure 3.34 is a comparison of the viral load with treatments of interferon, interferon and ribivarin, and interferon and amantadine. The delayed reaction of the interferon and

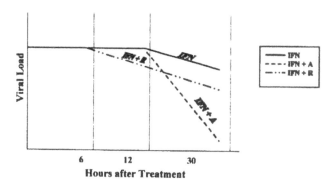

Fig. 3.34 Effect of IFN, IFN + Amantadine (IFN + A), and IFN + Ribavirin (IFN + R) on Influenza Viral Load.

amantadine indicates the combination may have no direct effect on viral replication (334). It may also indicate that amantadine alone can reduce the viral load, but not completely eliminate it (335). Amantadine may prevent the release of infectous viral nucleic acid by interfering with transmembrane function. Amantadine does not interfere with the immunogenicity of inactivated influenza A virus vaccine.

Clinical Studies that Support Treatment with Amantadine

The clinical safety and efficacy profile of amantadine is sketchy with positive and negative effects of most treatment therapies (331,332,336–349) (Table 3.30). A number of studies involving large complexes of military personnel or schools indicate that amantadine may be effective in reducing the effects of influenza, but may increase the number of adverse effects on the subject population. As the dosage of amantadine increases, there is an increased number of adverse effects. Patients treated with amantadine generally experience one day less fever than those who are untreated (Fig. 3.35). This translates to a significant economic advantage for workers who can return to work one day earlier.

Table 3.30 Studies that Support the Use of Amantadine

Topic	Findings	Reference
Chronic hepatitis C	100 mg amantadine HCl orally b.i.d. for 3–12 consecutive months. A 3-month administration for therapy is not as effective as previously indicated.	336
Use of amantadine and interferon-alpha to treat HCV	After three months of therapy, 73% of study subjects were considered to be HCV PCR-negative compared with only 46% of the controls.	337
Alopecia in Parkinson's patients	Amantadine in combination with other dopamine agonists may cause hair loss in Parkinson's patients.	338
Comparison of interferon, interferon and ribavirin, and interferon and amantadine	Viral loads for interferon alone 6–12 hours after treatment show no change while interferon and amantadine show a more rapid decline in the viral load. (See Fig. 3.34).	331
Reduced duration of fever in influenza patients treated with amantadine vs control	Patients treated with amantadine have a fever duration for approximately one day less than those who do not receive amantadine. (See Fig. 3.35).	339–341
Comparison of ribavirin with interferon alpha -2b and amantadine with interferon alpha -2b in hepatitis C monotherapy (interferon alpha -2b) non-responders	Treatment with interferon and amantadine was not associated with any sustained viral eradication.	342

(continued)

Table 3.30 (*Continued*)

Topic	Findings	Reference
Interferon and amantadine treatment of elderly Hepatitis C patients	Amantadine hydrochloride coadministered with interferon improved the negativization of HCV-RNA and decreased the malaise associated with interferon. Viral copies were observed in about 40% of amantadine patients.	332
Preventing and treating influenza A in adults (amantadine and rimantadine)		343
Efficacy and safety of amantadine given at 200 mg daily	Amantadine reduced the rate of influenza-like illness by 78% (91% when results of laboratory-documented cases are incorporated). Adverse effects were insomnia, difficulty in concentrating, and jitteriness.	344
Toxicity of amantadine vs rimantadine	Rimantidine is better tolerated in healthy young workers with significantly more CNS effects than placebo recipients. 61% of amantadine vs 29% of the rimantidine patients reported adverse effects.	345
Efficacy and safety of oral amantadine (100 mg/day as a preventive treatment)	Little influenza activity was observed, but adverse effects included difficulty in concentrating, insomnia, and impotence.	346

(*continued*)

Table 3.30   (*Continued*)

Topic	Findings	Reference
Amantadine to prevent influenza and withdrawal effects	Amantadine (100 mg twice daily, taken orally) prevents influenza and withdrawal of amantadine leads to an increased incidence of the illness.	347
Safety and efficacy of amantadine (100 mg twice daily for 14 days) combined with previous vaccination in subjects	Amantadine is an effective and safe way to prevent influenza outbreaks when used with immunizations for influenza. One case of urticaria was reported.	348
Efficacy of inhaled amantadine (20 mg daily)	Adverse effects were local and due to the aerosol with "nasal burning" being the most significant.	349

Treatment

Dosage for treatment is shown in Table 3.31.

Adverse Effects

Neurological presentations. Includes, but is not limited to, jitteriness, inability to concentrate, insomnia, tremors, confusion, depression, hallucinations, congestive heart failure, orthostatic hypotension, and urinary retention.

Rash or nausea. Symptoms usually disappear within a week.

Livedo reticularis. Purplish swelling of the ankles.

Neuroleptic malignant syndrome (NMS). Characterized by high fever, disturbance of consciousness, and increased muscular rigidity (350,351).

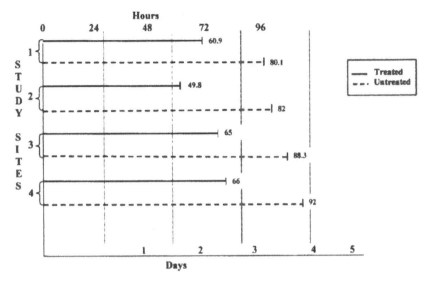

Fig. 3.35 Duration of fever after treatment of influenza with amantadine. Patients treated with amantadine for influenza experience approximately one day less fever than those with placebo.

Special Considerations

Patients with HIV. In vitro, high doses of amantadine increase HIV infectivity. However, normal levels of amantadine in the plasma of patients being treated (300 ng/ml) are not nearly as high as those that stimulate HIV activity (352).

Table 3.31 Treatment with Amantadine

Symptom	Treatment
Prophylaxis for viral disease—oral tablets	100 mg/day for adults. Children 1–9 years old: 4.4–8.8 mg/kg in 2–3 daily doses (not to exceed 150 mg/day). Children older than 9 years get the adult dosage.
Prophylaxis for viral disease—syrup	Syrup is 50 mg/5 ml. Dosage is 4.4–8.8 mg/kg of body weight in 2–3 daily doses.
Hepatitis C	Oral 100 mg amantadine HCl b.i.d. for 3–12 consecutive months.
Influenza	Oral
Influenza	Parenteral

Drug resistance. Drug-resistant H3N2-subtype influenza A viruses have been isolated during treatment with amantadine and rimantadine, especially in institutions (353).

Coadministration with anticholinergic and antiparkinsonian agents, thiazide-type diuretics, and triamterene. Amantadine will react with these medications with increased dry mouth, ataxia, blurred vision, slurred speech, and toxic psychosis as clinical manifestations.

Abrupt discontinuation. May cause a parkinsonian crisis.
Renal insufficiency.
Congestive heart failure.
Peripheral edema.
Orthostatic hypotension.

Rimantadine

Introduction

Rimantadine is a systemic antiviral agent that is used to prevent and treat influenza A viral infections. Rimantadine is taken as either a tablet or liquid by mouth. For maximum efficacy, it is usually coadministered with influenza vaccine. Rimantadine is not effective for the treatment of colds, other types of influenza, or other virus infections (Fig. 3.36).

Generic Name Rimantadine	Structure	Viral Diseases Treated (FDA Approved)
Brand Name(s) Flumadine **Other Name(s)**	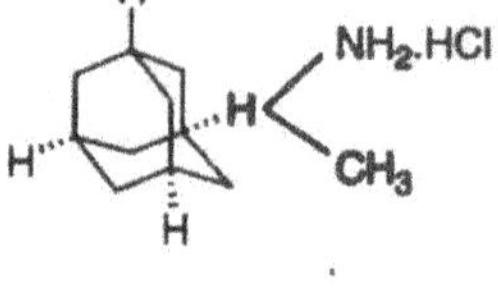	Influenza A virus

Fig. 3.36 Associated names, structure, and applicability of rimantadine.

Table 3.32 Clinical Studies of Rimantadine

Topic	Findings	References
Rimantadine for use as a prophylaxis in nursing homes	Among those vaccinated elderly, 100 mg/day of rimantadine is effective as a prophylaxis.	354
Resistance to rimantadine	Resistance is genetic—a single nucleotide sequence code.	355
Prophylaxis for children	Prophylaxis in children seems to be an effective way to prevent influenza A in children and their parents.	356

Mechanisms of Action

The mechanisms of action for rimantadine remain a mystery. It possibly affects the uncoating of the virus as inhibition occurs early during viral replication.

Clinical Studies that Support Treatment with Rimantadine

Numerous studies indicate that treatment with rimantadine is effective (354–356) (Table 3.32).

Treatment

Rimantadine is taken with food or milk as it may cause an upset stomach. Nervousness, tiredness, difficulty in sleeping or concentrating, and light-headedness are fairly common side effects (Table 3.33). Antiviral agents should be considered for the prophylaxis and treatment of influenza for the following

Table 3.33 Treatment of Influenza with Rimantadine

Symptom	Treatment
Influenza A (prevention and treatment	Adults and children 10 years of age or older: 100 mg 2 times daily. Elderly adults: 100 mg once a day. Children <10 years of age: 5 mg/kg of body weight once a day, not to exceed 150 mg/day as a prophylaxis.

individuals: 1) unvaccinated, high-risk persons; 2) high-risk persons when the vaccine/epidemic virus match is poor; 3) those who need protection during the 14-day period when the immune response is not fully developed after vaccination; 4) those with immunodeficiencies; 5) unvaccinated persons in close contact with a high-risk person; and 6) for outbreak control in long-term care facilities. Prophylaxis should be considered when there are others in the household who might be exposed to influenza and to increase the protection of vaccinated high-risk persons. Treatment is recommended for all high-risk persons with influenza or persons with severe influenza. Others with influenza also should be considered for treatment with an antiviral agent (357).

Adverse Effects

Skin rash.

Yellowing of the skin or eyes. Indication that there may be an effect on the liver.

Mood changes.

Mental confusion.

Vision changes.

Special Considerations

History of epilepsy or other seizures. Patients with a history of seizures or epilepsy may experience an increase in the frequency of convulsive events.

Kidney disease. Rimantadine is excreted through the kidneys. Patients with impaired kidney function must receive a lower dose of rimantadine.

Liver disease. Patients with liver disease may need to receive lower doses of rimantadine.

Zanamivir

Introduction

Zanamivir was the first neuraminidase inhibitor approved by the FDA. It is used to treat naturally occurring influenza A and B and is administered by oral inhalation only (Fig. 3.37).

Generic Name	Structure	Viral Diseases Treated
Zanamivir		(FDA Approved)
Brand Name(s) Relenza	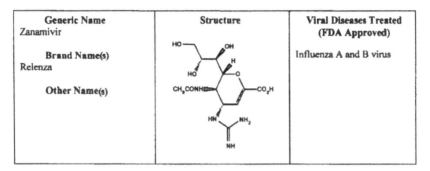	Influenza A and B virus
Other Name(s)		

Fig. 3.37 Associated names, structure, and applicability of zanamivir.

Mechanisms of Action

Zanamivir is a sialic acid analog. Antiviral activity occurs with inhibition of the influenza virus neuraminidase with some possibility that there is alteration of the virus particle aggregation and subsequent release of virions. By using herpes simplex virus translocating protein (VP22) to induce influenza into cells for the study of apoptosis, Morris, Smith, and Sweet were able to confirm that neuraminidase induces apoptosis and to indicate that other proteins may be involved as no single influenza virus protein is responsible for apoptosis (358).

Studies that Support Treatment with Zanamivir

A review of studies to address effectiveness of zanamivir in healthy and at-risk adults, adverse effects, and cost effectiveness was reported by Burls et al. (359). The review concluded that zanamivir could be especially useful in the at-risk population where fewer hospitalizations and complications and a lower death rate occur for those treated with zanamivir (360–362) (Table 3.34).

Treatment

Zanamivir reduces flu symptoms, such as weakness, headache, fever, cough, and sore throat, by 1.0 to 1.5 days. It does not,

Table 3.34 Studies that Support the Use of Zanamivir

Topic	Findings	References
Efficacy and safety of zanamivir in treating influenza in adults	In adults with influenza A or B virus infections, zanamivir, administered within 30 hours of onset of infection by inhalation therapy alone or in combination with intranasal therapy is safe and reduced symptoms if begun early.	360
Influenza in children undergoing therapy for acute lymphoblastic leukemia	Zanamivir used as influenza treatment in the immunocompromised is effective.	361
Efficacy of biocryst, zanamivir and oseltamivir on influenza A and B susceptibility	Biocryst (RWJ-270201) is most effective; oseltamivir was more effective than zanamivir.	362

however, prevent influenza infection. Therapy should begin within 2 days of the onset of flu symptoms. Zanamivir is administered as a dry-powder inhaler (10 mg twice daily for 5 days). Patients must be taught proper use of the inhaler for best efficacy of treatment. Treatment with zanamivir does not keep a patient from infecting others with the flu virus. Dosages are shown in Table 3.35.

Table 3.35 Treatment of Influenza A and B with Zanamivir

Symptom	Treatment
Adults and children over the age of 7 years of age	Two puffs twice daily (approximately 12 hours apart) for 5 days. Separate treatments by at least 2 hours and treat twice on the first day.

Adverse Effects

Adverse effects are difficult to assess in administration of zanamivir. Adverse events tend to be bronchial or gastrointestinal in nature. It is difficult to separate out what is a symptom of the influenza infection versus what is an adverse effect from the zanamivir or the method of administration (inhaled or intranasal). Nasal irritation, upper respiratory problems, and gastrointestinal distress occur with placebo (363).

> **Bronchial irritation in patients with asthma or airways disease.** Zanamivir should be discontinued immediately and medical treatment started for asthma or airways disease. Some patients without prior pulmonary disease may have respiratory abnormalities from acute respiratory infection that could resemble adverse drug reactions or increase vulnerability to drug reactions. Brochospasm and decline in lung function have been reported in some patients receiving zanamivir. Zanamivir is not generally recommended for treatment of patients with underlying airways disease, such as asthma or chronic obstructive pulmonary disease.
>
> **Cough.** Cough occurs in 2% of treatment cases.
>
> **Allergic reactions.** Oropharyngeal edema and serious rashes (facial edema or other cutaneous reactions) have been reported. Zanamivir should be stopped and appropriate treatment for allergy instituted.
>
> **Cardiac.** Arrhythmias, syncope.
>
> **Neurologic.** Seizures may occur.

Special Considerations

> **Drug interactions.** No drug interactions have been published to date.
>
> **No laboratory-documented influenza-virus infection.** Zanamivir is of no benefit in non-influenza cases. Before prescribing zanamivir, use rapid viral diagnosis when the likelihood of infection is not high.
>
> **Allergic reactions.** Zanamivir is contraindicated in patients with a known hypersensitivity to any component of the formulation.

Renal impairment. Patients with renal impairment do not require any dosage adjustment as there is low systemic availability of zanamivir.

Oseltamivir

Introduction

Oseltamivir is a neuraminidase inhibitor that has been introduced recently for influenza management and treatment (364). It has been marketed in the European Union for the prevention and treatment of suspected influenza during epidemics although one article questions the choices of oseltamivir, zanamivir, or amantadine as useful for the prevention and treatment of influenza (365). Oseltamivir may have antiviral implications for both influenza A and B. While other known influenza A antivirals appear to work with some efficacy, there have been few drugs (other than zanamivir) known to be effective for influenza B. Oseltamivir seems to provide prophylaxis, particularly in households where one or more high-risk, but vaccinated, patients live, or where vaccination is unsuitable for other members of a household (366,367). Secondary complications from influenza, such as otitis media, bronchitis, pneumonia, and sinusitis, are reduced with oseltamivir (368). Oseltamivir seems to have no severe adverse effects and clinical resistance in humans to oseltamivir by influenza virus has not been extensively reported (368). Influenza symptoms tend to improve within 24 hours if treatment begins within 24 hours of onset (369) (Fig. 3.38).

Generic Name Oseltamivir	Structure	Viral Diseases Treated (FDA Approved)
Brand Name(s) Tamiflu		Influenza A and B virus
Other Name(s)		

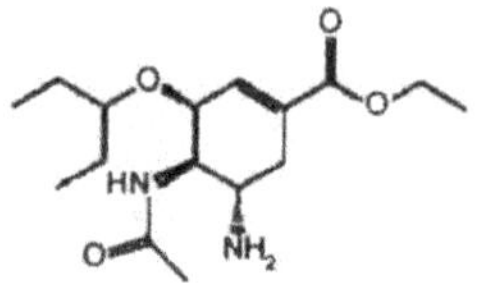

Fig. 3.38 Associated names, structure, and applicability of oseltamivir.

Mechanisms of Action

The antiviral oseltamivir is an ethyl ester prodrug of oseltamivir carboxylate, a selective inhibitor of influenza A and B (Fig. 3.39). It is metabolized in the liver where it then distributes throughout the body, including the upper and lower respiratory tracts, a major site of infection (370,371). The oseltamivir carboxylate is 3% bound to human plasma proteins and excreted through the kidneys.

Clinical Studies that Support Treatment with Oseltamivir

Oseltamivir appears to be effective for prevention of influenza with few side effects. A summary of clinical trials that support effective treatment with oseltamivir is shown in Table 3.36 (368,369,371–378).

Treatment

Oseltamivir has been shown to be over 85% effective in preventing influenza outbreaks among contacts within a household, even after exposure (372). It is considered to be a safe and effective prophylaxis of influenza for the frail and elderly as there are significantly fewer cases of laboratory-confirmed clinical influenza and fewer influenza complications in patients receiving oseltamivir than in the placebo group (347). In outbreaks of influenza A, after amantadine failed to control the outbreak, oseltamivir was used successfully for outbreak control (367). In children, oseltamivir treatment reduced cough, coryza, duration of fever, and new cases of otitis media (379). Dosages for children are higher than those for adults in that they metabolize and excrete oseltamivir more rapidly than adults (Table 3.37).

Adverse Effects

Gastrointestinal disorder. Tend to be mild and transient. Taking oseltamivir with food reduces the duration of the symptoms (371).

Nausea and vomiting. Most commonly reported side effects. Taking oseltamivir with food reduces the duration of the symptoms (371).

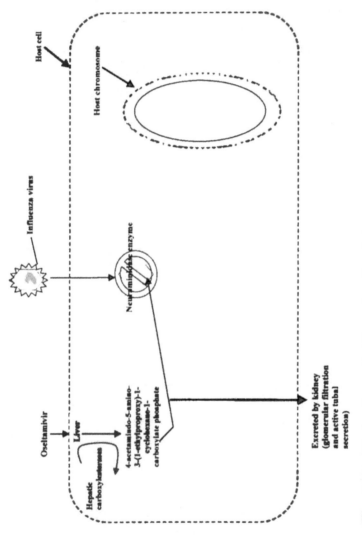

Fig. 3.39 Mechanisms of action of oseltamivir.

Table 3.36   Clinical Studies that Support the Efficacy of Oseltamivir

Topic	Findings	References
Preventing spread of influenza in households	Oseltamivir (75 mg oseltamivir once daily for 7 days) given within 48 hours of symptom onset reduces the spread of the influenza virus among household contacts.	372
Treatment of influenza with oseltamivir	75 mg of oseltamivir twice daily for 5 days reduced the illness from 95.0 to 91.6 hours.	373
Influenza prophylaxis in the frail and elderly	Long term use of oseltamivir in vaccinated frail and elderly.	374
Efficacy and safety of oral oseltamivir in treating influenza	Both doses (75 mg twice daily and 150 mg twice daily) significantly reduced the duration of influenza and patients were able to conduct normal business 2–3 days earlier than the placebo group. Bronchitis and sinusitis did occur in some of the oseltamivir patients.	375
Efficacy and safety of oseltamivir in treating acute influenza	Both doses of (75 mg twice daily and 150 mg twice daily) were associated with lower symptom scores, less viral shedding, and improved health, activity, and sleep quality with few adverse effects.	369
Efficacy of treatment with oseltamivir after onset of influenza	12 hours reduction in symptoms.	368,369
	24 hours reduction in symptoms.	371
	36 hours reduction in symptoms.	373,375

(continued)

Table 3.36 (*Continued*)

Topic	Findings	References
Pharmacokinetic interaction between oral oseltamivir and antacids	There are no measurable pharmacokinetic interactions between oseltamivir with antacids containing magnesium, aluminum, or calcium.	376
Effect of amoxicillin or cimetidine on pharmacokinetics of oseltamivir	Oseltamivir has a low drug to drug interaction potential at the renal tubular level.	377
Efficacy of treatment of influenza in children with oral oseltamivir	<33 lbs (15 kg) age 1–3 yrs: 30 mg oral suspension twice daily. 33–51 lbs (15–23 kg) age 4–7 yrs: 45 mg oral suspension twice daily. 51–88 lbs (23–40 kg) age 8–12 yrs: 60 mg oral suspension twice daily.	378

Neurological symptoms (373).

Phlegm-producing cough or wheezing. The patient should stop using this medicine and seek emergency help immediately.

Special Considerations

Co-administration with probenecid. May result in high blood levels of the active metabolite oseltamivir which may cause an increase in blood pressure.

Viral illnesses other than influenza A or B. Kidney, heart, lung, and liver diseases may affect the efficacy of oseltamivir.

Table 3.37   Treatment of Influenza with Oseltamivir

Symptom	Treatment
Oseltamivir as an influenza prophylaxis for the frail and elderly	75 mg once daily for 5 weeks.
Oseltamivir for prevention of flu (adults and teenagers >13 years of age	75 mg once daily for at least 7 days.
Oseltamivir for prevention of flu in children <13 years of age	Use and dosage to be determined by physician.
Oseltamivir to treat influenza in adults	75 mg 2 times a day for 5 days.
Oseltamivir to treat influenza in children	Dosage is based on body weight (2 mg/kg of body weight per day) and usually ranges from 30–75 mg 2 times a day for 5 days.
	Use capsular oseltamivir in children over the age of eight if they can tolerate solid capsules.

Children. Children may experience unexplained nose-bleeds or excessive watering or tearing of the eyes.

PYRIMIDINES

Pyrimidines inhibit enzymes in the DNA pathway and become incorporated into both cellular and viral DNA. This causes faulty transcription of messenger RNA and results in non-functioning viral proteins.

Trifluridine (1% Ophthalmic Solution)

Introduction

Trifluridine is effective against herpes simplex types 1 and 2, CMV, vaccinia virus, and some strains of adenovirus (380–382). Treatment of keratoconjunctivitis and recurrent

Generic Name	Structure	Viral Diseases Treated (FDA Approved)
Trifluridine		
Brand Name(s) Viroptic		Herpes simplex virus 1 (HSV-1) Herpes simplex virus 2 (HSV-2)
Other Name(s)		

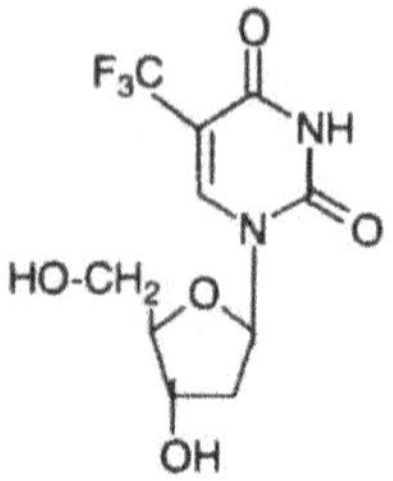

Fig. 3.40 Associated names, structure, and applicability of trifluridine ophthalmic solution, 1%.

epithelial keratitis from HSV-1 and HSV-2 with trifluridine is FDA approved (Fig. 3.40). Topical trifluridine has been suggested as an alternative medicine following treatment failure with acyclovir-related agents, particularly in HIV-positive women (382). Trifluridine ophthalmic solution (1%) is an antiviral drug for the treatment of epithelial keratitis caused by herpes simplex virus. Trifluridine can also be used to treat vaccinia of the cornea and may be useful in ocular complications from other poxviruses (383–386). A potential emerging problem is mass smallpox vaccination of 100 million persons where it is estimated that 1000–2000 cases of ocular vaccinia may occur.

Mechanism of Action

This compound is known to interfere with viral DNA synthesis in cultured mammalian cells. Trifluridine is a fluorinated pyrimidine nucleoside. Although the mechanism of action is not known, trifluridine administration results in non-functional viral proteins.

Clinical Studies that Support Treatment with Trifluridine

Trifluridine is effective in treating herpes simplex and ocular complications from vaccinia (303,383–387) (Table 3.38).

Table 3.38 Clinical Reports of Trifluridine Usage

Topic	Findings	Reference
Acyclovir-resistant mucocutaneous herpes simplex infections	Trifluridine is effective.	303,383
Vaccinia of the cornea	Trifluridine is effective.	384–387

Treatment

See Table 3.39 for treatment of eye disorders with trifluridine.

Table 3.39 Treatment with Trifluridine

Symptom	Treatment
Acyclovir-resistant mucocutaneous herpes simplex infections	One (1) drop of 1% trifluridine in aqueous solution in the affected eye every 2 hours while awake until the corneal ulcer is completely re-epithelialized (maximum 9 drops per day).
Vaccinia of the cornea	Eye drops (1% trifluridine) administered 5–10 times daily.

Adverse Effects

Ocular burning or stinging. Approximately 4.6 % of patients experience this adverse effect.

Palpebral edema. Palpebral edema occurs in 2.8% of treatments.

Superficial punctate keratopathy.

Special Considerations

The eyes of those persons who continue to touch a smallpox immunization site are at risk, particularly those who use contact lenses. Hand-washing and covering the vaccination site are important. Trifluridine can be used to treat these outbreaks.

Mutagenicity. Chromatid exchange occurs with trifluridine in human lymphocytes and fibroblasts. Teratogenicity occurs in injected eggs and chick embryos (388).

OTHER ANTIVIRALS AND MEDICATIONS

Foscarnet

Introduction

Foscarnet is used for the treatment of CMV retinitis in immunosuppressed patients (187). Forcarnet also has emerged as a replacement for acyclovir for herpes simplex infections that have become acyclovir-resistant (389). Approved for use by the FDA, foscarnet is an organic analog of inorganic pyrophosphate (Fig. 3.41). The unique mechanism of foscarnet makes it more effective against TK-negative viral strains. In addition, foscarnet has efficacy against VZV strains that are acyclovir resistant although this use of foscarnet is not FDA-approved. Other possible applications of foscarnet include HIV and HHV-8 (213,390–393).

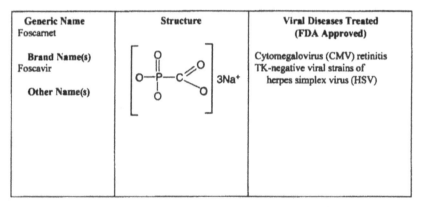

Generic Name Foscarnet	Structure	Viral Diseases Treated (FDA Approved)
Brand Name(s) Foscavir **Other Name(s)**		Cytomegalovirus (CMV) retinitis TK-negative viral strains of herpes simplex virus (HSV)

Fig. 3.41   Associated names, structure, and applicability of foscarnet.

Mechanism of Action

As an organic analog of inorganic pyrophosphate, foscarnet inhibits viral DNA polymerase by blocking its pyrophosphate binding site (Fig. 3.42). Foscarnet also inhibits HIV reverse transcriptase in the same manner. The nucleotide triphosphates are unable to cleave from the pyrophosphate and there is inhibition of further primer-template extension (392).

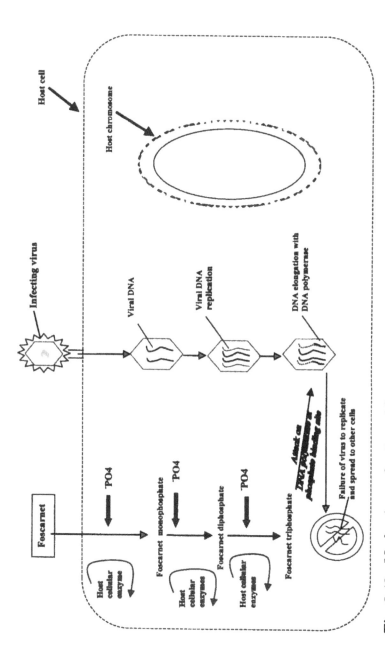

Fig. 3.42 Mechanisms of action of foscarnet.

Another asset of foscarnet is that it does not require phosphorylation by viral thymidine kinase (TK) for intracellular activation. This makes foscarnet effective against TK-negative viral strains.

Clinical Studies and Reports that Support the Use of Foscarnet

A diverse number of clinical studies and reports support the use of foscarnet as a major replacement therapy when acyclovir-resistant strains of specific viruses are present (186,211, 391–405) (Table 3.40).

Treatment

Currently, foscarnet is administered intravenously (Table 3.41) or by injection. Foscarnet does not cure CMV retinitis, but may help in preventing a worsening of symptoms. Foscarnet must be administered regularly as it works best when the blood titer does not vary. Foscarnet has been used for CMV infections in the lungs, esophagus, and intestines and for VZV infections that do not respond to acyclovir.

Adverse Effects

> **Anemia.** Foscarnet may cause or worsen anemia, dehydration, or kidney disease. Sores or ulcers in the mouth or throat are rare.
>
> **Most common side effects.** Some of the more common effects may not need medical attention and may go away as the body adjusts to foscarnet. These include:
>
> **Abdominal or stomach pain.**
> **Anxiety.**
> **Confusion.**
> **Dizziness.**
> **Loss of appetite.**
> **Nausea and vomiting.**
> **Unusual tiredness or weakness.**
> **Headache.**
> **Anemia without neutropenia.**

Table 3.40 Clinical Studies and Reports of Foscarnet Usage

Topic	Findings	Reference
Treatment of AIDS patients who have acyclovir-resistant HSV	Given foscarnet (120–180 mg/kg/day), 21 of 26 patients had a clinical response to the treatment, and 19 of those had complete re-epithelialization.	391
Effect of foscarnet on VZV, HHV-8, and HIV	Foscarnet is efficacious for acyclovir-resistant VZV and other applications.	392
Effect of foscarnet on HIV-1 RNA plasma loads	HIV-1 RNA plasma loads were reduced with foscarnet, independent of CMV infection.	393
Effect of foscarnet on acyclovir-resistant VZV	Successful treatment has been reported, although foscarnet is not FDA approved for acyclovir-resistant VZV.	394–396
Foscarnet 1% cream[a] for use on AIDS patients with HSV lesions	In a phase I/II open-label, nonrandomized trial, 65% of lesions had a good response with no pain in 73% who previously reported pain; 25% of patients developed new HSV lesions at untreated sites.	397
Treatment of CMV retinitis	Foscarnet can be used for the treatment of CMV retinitis in the immunocompromised. However, ganciclovir is usually preferred due to less severe side effects.	186
Treatment of HHV-8	Ganciclovir and foscarnet (used to treat CMV retinitis) are associated with a reduced risk of AIDS-related Kaposi's sarcoma.	398–401
Foscarnet vs ganciclovir to reduce length of time for progression of AIDS-related Kaposi's sarcoma	Patients on foscarnet had an average of 211 days for progression to Kaposi's sarcoma vs ganciclovir, which was 22 days.	402

(continued)

Table 3.40 (*Continued*)

Topic	Findings	Reference
Test of cidofovir as a preemptive therapy	Foscarnet is a rational choice for patients who fail cidofovir therapy.	211
CMV in a heart transplant patient treated with ganciclovir	Foscarnet reduced CMV antigenemia levels and prevented the development of CMV-associated disease after ganciclovir therapy was unsuccessful.	403
HHV-6 in vitro	Foscarnet is highest in antiviral activity.	404
HHV-7 in vitro	Foscarnet is the third most active antiviral against HHV-7. Cidofovir is the 2nd choice.	404
Ganciclovir-resistant cytomegalovirus retinitis	After failure of ganciclovir therapy, foscarnet therapy promoted quick resolution. Assay by an NASBA technique, amplifying B2.7 transcripts, provided a more rapid and sensitive assay than PCR for CMV DNA.	405

ᵃ Compounded; not FDA approved in topical formulation

Electrolytic imbalances. Patients may experience increased thirst and a change in frequency of urination. Foscarnet may cause genital ulcerations. Washing the genitals after urination may decrease the extent of this problem.

Nausea and vomiting.

Headache.

Central nervous system disturbances. Convulsions, muscle twitching, and tremors are less common.

Renal dysfunction. Renal dysfunction is usually reversible provided there is frequent monitoring of serum creatinine levels and adequate hydration.

Table 3.41 Treatment with Foscarnet

Symptom	Treatment
Acyclovir-resistant mucocutaneous HSV	Foscarnet (40mg/kg) is infused over at least 1 hour and repeated every 8 or 12 hours for 2–3 weeks, or until healing occurs.
CMV retinitis initial (induction) therapy	180 mg/kg/day (3×60 mg/kg/day, every 8 hours) for 14–21 days. Each dose infused over a period of 1 hour.
CMV retinitis maintenance therapy	120 mg/kg/day (3×40 mg/kg/day, every 8 hours). Each dose infused over a period of at least 2 hours. Maintenance therapy should be continued until the infection is controlled by the patient's immune system.
Herpes simplex	40 mg/kg 2 or 3 times a day. Each dose is infused over a period of 1 hour. Continue treatment for 2–3 weeks or until infection is healed.
Failed monotherapy for CMV retinitis	Foscarnet and ganciclovir combination therapy.

Renal toxicity. Risk of renal toxicity is increased when other nephrotoxic medications are concurrently administered. Dose adjustments should be made if changes in renal function occur.

Tingling, pain, or numbness. A tingling sensation around the mouth or pain or numbness in hands or feet while receiving medication may indicate a drop in normal calcium levels.

Special Considerations

Foscarnet-resistance. Six patients with AIDS have been reported to have foscarnet-resistant HSV. Five of these cases had been previously treated with foscarnet (391,392). Some of these cases responded to acyclovir, but there are reports of resistance to both acyclovir and foscarnet (406).

Monotherapy failure with foscarnet or ganciclovir.
Combination therapy of both foscarnet and ganciclovir
is indicated.

Aminoglycoside antibiotics coadministration. Coadministration of foscarnet with aminoglycoside antibiotics increases the risk of renal toxicity.

Amphotericin B coadministration. Coadministration
with foscarnet increases the risk of renal toxicity.

Other drug contraindications or dosage concerns:

- Carmustine;
- Cisplatin;
- Combination pain medicine containing acetaminophen
  and aspirin or other salicylates (with large amounts
  taken regularly);
- Cyclosporine;
- Deferoxamine (with long-term use);
- Gold salts (medicine for arthritis);
- Inflammation or pain medicine, except narcotics;
- Lithium;
- Methotrexate;
- Other anti-infectives (e.g., noted above);
- Penicillamine;
- Plicamycin;
- Streptozocin; or
- Tiopronin.
  Use of these medications may increase chances for
  renal dysfunction.
- **Pentamidine**

Use of pentamidine injection with foscarnet may lower the
level of calcium and magnesium in the blood. This increases
the chance for kidney problems.

Pregnant women. Not indicated for use in pregnant wom-
en. Foscarnet causes birth defects in studies in animals.

Breast-feeding. It is not known to what degree foscarnet appears in breast milk and what effect there might
be on the breast-feeding infant.

Children. No studies of risk or efficacy in children.

Hydration. Unless otherwise indicated, patients should drink several glasses of water each day to help prevent some unwanted effects foscarnet may have on the kidneys.

Docosonal

Introduction

1-Docosanol (n-docosanol) is an alcohol that exerts an inhibitory effect on the replication of viruses, such as herpes simplex and respiratory syncytial virus. Combination of docosanol and antiviral nucleoside analogs (e.g., acyclovir) can have a synergistic effect with few toxic side effects (Fig. 3.43).

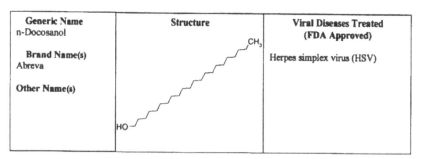

Generic Name n-Docosanol Brand Name(s) Abreva Other Name(s)	Structure	Viral Diseases Treated (FDA Approved) Herpes simplex virus (HSV)

Fig. 3.43 Associated names, structure, and applicability of n-docosanol.

Mechanism of Action

n-Docosanol is a 22-carbon, straight-chain, saturated alcohol formulated for topical applications as a cream. The mechanism of action is unclear. Pope et al. have reported that n-docosanol inhibits viral entry (407). Spruance reports that n-docosanal is a suspension as it is insoluble in water, does not inactivate the virus directly, and is not cytotoxic (408). For n-docosanal to be most effective, it should be applied before infection occurs (409,410). Spruance further reports that n-docosanal may be an anti-inflammatory agent in the murine model and a clinical trial supports the idea (411).

Treatment

Topical docosanol is used to treat symptoms of herpes simplex viral infections on the lips and around the mouth. Topical docosanol does not cure herpes simplex but relieves the pain and may help lesions heal faster.

IMPLICATIONS FOR NEW ANTIVIRAL AGENTS

As new viral diseases emerge and medicines that task the immune system become more common practice, challenges for developing new and better antivirals as alternative treatment strategies gain more importance. DNA-based viruses are a frequent cause of infection as they are able to develop long-term latency after the initial infection and are opportunistic when the patient's immune system is challenged (196).

Detection of viral diseases at an early stage via various diagnostic tests enables clinicians to make immediate decisions on treatment options. It is inappropriate to treat a disease with antivirals if the disease is not virus-based. Toxicity of many antivirals is a concern as it may place several components of a patient population at risk to the point that the risks outweigh the benefits.

REFERENCES

1. Pitre, C., G. Piriou, P. Assicot, E. Petit, C. L'Eilde, and N. Borgnis-Desbordes. 1999. Bell's palsy treatment with acyclovir. *J. de Pharmacie Clinique* 18:190–193.

2. Leclair, J. M., J. A. Zaia, M. J. Levin, R. G. Congdon, and D. A. Goldmann. 1980. Airborne transmission of chickenpox in a hospital. *N. Engl. J. Med.* 302:450–453.

3. Brentjens, M. H., G. Torres, P. Lee, and S. K. Tyring. 2003. Reduction of postherpetic neuralgia in herpes zoster: a study of the effects of gabapentin with valacyclovir during acute zoster outbreaks [poster presentation]. 61st Annual Meeting of American Academy of Dermatology, San Francisco, CA, March 2003, Poster P38.

4. Epstein, M. A., B. G. Achong, and Y. M. Barr. 1964. Virus particles in cultured lymphocytes Burkitt's lymphoma. *Lancet* 1:702–703.

5. Kieff, E. Epstein-Barr virus and its replication. 1996. In: B. C. Fields, D. M. Knipe, P. M. Howley, Eds. *Fields Virology*, 3rd ed. Philadelphia: Lippincott-Raven Press, 1996, pp. 2343–2396.

6. Young, L. S., and M. Rowe. 1992. Epstein-Barr virus, lymphomas and Hodgkin's disease. *Semin. Cancer Biol.* 3:273–284.

7. Junker, U., J. Baker, C. S. Kalfoglou, G. Veres, H. Kaneshima, and E. Bohnlein. 1997. Antiviral potency of drug-gene therapy combinations against human immunodeficiency virus type 1. *AIDS Res. Hum. Retroviruses* 13:1395–1402.

8. Walling, D. M., and S. D. Hudnall. 2002. Epstein-Barr Virus. In: S. K. Tyring, Ed. *Mucocutaneous Manifestations of Viral Disease*. New York: Marcel Dekker, 2002, p. 155.

9. Bonnet, M., J.-M. Guinebretiere, E. Kremmer, V. Grunewald, E. Benhamou, G. Contesso, and I. Joab. 1999. Detection of Epstein-Barr virus in invasive breast cancers. *J. Natl. Cancer Inst.* 92:1376–1381.

10. Labrecque, L., D. Barnes, I. Fentiman, and B. Griffin. 1995. Epstein-Barr viruses in epithelial cell tumors: a breast cancer study. *Cancer Res.* 55:39–45.

11. Luqmani, Y., S. Shousha. 1995. Presence of Epstein-Barr virus in breast carcinoma. *Int. J. Oncol.* 6:899–903.

12. Pari, G. S., and D. G. Anders. 1993. Eleven loci encoding transacting factors are required for transient complementation of human cytomegalovirus oriLyt-dependent DNA replication. *J. Virol.* 67:6979–6988.

13. Griffiths, P., and V. Emery. 2002. Cytomegalovirus. In: D. D. Richman, R. J. Whitley, and F. G. Hayden, Eds. *Clinical Virology*, 2nd ed. Washington, DC: ASM Press, 2002, pp. 433–461.

14. Kilgore, P. E., and R. I. Glass. 2002. Viral Gastroenteritis. In: D. D. Richman, R. J. Whitley, and F. G. Hayden, Eds. *Clinical Virology*, 2nd ed. New York: Churchill Livingstone, 2002, pp. 45.

15. Bell, W. R., J. D. Chulay, and J. E. Reinberg. 1997. Manifestations resembling thrombotic microangiopathy in patients with

advanced human immunodeficiency virus (HIV) disease in cytomegalovirus prophylaxis trial (ACTG 204). *Medicine* 76:369–380.

16. Maslo, C., M. N. Peraldi, J. C. Desenclor, J. D. Srarer, and W. E. Rozenbaum. 1995. Evidence for the role of cytomegalovirus in thrombotic microangiopathy in HIV-infected patients [abstract]. Programs and abstracts of the 2nd National Conference on Human Retroviruses and Related Infections. Washington, DC, January 29–February 2, 1995, LB22.

17. Wathen, M. W. 2002. Non-nucleoside inhibitors of herpesviruses. *Rev. Med. Virol.* 12:167–178.

18. Brown, T. J., A. Yen-Moore, and S. K. Tyring. 2002. Human herpesvirus 8. In: S. K. Tyring, Ed. *Mucocutaneous Manifestations of Viral Disease*. New York: Marcel Dekker, 2002, pp. 219–234.

19. Lane, H. C., J. A. Kovacs, J. Feinberg, B. Herpin, V. Davey, R. Walker, L. Deyton, J. A. Metcalf, M. Baseler, N. Salzman, et al. 1988. Anti-retroviral effects of interferon-alpha in AIDS-associated Kaposi's sarcoma. *Lancet* 2:1218–1222.

20. De Wit, R., J. K. M. E. Schattenkerk, C. A. B. Boucher, P. J. M. Bakker, K. H. N. Veenhof, and S. A. Danner. 1988. Clinical and virological effects of high-dose recombinant interferon-alpha in disseminated AIDS-related Kaposi's sarcoma. *Lancet* 2:1214–1217.

21. Geraminejad, P., O. Memar, I. Aronson, P. L. Rady, U. Hengge, and S. K. Tyring. 2002. Kaposi's sarcoma and other manifestations of human herpesvirus 8. *J. Am. Acad. Derm.* 47:641–655.

22. Humphrey, R. W., D. A. Davis, F. M. Newcomb, and R. Yarchoan. 1998. Human herpesvirus 8 (HHV-8) in the pathogenesis of Kaposi's sarcoma and other diseases. *Leuk. Lymphoma* 28:255–264.

23. Hammound, Z., D. M. Parenti, and G. L. Simon. 1998. Abatement of cutaneous Kaposi's sarcoma associated with cidofovir treatment [letter]. *Clin. Infect. Dis.* 26:1233.

24. Badiaga, S., P. Parola, C. Zandotti, and P. Brouqui. 1988. Successful treatment of Kaposi's sarcoma with a combination of antiviral drug therapy and chemotherapy: two case reports [letter]. *Clin. Infect. Dis.* 27:1558.

25. Simonart, T., J. C. Noel, G. De Dobbeleer, D. Parent, J. P. Van Vooren, E. DeClercq, and R. Snoeck. 1998. Treatment of classical Kaposi's sarcoma with intralesional injections of cidofovir: report of a case. *J. Med. Virol.* 55:215–218.

26. Krown, S. E., F. X. Real, S. Cunningham-Rundles, P. L. Myskowski, B. Koziner, S. Fein, A. Mittelman, H. F. Oettgen, and B. Safai. 1983. Preliminary observations on the effect of recombinant leukocyte A interferon in homosexual men with Kaposi's sarcoma. *N. Engl. J. Med.* 308:1071–1076.

27. Ylitalo, N., P. Sorensen, A. M. Josefsson, P. K. E. Magnusson, P. K. Andersen, J. Ponten, H. O. Adami, U. B. Gyllensten, and M. Melbye. 2000. Consistent high viral load of human papillomavirus 16 and risk of cervical carcinoma in situ: a nested case control study. *Lancet* 355:2194–2198.

28. Bergbrant, I.-M., L. Samuelsson, S. Olofsson, F. Jonassen, and A. Ricksten. 1994. Polymerase chain reaction for monitoring human papillomavirus contamination of medical personnel during treatment of genital warts with CO_2 laser and electrocoagulation. *Acta Dermatol. Venereol.* (Stockholm) 74:393–395.

29. Jablonska, S., S. Majewski, S. Obalek, and G. Orth. 1997. Cutaneous warts. *Clin. Dermatol.* 15:309–319.

30. Majewski, S., and S. Jablonska. 1997. Human papillomavirus-associated tumors of the skin and mucosa. *J. Am. Acad. Dermatol.* 36:659–685.

31. Beutner, K. R., D. J. Wiley, J. M. Douglas, S. K. Tyring, K. Fife, K. Trofatter, and K. M. Stone. 1999. Genital warts and their treatment. *Clin. Infect. Dis.* 28:S37–56.

32. Bonnez, W. 1999. Diseases due to human papillomavirus (sexually transmitted). In: R. Dolin, H. Masur, M. Saag, Eds. *Aids Therapy*. Philadelphia: WB Saunders, pp. 530–564.

33. Divan, D. G. 2002. Poxviruses. In: S. K. Tyring, Ed. *Mucocutaneous Manifestations of Viral Diseases*. New York: Marcel Dekker, 2002, pp. 50.

34. DeClercq, E. 2002. Cidofovir in the treatment of poxvirus infections. *Antiviral Res.* 55:1–13.

35. Koff, R. S. 2004. Hepatitis B virus and hepatitis D virus. In: S. L. Gorbach, J. G. Bartlett, and N. R. Blacklow, Eds. *Infectious*

Diseases, 3rd ed. Philadelphia: Lippincott Williams and Wilkins, 2004, pp. 1974–1980.

36. Alexander, G. J., J. Brahm, E. A. Fagan, H. M. Smith, H. M. Daniels, A. L. Eddleston, and R. Williams. 1987. Loss of HBsAg with interferon therapy in chronic hepatitis B virus infection. *Lancet* 2:66–69.

37. Redeker, A. G. 1975. Viral hepatitis: clinical aspects. *Am. J. Med. Sci.* 270:9–16.

38. Wright, T. L., and J. Y. Lau. 1993. Clinical aspects of hepatitis B virus infection. *Lancet* 342:1340–1344.

39. Zarski, J.-P., D. Ganem, and T. L. Wright. 2002. Hepatitis B Virus. In: D. D. Richman, R. J. Whitley, and F. G. Hayden, Eds. *Clinical Virology*. Washington, DC: ASM Press, 2002, pp. 623–657.

40. Perrillo, R. P., E. R. Schiff, G. L. Davis, H. C. Bodenheimer Jr., K. Lindsay, J. Payne, C. O'Brien, C. Tamburro, and I. M. Jacobson, for the Hepatitis Interventional Therapy Group. 1990. A randomized, controlled trial of interferon alpha-2b alone and after prednisone withdrawal for the treatment of chronic hepatitis B. *N. Engl. J. Med.* 323:295–301.

41. Lok, A. S. F., P. C. Wu, C. L. Lai, J. Y. Lau, E. K. Leung, L. S. Wong, O. C. Ma, I. J. Lauder, C. P. Ng, and H. T. Chung. 1992. A controlled trial of interferon with or without prednisone priming for chronic hepatitis B. *Gastroenterology* 102: 2091–2097.

42. Hoofnagle, J. H., M. G. Peters, K. D. Mullen, D. B. Jones, V. Rustgi, A. Di Bisceglie, C. Hallahan, Y. Park, C. Meschievitz, and E. A. Jones. 1988. Randomized controlled trial of recombinant human alpha-interferon in patients with chronic hepatitis B. *Gastroenterology* 95:1318–1325.

43. Eyster, M. E., K. E. Sherman, J. J. Goedert, and A. Katsoulidou. 1999. Prevalence and changes in hepatitis C virus genotypes among multitransfused persons with hemophilia. *J. Infect. Dis.* 179:1062–1069.

44. Jarvis, L. M., C. A. Ludlam, and P. Simmonds. 1995. Hepatitis C virus genotypes in multitransfused individuals. *Hemophilia* 1:3–7.

45. Di Bisceglie, A. M., T. L. Fong, M. W. Fried, M. G. Swain, B. Baker, J. Korenman, N. V. Bergasa, J. G. Waggoner, Y. Park, and J. H. Hoofnagle. 1993. A randomized controlled trial of recombinant alpha interferon therapy for chronic hepatitis B. *Am. J. Gastroenterol.* 88:1887–1892.

46. Wong, D. K., A. M. Cheung, K. O'Rourke, C. D. Naylor, A. S. Detsky, and J. Heathcote. 1993. Effect of alpha-interferon treatment in patients with hepatitis B e antigen-positive chronic hepatitis B: A meta-analysis. *Ann. Intern. Med.* 119:312–323.

47. Sharma, V., M. D. Dowd, A. J. Slaughter, and S. D. Simon. 2002. Effect of rapid diagnosis of influenza virus type a on the emergency department management of febrile infants and toddlers. *Arch. Ped. Adolesc. Med.* 156:41–43.

48. Smith, K. J., and M. S. Roberts. 2002. Cost-effectiveness of newer treatment strategies for influenza. *Am. J. Med.* 113:300–307.

49. Morens, D. M., and V. M. Rash. 1995. Lessons from a nursing home outbreak of influenza A. *Infect. Control Hosp. Epdemiol.* 16:275–280.

50. Gomolin, I. H., and R. K. Kathpalia. 2002. Influenza: how to prevent and control nursing home outbreaks. *Geriatrics* 57:28–34.

51. Sethi, S. 2002. Bacterial pneumonia. Managing a deadly complication of influenza in older adults with comorbid disease. *Geriatrics* 57:56–61.

52. Coonrod, J. D. 2001. Influenza: will new diagnostic tests and antiviral drugs make a difference? *Chest* 119:1630–1632.

53. Disease Prevention News [Texas Department of Health] 62 (7 October 2002):1.

54. Wray, S. K., B. E. Gilbert, M. W. Noall, and V. Knight. 1985. Mode of action of ribavirin: effect of nucleotide pool alterations on influenza virus ribonucleoprotein synthesis. *Antiviral Res.* 5:29–37.

55. Hall, C. B., J. T. McBride, E. E. Walsh, D. M. Bell, C. L. Gala, S. Hildreth, L. G. Ten Eyck, and W. J. Hall. 1983. Aerosolized ribovirin treatment of infants with respiratory syncytial virus

infection: a randomized double-blind study. *N. Engl. J. Med.* 308:1443–1447.

56. Levy, B. T., and M. A. Graber. 1997. Respiratory syncytial virus infection in infants and young children. *J. Fam. Pract.* 45:473–481.

57. LaVia, W. V., M. I. Marks, and H. R. Stutman. 1992. Respiratory syncytial virus puzzle: clinical features, pathophysiology, treatment, and prevention. *J. Pediatrics* 121:503–510.

58. Karron, R. A., R. J. Singleton, L. Bulkow, A. Parkinson, D. Kruse, I. De Smet, C. Indorf, K. M. Petersen, D. Leombruno, D. Hurlburt, M. Santosham, and L. H. Harrison, for the RSV Alaska Study Group. 1999. Severe respiratory syncytial virus disease in Alaska native children. *J. Infect. Dis.* 180:41–49.

59. Williams, R. B., and J. M. Gwaltney. 1972. Allergic rhinitis or virus cold? Nasal smear eosinophilia in differential diagnosis. *Ann. Allergy* 80:189–194.

60. Wutzler, P., and R. Thust. Genetic risks of antiviral nucleosdie analogues—a survey. 2001. *Antiviral Res.* 49:55–74.

61. Miller, W. H., R. L. Miller. 1980. Phosphorylation of acyclovir (acycloguanosine) monophosphate by GMP kinase. *J. Biol. Chem.* 255:7204–7207.

62. Fyfe, J. A., P. M. Keller, P. A. Furman, R. L. Miller, and G. B. Elion. 1978. Thymidine kinase from herpes simplex virus phosphorylates the new antiviral compound 9-(2-hydroxyethoxymethyl)guanine. *J. Biol. Chem.* 253:8721–8727.

63. Elion, G. B., P. H. Furman, J. A. Fyfe, P. De Miranda, L. Beauchamp, and H. J. Schaeffer. 1977. Selectivity of action of an antiherpetic agent 9-(2-hydroxyethoxymethyl)guanine. *Proc. Natl. Acad. Sci. USA* 74:5716–5720.

64. Spruance, S. L., J. C. Steward, N. H. Rowe, M. B. McKeough, G. Wenerstrom, and D. J. Freeman. 1990. Treatment of recurrent herpes simplex labialis with oral acyclovir. *J. Infect. Dis.* 161:185–190.

65. Fiddian, A. P., D. Brigden, J. M. Yeo, and E. A. Hickmott. 1984. Acyclovir: an update on the clinical applications of this antiherpes agent. *Antiviral Res.* 4:99–117.

66. Brand, G., G. F. Schiavano, E. Balestra, B. Tavazzi, C. F. Perno, and M. Magnani. 2001. The potency of acyclovir can be markedly different in different cell types. *Life Sci.* 69:1285–1290.

67. Goldberg, L. H., R. Kaufman, T. O. Kurtz, M. A. Conant, L. J. Eron, R. L. Batenhorst, and G. S. Boone. 1993. Long-term suppression of recurrent genital herpes with acyclovir: a 5-year benchmark. The Acyclovir Study Group. *Arch. Dermatol.* 129:582–587.

68. Wald, A., J. Zeh, G. Barnum, L. G. Davis, and L. Corey. 1996. Suppression of subclinical shedding of herpes simplex virus type 2 with acyclovir. *Ann. Intern. Med.* 124:8–15.

69. Whitley, R. J., M. Levin, N. Barton, B. J. Hershey, G. Davis, R. E. Keeney, J. Whelchel, A. G. Diethelm, P. Kartus, and S. J. Soong. 1984. Infections caused by herpes simplex virus in the immunocompromised host: natural history and topical acyclovir therapy. *J. Infect. Dis.* 150:323–329.

70. Spruance, S. L., C. S. Crumpacker, L. E. Schnipper, E. R. Kern, S. Marlowe, K. A. Arndt, and J. C. Overall Jr. 1984. Early, patient-initiated treatment of herpes labialis with topical 10% acyclovir. *Antimicrob. Agents Chemother.* 25:553–535.

71. Raborn, G. W., W. T. McGaw, M. Grace, and L. Houle. 1989. Herpes labialis treatment with acyclovir 5 percent ointment. *J. Can. Dent. Assoc.* 55:135–137.

72. Fiddian, A. P., and L. Ivanyi. 1983. Topical acyclovir in the management of recurrent herpes labialis. *Br. J. Dermatol.* 109:321–326.

73. Spruance, S. L., R. Nett, T. Marbury, R. Wolff, J. Johnson, and T. Spaulding. 2002. Acyclovir cream for treatment of herpes simplex labialis: results of two randomized, double-blind, vehicle-controlled, multicenter clinical trials. *Antimicrob. Agents Chemother.* 46:2238–2243.

74. Wallace, M. R., W. A. Bowler, N. B. Murray, S. K. Brodine, and E. C. Oldfield 3d. 1992. Treatment of adult varicella with oral acyclovir: a randomized, placebo-controlled trial. *Ann. Intern. Med.* 117:358–363.

75. Balfour, H. H. Jr., J. M. Kelly, C. S. Suarez, R. C. Heussner, J. A. Englund, D. D. Crane, P. V. McGuirt, A. F. Clemmer, and

D. M. Aeppli. 1990. Acyclovir treatment of varicella in otherwise healthy children. *J. Pediatr.* 116:633–639.

76. Dunkle, L. M., A. M. Arvin, R. J. Whitley, H. A. Rotbart, H. M. Feder Jr., S. Feldman, A. A. Gershon, M. L. Levy, G. F. Hayden, P. V. McGuirt, et al. 1991. A controlled trial of acyclovir for chickenpox in normal children. *N. Engl. J. Med.* 325:1539–1544.

77. Bean, B. C. Braun, and H. H. Balfour Jr. 1982. Acyclovir therapy for acute herpes zoster. *Lancet* 2:118–121.

78. Peterslund, N. A., K. Seyer-Hansen, J. Ipsen, V. Esmann, H. Schonheyder, and H. Juhl. 1981. Acyclovir in herpes zoster. *Lancet* 2:827–830.

79. McGill, J., D. R. MacDonald, C. Fall, G. D. W. McKendrick, and A. Copplestone. 1983. Intravenous acyclovir in acute herpes zoster infection. *J. Infect. Dis.* 6:157–161.

80. Wood, M. J., P. H. Ogan, M. W. McKendrick, C. D. Care, J. I. McGill, and E. M. Webb. 1988. Efficacy of oral acyclovir treatment of acute herpes zoster. *Am. J. Med.* 85 (Supl 2A):79–83.

81. Morton, P., A. N. Thomson. 1989. Oral acyclovir in the treatment of herpes zoster in general practice. *N. Z. Med. J.* 102:93–95.

82. Huff, J. C., B. Bean, H. H. Balfour Jr., O. L. Laskin, J. D. Connor, L. Corey, Y. J. Bryson, and P. McGuirt. 1988. Therapy of herpes zoster with oral acyclovir. *Am. J. Med.* 85(Supl 2A): 84–89.

83. Huff, J. C., J. L. Drucker, A. Clemmer, O. L. Laskin, J. D. Connor, Y. L. Bryson, and H. H. Balfour Jr. 1993. Effect of oral acyclovir on pain resolution in herpes zoster: a re-analysis. *J. Med. Virol.* Suppl. 1:93–96.

84. van den Broek, P. J., J. W. van der Meer, J. D. Mulder, J. Versteeg, and H. Mattie. 1984. Limited value of acyclovir in the treatment of uncomplicated herpes zoster: a placebo-controlled study. *Infection* 12:338–341.

85. Jackson, J. L., R. Gibbons, G. Meyer, and L. Inouye. 1997. The effect of treating herpes zoster with oral acyclovir in preventing postherpetic neuralgia. A meta-analysis. *Arch. Intern. Med.* 157:909–912.

86. Merayo-Lloves, J., S. Baltatzis, and C. S. Foster. 2001. Epstein-Barr virus dacryoadenitis resulting in keratoconjunctivitis sicca in a child. *Am. J. Ophthalmol.* 132:922–923.

87. Wood, M. J., R. W. Johnson, M. W. McKendrick, J. Taylor, B. K. Mandal, and J. Crooks. 1994. A randomized trial of acyclovir for 7 days or 21 days with and without prednisolone for treatment of acute herpes zoster. *N. Engl. J. Med.* 330:896–900.

88. Whitley, R. F., H. Weiss, J. W. Gnann Jr., S. Tyring, G. J. Mertz, P. G. Pappas, C. J. Schleupner, F. Hayden, J. Wolf, and S. J. Soong, for the National Institute of Allergy and Infectious Diseases Collaborative Antiviral Study Group. 1996. Acyclovir with and without prednisone for the treatment of herpes zoster. A randomized, placebo-controlled trial. *Ann. Intern. Med.* 125:376–383.

89. Lau, R. J., M. G. Emery, and R. E. Galinsky. 1987. Unexpected accumulation of acyclovir in breast milk with estimation of infant exposure. *Obstet. Gynecol.* 69:468–471.

90. Meyer, L. J., P. De Miranda, N. Sheth, and S. Spruance. 1988. Acyclovir in human breast milk. *Am. J. Obstet. Gynecol.* 158:586–588.

91. Taddio, A., J. Klein, and G. Koren. 1994. Acyclovir excretion in human breast milk. *Ann. Pharmacother.* 28:585–587.

92. Erlich, K. S., J. Mills, P. Chatis, G. J. Mertz, D. F. Busch, S. E. Follansbee, R. M. Grant, and C. S. Crumpacker. 1989. Acyclovir-resistant herpes simplex virus infections in patients with the acquired immunodeficiency syndrome. *N. Engl. J. Med.* 320:293–296.

93. Hill, E. L., G. A. Hunter, and M. N. Ellis. 1991. In vitro and in vivo characterization of herpes simplex virus clinical isolates recovered from patients infected with human immunodeficiency virus. *Antimicrob. Agents Chemother.* 35:2322–2328.

94. Wade, J. C., B. Newton, C. McLaren, N. Flournoy, R. E. Keeney, and J. D. Meyers. 1982. Intravenous acyclovir to treat mucocutaneous herpes simplex virus infection after marrow transplantation: a double-blind test. *Ann. Intern. Med.* 96:265–269.

95. Englund, J. A., M. E. Zimmerman, E. M. Swierkosz, J. L. Goodman, D. R. Scholl, and H. H. Balfour Jr. 1990. Herpes

simplex resistance to acyclovir: a study in a tertiary care center. *Ann. Intern. Med.* 112:416–422.

96. Reusser, P. 1994. Virostatika-Resistenz bei Herpesviren: Mechanismen, Haufigkeit und klinische Bedeutung. *Schweiz. Med. Wochenschr.* 124:152–158.

97. Christophers, J., J. Clayton, J. Craske, R. Ward, P. Collins, M. Trowbridge, and G. Darby. 1998. Survey of resistance of herpes simplex virus to acyclovir in northwest England. *Antimicrob. Agents Chemother.* 42:868–872.

98. Patel, R., and S. E. Barton. 1995. Antiviral chemotherapy in genital herpes simplex virus infections. *Int. J. STD AIDS* 6:320–328.

99. McGrath, B. J., and C. L. Newman. 1994. Genital herpes simplex infections in patients with the acquired immunodeficiency syndrome. *Pharmacotherapy* 14:529–542.

100. Easterbrook, P., and M. J. Wood. 1994. Successors to acyclovir. *J. Antimicrob. Chemother.* 34:307–311.

101. van der Horst, C., J. Joncas, G. Ahronheim, N. Gustafson, G. Stein, M. Gurwith, G. Fleisher, J. Sullivan, J. Sixbey, S. Roland, et al. 1991. Lack of effect on peroral acyclovir for the treatment of infectious mononucleosis. *J. Infect. Dis.* 164:788–792.

102. Andersson, J., and I. Ernberg. 1988. Management of Epstein-Barr virus infections. *Am. J. Med.* 85:107–115.

103. Straus, S. E., moderator. 1992. Epstein-Barr virus infections: biology, pathogenesis, and management. *Ann. Intern. Med.* 118:45–58.

104. Naher, H., S. Helfrich, M. Hartmann, and U. K. Freese. 1990. EBV-Replikation und Therapie der oralen Haarleukoplakie mit Acyclovir. *Hautarzt* 41:680–682.

105. Glick, M., and M. E. Pliskin. 1990. Regression of oral hairy leukoplakia after oral administration of acyclovir. *Gen. Dent.* 38:374–375.

106. Ochsendorf, F. R., H. Schofer, U. Runne, and R. Milbradt. Therapie der oralen Haarlenkoplakie mit Acyclovir. *Hautarzt* 39:736–738, 1988.

107. Whitley, R. J., C. A. Alford, Jr., M. S. Hirsch, R. T. Schooley, J. P. Luby, F. Y. Aoki, D. Hanley, A. J. Nahmias, and S. J. Soong.

1986. Vidarabine versus acyclovir therapy in herpes simplex encephalitis. *N. Engl. J. Med.* 314:144–149.

108. McGrath, N., N. E. Anderson, M. C. Croxson, and K. F. Powell. 1997. Herpes simplex encephalitis treated with acyclovir: diagnosis and long term outcome. *J. Neurol. Neurosurg. Psychiatry* 63:321–326.

109. Evans, T. G., D. I. Bernstein, G. W. Raborn, J. Harmenberg, J. Kowalski, and S. L. Spruance. 2002. Double-blind, randomized, placebo-controlled study of topical 5% acyclovir-1% hydrocortisone cream (ME-609) for treatment of UV radiation-induced herpes labialis. *Antimicrob. Agents Chemother.* 46:1870–1874.

110. McKeough, M. B., and S. L. Spruance. 2001. Comparison of new topical treatments for herpes labialis: efficacy of penciclovir cream, acyclovir cream, and n-docosanol cream against experimental cutaneous herpes simplex virus type 1 infection. *Arch. Derm.* 137:1153–1158.

111. Acosta, E. P., and H. H. Balfour. 2001. Acyclovir for treatment of postherpetic neuralgia: efficacy and pharmacokinetics. *Antimicrob. Agents Chemother.* 45:2771–2774.

112. Murakami, S., N. Hato, J. Horiuchi, et al. 1997. Treatment of Ramsey Hunt syndrome with acyclovir-prednisone: significance of early diagnosis and treatment. *Ann. Neurol.* 41:353–357.

113. Ramanathan, J., M. Rammouni, J. Baran Jr., and R. Khatib. 2000. Herpes simplex virus esophagitis in the immunocompetent host: an overview. *Am. J. Gastroent.* 95: 2171–2175.

114. Zheng, Y. T., W. L. Chan, P. Chan, H. Huang, and S. C. Tam. 2001. Enhancement of the anti-herpetic effect of trichosanthin by acyclovir and interferon. *FEBS Lett.* 496:139–142.

115. Kimberlin, D. W. 2001. Advances in the treatment of neonatal herpes simplex infections. *Rev. Med. Virol.* 11:157–163.

116. Kuo, Y. H., Y. Yip, and S. N. Chen. 2001. Retinal vasculitis associated with chickenpox. *Am. J. Ophthalmol.* 132:584–585.

117. Szinnai, G., U. B. Schaad, and U. Heininger. 2001. Multiple herpetic whitlow lesions in a 4-year-old girl: case report and review of the literature. *Eur. J. Pedia.* 160:528–533.

118. Hoglund, M., P. Ljungman, and S. Weller. 2001. Comparable aciclovir exposures produced by oral valaciclovir and intravenous aciclovir in immunocompromised cancer patients. *J. Antimicrob. Chemother.* 47:855–861.

119. Levin, M. J., A. Weinberg, J. J. Leary, and R. T. Sarisky. 2001. Development of acyclovir-resistant herpes simplex virus early during the treatment of herpes neonatorum. *Pediatr. Infect. Dis. J.* 20:1094–1097.

120. Harivada, V., and M. C. Paffett. 2001. Recurrent eczema herpeticum: an underrecognised condition. *Sex. Transm. Infect.* 77:76.

121. Nyerges, G., Z. Meszner, E. Gyarmati, and S. Kerpel-Fronius. 1988. Acyclovir prevents dissemination of varicella in immunocompromised children. *J. Infect. Dis.* 157:309–313.

122. Meszner, Z., G. Nyerges, and A. R. Bell. 1993. Oral acyclovir to prevent dissemination of varicella in immunocompromised children. *J. Infect.* 26:9–15.

123. Tucker, W. E., H. C. Krasny, P. de Miranda, E. I. Goldenthal, G. B. Elion, G. Hajian, and G. M. Szczech. 1983. Preclinical studies with acyclovir: carcinogenicity bioassays and chronic toxicity tests. *Fund Appl. Toxicol.* 3:579–586.

124. Delume, S., B. DeJonghe, O. Prost, and H. Outin. 2002. Acyclovir-induced coma in a young patient without preexisting renal impairment. *Intensive Care Med.* 28:661–662.

125. Blossom, A. P., J. D. Cleary, and W. P. Daley. 2002. Acyclovir-induced crystalluria. *Ann Pharm* 36:526.

126. Lyon AW, A Mansoor, MJ Trotter. 2002. Urinary gems: acyclovir crystalluria. *Arch. Path. Lab. Med.* 126:753–754.

127. Pottage, J. C., and H. A. Kessler. 1995. Herpes simplex virus resistance to acyclovir: clinical relevance. *Infect. Agents Dis.* 4:115–124.

128. Shin, Y. K., G. Y. Cai, A. Weinberg, J. J. Leary, and M. J. Levin. 2001. Frequency of acyclovir-resistant herpes simplex virus in clinical specimens and laboratory isolates. *J. Clin. Microbiol.* 39:913–917.

129. Snoeck, R., M. Gerard, C. Sadzot-Delvaux, G. Andrei, J. Balzarini, D. Reymen, N. Ahadi, J. M. De Bruyn, J. Piette, B. Rentier, et al. 1994. Meningoradiculoneuritis due to acyclovir-resistant

varicella zoster virus in an acquired immune deficiency syndrome patient. *J. Med. Virol.* 42:338–347.

130. Pahwa, S., K. Biron, W. Lim, P. Swenson, M. H. Kaplan, N. Sadick, and R. Pahwa. 1988. Continuous varicella-zoster infection associated with acyclovir resistance in a child with AIDS. *J. Am. Med. Assoc.* 260:2879–2882.

131. Linnemann, C. C. Jr., K. K. Biron, W. G. Hoppenjans, and A. M. Solinger. 1990. Emergence of acyclovir-resistant varicella zoster virus in an AIDS patient on prolonged acyclovir therapy. *AIDS* 4:577–579.

132. Jacobson, M. A., T. G. Berger, S. Fikrig, P. Becherer, J. W. Moohr, S. C. Stanat, and K. K. Biron. 1990. Acyclovir-resistant varicella zoster virus infection after chronic oral acyclovir therapy in patients with the acquired immunodeficiency syndrome (AIDS). *Ann. Intern. Med.* 112:187–191.

133. Alcorn, J., and P. J. McNamara. 2002. Acyclovir, ganciclovir, and zidovudine transfer into rat milk. *Antimicrob. Agents Chemother.* 46:1831–1836.

134. Cooper, D. A., P. O. Pehrson, C. Pedersen, M. Moroni, E. Oksenhendler, W. Rozenbaum, N. Clumeck, V. Faber, W. Stille, and B. Hirschel, for the European-Australian Collaborative Group. 1993. The efficacy and safety of zidovudine alone or as cotherapy with acyclovir for the treatment of patients with AIDS and AIDS-related complex: a double-blind, randomized trial. *AIDS* 7:197–207.

135. Erbelding, E. J., R. E. Chaisson, J. E. Gallant, and R. D. Moore. 1997. Acyclovir in combination with zidovudine does not prolong survival in advanced HIV disease. *Antiviral Therapy* 2:71–77.

136. Soul-Lawton, J., E. Seaber, N. On, R. Wooton, P. Rolan, and J. Posner. 1995. Absolute bioavailability and metabolic disposition of valaciclovir, the L-valyl ester of acyclovir, following oral administration to humans. *Antimicrob. Agents Chemother.* 39:2759–2764.

137. Naesens, L., and E. DeClercq. 2001. Recent developments in herpesvirus therapy. *Herpes* 8:12–16.

138. Beutner, K. R., D. J. Friedman, C. Forszpaniak, P. L. Andersen, and M. J. Wood. 1995. Valaciclovir compared with acyclovir for

improved therapy for herpes zoster in immunocompetent adults. *Antimicrob. Agents Chemother.* 39:1546–1553.

139. Fife, K. H., R. A. Barbarash, T. Rudolph, B. Degregario, and R. Roth. 1997. Valaciclovir versus acyclovir in the treatment of first-episode genital herpes infection. Results of an international, multicenter, double-blind, randomized clinical trial. The Valaciclovir International Herpes Simplex Virus Study Group. *Sex. Trans. Dis.* 24:481–486.

140. Leone, P. A., S. Trottier, and J. M. Miller. 1998. A comparison of oral valaciclovir 500 mg twice daily for three or five days in the treatment of recurrent genital herpes. In: Program and Abstracts of the 8th International Congress of Infectious Disease, 15–18 May 1998, Boston, MA, p. 90, Poster 22.012.

141. Reitano, M., S. K. Tyring, W. Lang, C. Thoming, A. M. Worm, S. Borelli, L. O. Chambers, J. M. Robinson, and L. Corey. 1998. Valaciclovir for the suppression of recurrent genital herpes simplex virus infection: a large-scale dose range-finding study. International Valaciclovir HSV Study Group. *J. Infect. Dis.* 178:603–610.

142. Corey, L., A. Wald, R. Patel, S. L. Sacks, S. K. Tyring, T. Warren, J. M. Douglas Jr., J. Paavonen, R. A. Morrow, K. R. Beutner, L. S. Sratchounsky, G. Mertz, O. N. Keene, H. A. Watson, D. Tait, and M. Vargas-Cortes, for the Valacyclovir HSV Transmission Study Group. 2004. Once-daily valacyclovir to reduce the risk of transmission of genital herpes. *N. Engl. J. Med.* 350:11–20.

143. Alster, T. S., and C. A. Nanni. 1999. Famciclovir prophylaxis of herpes simplex virus reactivation after laser resurfacing. *Dermatol. Surg* 25:242–246.

144. Nanni, C. A., and T. S. Alster. 1998. Herpes simplex virus prophylaxis for cutaneous laser resurfacing: a comparison of acyclovir, valacyclovir and famciclovir. *Laser Surg. Med. Suppl.* 10:66.

145. Hoglund, M., P. Ljungman, and S. Weller. 2001. Comparable aciclovir exposures produced by oral valaciclovir and intravenous aciclovir in immunocompromised cancer patients. *J. Antimicrob. Chemother.* 47:855–861.

146. Sarkany, I. 1988. The skin-liver connection. *Clin. Exp. Dermatol.* 13:151–159.

147. Desmond, R. A., H. L. Weiss, R. B. Arani, S. J. Soong, M. J. Wood, P. A. Fiddian, J. W. Gnann, and R. J. Whitley. 2002. Clinical applications for change-point analysis of herpes zoster pain. *J. Pain Symptom Manage.* 23:510–516.

148. Peyriere, H., B. Branger, C. Bengler, F. Vecina, V. Pinzani, and D. Hillaire-Buys. 2001. Neurologic toxicity caused by zelitrex (valaciclovir) in 3 patients with renal failure. Is overdose associated with improvement of product bioavailability improvement? *Rev. Med. Intern.* 22:297–303.

149. Bell's Palsy Information Site. www.bellspalsy.ws (accessed 20 August 2002).

150. Adour, K. K. 1998. Combination treatment with acyclovir and prednisone for Bell palsy. *Arch. Otolaryngol. Head Neck Surg.* 124:824.

151. Spruance, S. L., T. L. Rea, C. Thoming, R. Tucker, R. Saltzman, and R. Boon. 1997. Penciclovir cream for the treatment of herpes simplex labialis. A randomized, multicenter, double-blind, placebo-controlled trial. The Topical Penciclovir Collaborative Study Group. *J. Am. Med. Assoc.* 277:1374–1379.

152. Cohen, J. I., P. A. Brunell, S. E. Staus, and P. R. Krause. 1999. Recent advances in varicella-zoster virus infection. *Ann. Intern. Med.* 130:922–923.

153. Tyring, S., R. Engst, C. Corriveau, N. Robillard, S. Trottier, S. Van Slycken, R. A. Crann, L. A. Locke, R. Saltzman, and A. G. Palestine, for the Collaborative Famciclovir Ophthalmic Zoster Research Group. 2001. Famciclovir for ophthalmic zoster: a randomized acyclovir controlled study. *Br. J. Ophthalmol.* 85:576–581.

154. Huse, D. M., S. Schainbaum, A. J. Kirsch, and S. Tyring. 1997. Economic evaluation of famciclovir in reducing the duration of postherpetic neuralgia. *Am J. Health Syst. Pharm.* 54: 1180–1184.

155. Leon, P., F. Pozo, and J. M. Echevarria. 2004. Detection of hepatitis B virus variants resistant to lamivudine and famciclovir among randomly selected chronic carriers from Spain. *Enferm. Infecc. Microbiol. Clin.* 22:133–137.

156. Vere Hodge, R. A. 1993. Famciclovir and penciclovir: the mode of action of famciclovir including into conversion to penciclovir. *Antivir. Chem. Chemother.* 4:67–84.

157. Spruance, S. L., N. H. Rowe, G. W. Roborn, E. A. Thibodeau, J. A. D'Ambrosio, and D. I. Bernstein. 1999. Peroral famciclovir in the treatment of experimental ultraviolet radiation-induced herpes simplex labialis: a double-blind, dose-ranging placebo-controlled, multicenter trial. *J. Infect. Dis.* 179:303–310.

158. Sacks, S. L., F. Aoki, F. Diaz-Mitoma, J. Sellors, and S. D. Shafran. 1996. Patient-initiated, twice-daily oral famciclovir for early recurrent genital herpes: a randomized, double-blind multicenter trial. Canadian Famciclovir Study Group. *J. Am. Med. Assoc.* 276:44–49.

159. Diaz-Mitoma, F., R. G. Sibbald, S. D. Shafran, R. Boon, and R. L. Saltzman. 1998. Oral famciclovir for the suppression of recurrent genital herpes: a randomized controlled trial. Collaborative Famciclovir Genital Herpes Research Group. *J. Am. Med. Assoc.* 280:887–892.

160. Frechette, G., and B. Ramanawski, on behalf of the Famciclovir Study Group. 1997. Efficacy and safety of famciclovir for the treatment of HSV infection in HIV+ patients. Sixth Annual Canadian Conference on HIV/AIDS Research. Ottawa, Ontario, 22–25 May 1997, Oral Presentation 301.

161. Schacker, T., H. L. Hu, D. M. Koelle, J. Zeh, R. Saltzman, R. Boon, M. Shaughnessy, G. Barnum, and L. Corey. 1998. Famciclovir for the suppression of symptomatic and asymptomatic herpes simplex virus reactivation in HIV-infected persons: a double-blind, placebo-controlled trial. *Ann. Intern. Med.* 128:21–28.

162. Degreef, H. 1994. Famciclovir, a new oral antiherpes drug: results of the first controlled clinical study demonstrating its efficacy and safety in the treatment of uncomplicated herpes zoster in immunocompetent patients. Famciclovir Herpes Zoster Clinical Study Group. *Int. J. Antimicrob. Agents* 4:241–246.

163. Tyring, S. K., R. A. Barbarash, J. E. Nahlik, A. Cunningham, J. Marley, M. Heng, T. Jones, T. Rea, R. Boon, and R. Saltzman, for the Collaborative Famciclovir Herpes Zoster Study Group. 1995. Famciclovir for the treatment of acute herpes zoster:

effects on acute disease and postherpetic neuralgia: a randomized, double-blind, placebo-controlled trial. *Ann. Intern. Med.* 123:89–96.

164. Tyring, S. K., K. R. Beutner, B. A. Tucker, W. C. Anderson, and J. Crooks. 2000. Antiviral therapy for herpes zoster. *Arch. Fam. Med.* 9:863–869.

165. Sweeney, C. J., and D. J. Gilden. 2001. Ramsay Hunt syndrome. *J. Neurol. Neurosurg. Psychiatry* 71:149–154.

166. Tyring, S. K., R. Belanger, W. Bezwoda, P. Ljungman, R. Boon, and R. L. Saltzman, 2001. A randomized, double blind trial of famciclovir versus acyclovir for the treatment of localized dermatomal herpes zoster in immunocompromised patients. *Cancer Invest.* 19:13–22.

167. deMan, R. A., P. Marcellin, F. Habal, P. Desmond, T. Wright, T. Rose, and R. Jurewicz. 2000. A randomized, placebo-controlled study to evaluate the efficacy of 12-month famciclovir treatment in patients with chronic hepatitis B and antigen-positive hepatitis B. *Hepatology* 32:413–417.

168. Hadziyannis, S. J., E. G. Manesis, and A. Papakonstantinou. 1999. Oral ganciclovir treatment in chronic hepatitis B virus infection: a pilot study. *J. Hepatol.* 31:210–214.

169. Wolters, L. M. M., H. G. M. Niester, and R. A. de Man. 2001. Nucleoside analogues for chronic hepatitis B. *Euro. J. Gastroenterol. Hepatol.* 13:1499–1506.

170. Berenguer, M., M. Prieto, M. Rayon, M. Bustamante, D. Carrasco, A. Moya, M. A. Pastor, M. Gobernado, J. Mir, and J. Berenguer. 2001. Famciclovir treatment in transplant recipients with HBV-related liver disease: disappointing results. *Am. J. Gastroenterol.* 96:526–533.

171. Aoki, F. Y. 2001. Management of genital herpes in HIV-infected patients. *Herpes* 8:41–45.

172. Gershon, A. A. 2001. Prevention and treatment of VZV infections in patients with HIV. *Herpes* 8:32–36.

173. Lai, C. W., M. F. Yuen, C. K. Hui, S. Garrido-Lestache, C. T. Cheng, and Y. P. Lai. 2002. Comparison of the efficacy of lamivudine and famciclovir in Asian patients with chronic hepatitis B: results of 24 weeks of therapy. *J. Med. Virol.* 67:334–338.

174. Lazarus, H. M., R. Belanger, A. Candoni, M. Aoun, R. Jurewicz, and L. Marks, for the Penciclovir Immunocompromised Study Group. 1999. Intravenous penciclovir for treatment of herpes simplex infections in immunocompromised patients: results of a multicenter, acyclovir-controlled trial. *Antimicrob. Agents Chemother.* 43:1192–1197.

175. Boyd, M. R., S. Safrin, and E. R. Kern. 1993. Penciclovir: a review of the spectrum of activity, selectivity, and cross resistance pattern. *Antivir. Chem. Chemother.* 4(Suppl 1):3–11.

176. Earnshaw, D. L., T. H. Bacon, S. J. Darlison, K. Edmonds, R. M. Perkins, and R. A. Vere Hodge. 1992. Mode of antiviral action of penciclovir in MRC-5 cells infected with herpes simplex virus type 1 (HSV-1), HSV-2, and varicella-zoster virus. *Antimicrob. Agents Chemother.* 36:2747–2757.

177. Erice, A., M. C. Jordan, B. A. Chace, C. Fletcher, B. J. Chinnook, and H. H. Balfour Jr. 1987. Ganciclovir treatment of cytomegalovirus disease in transplant recipients and other immunocompromised hosts. *J. Am. Med. Assoc.* 257:3082–3087.

178. Winston, D. J., D. Wirin, A. Shaked, and R. W. Busuttil. 1995. Randomized comparison of ganciclovir and high-dose acyclovir for long-term cytomegalovirus prophylaxis in liver-transplant recipients. *Lancet* 346:69–74.

179. Goodrich, J. M., M. Mori, C. A. Gleaves, C. Du Mond, M. Cays, D. F. Ebeling, W. C. Buhles, B. DeArmond, and J. D. Meyers. 1991. Early treatment with ganciclovir to prevent cytomegalovirus disease after allogeneic bone marrow transplantation. *N. Engl. J. Med.* 325:1601–1607.

180. Biron, K. K., S. C. Stanat, J. B. Sorrell, J. A. Fyfe, P. M. Keller, C. U. Lambe, and D. J. Nelson. 1985. Metabolic activation of the nucleoside analog 9-[(2-hydroxy-1-(hydroxymethyl) ethoxy]methyl)guanine in human diploid fibroblasts infected with human cytomegalovirus. *Proc. Natl. Acad. Sci. USA* 82: 2473–2477.

181. Sullivan, V., C. L. Talarico, S. C. Stanat, M. Davis, D. M. Coen, and K. K. Biron. 1992. A protein kinase homologue controls phosphorylation of ganciclovir in human cytomegalovirus-infected cells. *Nature* 358:162–14. [Errata: *Nature* 359:85, 1992; and 366:756, 1993.]

182. Littler, E., A. D. Stuart, and M. S. Chee. 1992. Human cytome-galovirus UL97 open reading frame encodes a protein that phosphorylates the antiviral nucleoside analogue ganciclovir. *Nature* 358:160–162.

183. Anderson, R. D., K. G. Griffy, D. Jung, A. Dorr, J. D. Hulse, and R. B. Smith. 1995. Ganciclovir absolute bioavailability and steady-state pharmacokinetics after oral administration of two 3000-mg/d dosing regimens in human immunodeficiency virus and cytomegalovirus-seropositive patients. *Clin. Ther.* 17: 425–432.

184. Zhou, L., T. C. Harder, U. Ullmann, and P. Rautenberg. 1999. Rapid detection by reverse hybridization of mutations in the UL97 gene of human cytomegalovirus conferring resistance to ganciclovir. *J. Clin. Virol.* 13:53–59.

185. Martin, D. F., B. D. Kuppermann, R. A. Wolitz, A. G. Palestine, H. Li, and C. A. Robinson. 1999. Oral ganciclovir for patients with cytomegalovirus retinitis treated with a ganciclovir im-plant. *N. Engl. J. Med.* 340:1063–1070.

186. Studies of Ocular Complications of AIDS Research Group, in collaboration with the AIDS Clinical Trials Group. 1992. Mor-tality in patients with the acquired immunodeficiency syndrome treated with either foscarnet or ganciclovir for cytomegalovirus retinitis. *N. Engl. J. Med.* 326:213–220. [Erratum: *N. Engl. J. Med.* 326:1172, 1992.]

187. Faller, D. V., S. J. Mentzer, and S. P. Perrine. 2001. Induction of the Epstein-Barr virus thymidine kinase gene with concomitant nucleoside antivirals as a therapeutic strategy for Epstein-Barr virus-associated malignancies. *Curr. Opin. Oncol.* 13:360–367.

188. Mendez, J. C., D. H. Dockrell, M. J. Espy, T. F. Smith, J. A. Wilson, W. S. Harmsen, D. Ilstrup, and C. V. Paya. 2001. Human beta-herpesvirus interactions in solid organ transplant recipi-ents. *JID* 183:179–184.

189. Castagnola, E., E. Cristina, and C. Dufour. 2002. High-dose oral ganciclovir for management of CMV-symptomatic infection in a child with acute lymphoblastic leukemia. *Med. Pediatr. Oncol.* 38:295–296.

190. Mannerstrom, M., M. Zorn-Kruppa, H. Diehl, M. Engelke, T. Toimela, H. Maenpaa, A. Huhtala, H. Uusitalo, L. Salminen,

P. Pappas, M. Marselos, M. Mantyla, E. Mantyla, and H. Tahti. 2002. Evaluation of the cytotoxicity of selected systemic and intravitreally dosed drugs in the cultures of human retinal pigment epithelial cell line and of pig primary retinal pigment epithelial cells. *Toxicology in Vitro* 16:193–200.

191. Van der Boj, W., and R. Sperch. 2001. Management of cytomegalovirus infection and disease after solid-organ transplantatioin. *Clin. Infect. Dis.* 33:S33–37.

192. Snydman, D. R., M. E. Falagas, R. Avery, C. Perlino, R. Ruthazer, R. Freeman, R. Rohrer, R. Fairchild, E. O'Rourke, P. Hibberd, and B. G. Werner. 2001. Use of combination cytomegalovirus immune globulin plus ganciclovir for prophylaxis in CMV-seronegative liver transplant recipients of a CMV-seropositive donor organ: a multicenter, open-label study. *Transplant Proc.* 33:2571–2575.

193. Lopez-Cortes, L. F., T. Pastor-Ramos, E. Cordero, F. J. Caballero-Granado, P. Viciana, and J. Pachon. 2001. Influence of the response to induction therapy on the rate of progression of cytomegalovirus retinitis in AIDS patients on intravitreal maintenance therapy. *Eur. J. Clin. Microbiol. Inf. Dis.* 20:385–388.

194. Nichols, W. G., and M. Boeckh. 2000. Recent advances in the therapy and prevention of CMV infections. *J. Clin. Virol.* 16:25–40.

195. Razonable, R. R., A. Rivero, A. Rodriguez, J. Wilson, J. Daniels, G. Jenkins, T. Larson, W. C. Hellinger, J. R. Spivey, and C. V. Paya. 2001. Allograft rejection predicts the occurrence of late-onset cytomegalovirus (CMV) disease among CMV-mismatched solid organ transplant patients receiving prophylaxis with oral ganciclovir. *J. Infect. Dis.* 184:1461–1464.

196. Reusser, P. 2002. Challenges and options in the management of viral infections after stem cell transplantation. *Support Care Cancer* 10:197–203.

197. Saran, B. R., and A. M. McGuire. 1994. Retinal toxicity of high dose intravitreal ganciclovir. *Retina* 14:248–252.

198. Jabs, D. A., B. K. Martin, M. S. Forman, J. P. Dunn, J. L. Davis, D. V. Weinberg, K. K. Biron, and F. Baldanti, for the Cytomegalovirus Retinitis and Viral Resistance Study Group. 2001. Mutations conferring ganciclovir resistance in a cohort of

patients with acquired immunodeficiency syndrome and cytomegalovirus retinitis. *J. Infect. Dis.* 183:333–337.

199. Flexman, J., I. Kay, R. Fonte, R. Herrmann, E. Gabbay, and S. Palladino. 2001. Differences between the quantitative antigenemia assay and the cobas amplicor monitor quantitative PCR assay for detecting CMV viraemia in bone marrow and solid organ transplant patients. *J. Med. Virol.* 64:275–282.

200. Tong, C. Y., L. Cuevas, H. Williams, and A. Bakran. 1999. Use of laboratory assays to predict cytomegalovirus disease in renal transplant recipients. *J. Clin. Microbiol.* 36:2681–2685.

201. Pescovitz, M. D. 1999. Absence of teratogenicity of oral ganciclovir used during early pregnancy in a liver transplant recipient. *Transplantation* 67:758–759.

202. Whitley, R. J., G. Cloud, W. Gruber, G. A. Storch, G. J. Demmler, R. F. Jacobs, W. Dankner, S. A. Spector, S. Starr, R. F. Pass, S. Stagno, W. J. Britt, C. Alford Jr., S. Soong, X. J. Zhou, L. Sherrill, J. M. FitzGerald, and J. P. Sommadossi. 1997. Ganciclovir treatment of symptomatic congenital cytomegalovirus infection: results of a phase II study. National Institute of Allergy and Infectious Diseases Collaborative Antiviral Study Group. *J. Infect. Dis.* 175:1080–1086.

203. Nichols, W. G., L. Corey, T. Gooley, W. L. Drew, R. Miner, M. Huang, C. Davis, and M. Boeckh. 2001. Rising pp65 antigenemia during preemptive anticytomegalovirs therapy after allogeneic hematopoietic stem cell transplantation: risk factors, correlation with DNA load, and outcomes. *Blood* 97:867–874.

204. Nichols, W. G., and M. Boeckh. 2001. Response: Parainfluenza viral infections after hematopoietic stem cell transplantation: risk factors, response to antiviral therapy. *Blood* 98:1629.

205. Boivin, G., C. Gilbert, A. Gaudreau, I. Greenfield, R. Sudlow, and N. A. Roberts. 2001. Rate of emergence of cytomegalovirus (CMV) mutations in leukocytes of patients with acquired immunodeficiency syndrome who are receiving valganciclovir as induction and maintenance therapy for CMV retinitis. *J. Infect. Dis.* 184: 1598–602.

206. Gavin, P. J., and B. Z. Katz. 2002. Intravenous ribavirin treatment for severe adenovirus disease in immunocompromised children. *Pediatrics* 110:e9.

207. Graci, J. D., and C. E. Cameron. 2002. Quasispecies, error catastrophe, and the antiviral activity of ribavirin. *Virology* 298: 175–180.

208. Crotty, S., C. E. Cameron, and R. Andino. 2001. RNA virus error catastrophe: direct molecular test by using ribavirin. *Proc. Natl. Acad. Sci. USA* 98:6895–6900.

209. Smee, D. F., M. Bray, and J. W. Huggins. 2001. Antiviral activity and mode of action studies of ribavirin and mycophenolic acid against orthopoxviruses in vitro. *Antivir. Chem. Chemother.* 12: 327–335.

210. MedlinePlus Drug Information: Ribavirin (Systemic). Revised 10 July 2002.

211. Chakrabarti, S., K. E. Collingham, H. Osman, C. D. Fegan, and D. W. Milligan. 2001. Cidofovir as primary pre-emptive therapy for post-transplant cytomegalovirus infections. *Bone Marrow Transplant* 28(9):879–881.

212. Smee, D. F., R. W. Sidwell, D. Kefauver, M. Bray, and J. W. Huggins. 2002. Characterization of wild-type and cidofovir-resistant strains of camelpox, cowpox, monkeypox, and vaccinia viruses. *Antimicrob. Agents Chemother.* 46:1329–1335.

213. DeClercq, E. 2001. Antiviral drugs: current state of the art. *J. Clin. Virol.* 22:73–89.

214. Hall, C. D., U. Dafni, D. Simpson, D. Clifford, P. E. Wetherill, B. Cohen, J. McArthur, H. Hollander, C. Yainnoutsos, E. Major, L. Millar, and J. Timpone. 1998. Failure of cytarabine in progressive multifocal leukoencephalopathy associated with human immunodeficiency virus infection. AIDS Clinical Trials Group 243 Team. *N. Engl. J. Med.* 338:1345–1351.

215. Ljungman, P., G. L. Deliliers, U. Platzbecker, S. Matthes-Martin, A. Bacigalupo, H. Einsele, J. Ullmann, M. Musso, R. Trenschel, P. Ribaud, M. Bornhäuser, S. Cesaro, B. Crooks, A. Dekker, N. Gratecos, T. Klingebiel, E. Tagliaferri, A. J. Ullmann, P. Wacker, and C. Cordonnier, for the Infectious Diseases Working Party of the European group for Blood and Marrow Transplantation. 2001. Cidofovir for cytomegalovirs infection and disease in allogeneic stem cell transplant recipients. *Blood* 97:388–392.

216. Snoeck, R., M. Bossens, D. Parent, B. Delaere, H. Degreef, M. Van Ranst, J. C. Noel, M. S. Wulfsohn, J. F. Rooney, H. S. Jaffe,

and E. DeClercq. 2001. Phase II double-blind, placebo-controlled study of the safety and efficacy of cidofovir topical gel for the treatment of patients with human papillomavirus infection. *Clin. Infect. Dis.* 33:597–602.

217. Xiong, X., J. L. Smith, M. S. Chen. 1997. Effect of incorporation of cidofovir into DNA by human cytomegalovirus DNA polymerase on DNA elongation. *Antimicrob. Agents Chemother.* 41:594–595.

218. Ho, H. T., K. L. Woods, J. J. Bronson, H. DeBoeck, J. C. Martin, and M. J. Hitchcock. 1992. Intracellular metabolism of the antiherpes agent (S)-1-[3-hydroxy-2-(phosphonylmethoxy)propyl]cytosine. *Mol. Pharmacol.* 41:197–202.

219. Safrin, S., J. Cherrington, and H. S. Jaffe. 1997. Clinical uses of cidofovir. *Rev. Med. Virol.* 7:145–146.

220. Lalezari, J. P., C. Kemper, and R. Stagg. 1996. A randomized, controlled study of the safety and efficacy of intravenous cidofovir (CDV, HPMPC) for the treatment of relapsing cytomegalovirus retinitis in patients with AIDS [abstract]. XI. International Conference on AIDS, Vancouver, British Columbia, 7–12 July 1996.

221. Studies, of Ocular Complications of AIDS Research Group, in collaboration with the AIDS Clinical Trials Group. 1997. Parenteral cidofovir for cytomegalovirus retinitis in patients with AIDS: the HPMPC peripheral cytomegalovirus retinitis trial. *Ann. Intern. Med.* 126:264–274.

222. Kirsch, L. S., J. F. Arevalo, E. Chavez de la Paz, D. Munguia, E. DeClercq, and W. R. Freeman. 1995. Intravitreal cidofovir (HPMPC) treatment of cytomegalovirus retinitis in patients with acquired immune deficiency syndrome. *Ophthalmology* 102:533–542.

223. Rahhal, F. M., J. F. Arevalo, E. Chavez de la Paz, D. Munguia, S. P. Azen, and W. R. Freeman. 1996. Treatment of cytomegalovirus retinitis with intravitreous cidofovir in patients with AIDS. *Ann. Intern. Med.* 125:98–103.

224. Marwick, C. 1998. First "antisense" drug will treat CMV retinitis. *J. Am. Med. Assoc.* 280:871.

225. Krown, S. E. 1991. Interferon and other biologic agents for the treatment of Kaposi's sarcoma. *Hematol. Oncol. Clin. North Am.* 5:311–322.

226. Abrams, D. I., and P. A. Volberding. 1987. Alpha interferon therapy of AIDS-associated Kaposi's sarcoma. *Semin. Oncol.* 14(2 Suppl 2):43–47.

227. Groopman, J. E., M. S. Gottlieb, J. Goodman, R. T. Mitsuyasu, M. A. Conant, H. Prince, J. L. Fahey, M. Derezin, W. M. Weinstein, C. Casavante, et al. 1984. Recombinant alpha-2 interferon therapy for Kaposi's sarcoma associated with the acquired immunodeficiency syndrome. *Ann. Intern. Med.* 100:671–676.

228. Sacks, S. L., R. Fox, P. Levendusky, H. G. Stiver, S. Roland, S. Nusinoff-Lehrman, and R. Keeney. 1988. Chronic suppression for six months compared with intermittent lesional therapy of recurrent genital herpes using oral acyclovir: effects on lesions and nonlesional prodromes. *Sex. Transm. Dis.* 15:58–62.

229. Sacks, S., S. Shafran, and D. Francisco. 1997. A randomized, double-blind, placebo controlled pilot study of cidofovir topical gel for recurrent genital herpes infection [abstract]. American Academy of Dermatology, 55th Annual Meeting, San Francisco, 21–26 March 1997, Abstract 290.

230. Sacks, S. L., S. D. Shafran, F. Diaz-Mitoma, S. Trottier, R. G. Sibbald, A. Hughes, S. Safrin, J. Rudy, B. McGuire, and H. S. Jaffe. 1998. A multicenter phase I/II dose escalation study of single-dose cidofavir gel for treatment of recurrent genital herpes. *Antimicrob. Agents Chemother.* 42:2996–2999.

231. Meadows, K. P., S. K. Tyring, A. T. Pavia, and T. M. Rallis. 1997. Resolution of recalcitrant molluscum contagiosum lesions in human immunodeficiency virus-infected patients treated with cidofovir. *Arch. Dermatol.* 133(8):987–990.

232. Davies, E. G., A. Thrasher, K. Lacey, and J. Harper. 1999. Topical cidofovir for severe molluscum contagiosum [letter]. *Lancet* 353:2042.

233. Smith, K. J., E. Liota, J. Yager, and P. Menon. 1999. Treatment of molluscum contagiosum with topical imiquimod [poster presentation]. 57th Annual Meeting of the American Academy of Dermatology, 19–24 March 1999, New Orleans, L A, p. 352.

234. Eron, L. J., F. Judson, S. Tucker, S. Prawer, J. Mills, K. Murphy, M. Hickey, M. Rogers, S. Flannigan, N. Hien, et al. 1986. Interferon therapy for condyloma acuminata. *N. Engl. J. Med.* 315:1059–1064.

235. Orlando, G., M. M. Fasolo, R. Beretta, S. Merli, and A. Cargnel. 2002. Combined surgery and cidofovir is an effective treatment for genital warts in HIV-infected patients. *AIDS* 16:447–450.

236. Douglas, J., T. Carey, and S. Tyring. 1997. A phase I/II study of cidofovir topical gel for refractory condyloma acuminatum in patients with HIV infection [poster presentation]. 4th Conference on Retroviruses and Opportunistic Infections, Washington, D. C., 22–26 January 1997, Poster 334.

237. Beadle, J. R., C. Hartline, K. A. Aldern, N. Rodriquez, E. Harden, E. R. Kern, and K. Y. Hostetler. 2002. Alkoxyalkyl esters of cidofovir and cyclic cidofovir exhibit multiple-log enhancement of antiviral activity against cytomegalovirus and herpesvirus replication in vitro. *Antimicrob. Agents Chemother.* 46:2381–2386.

238. Van, Valckenborgh. I., W. Wellens, K. De Boeck, R. Snoeck, E. DeClercq, and L. Feenstra. 2001. Systemic cidofovir in papillomavirus. *Clin. Infect. Dis.* 32:e62–64.

239. Bordigoni, P., A.-S. Carret, V. Venard, F. Witz, and A. Le Faou. 2001. Treatment of adenovirus infections in patients undergoing allogeneic hematopoietic stem cell transplantation. *CID* 32:1290–1297.

240. Legrand, F., D. Berrebi, N. Houhou, F. Freymuth, A. Faye, M. Duval, J. F. Mougenot, M. Peuchmaur, and E. Vilmer. 2001. Early diagnosis of adenovirus infection and treatment with cidofovir after bone marrow transplantation in children. *Bone Marrow Transplantation* 27:621–626.

241. Held, T. K., S. S. Biel, A. Nitsche, A. Kurth, S. Chen, H. R. Gelderblom, and W. Siegert. 2000. Treatment of BK virus-associated hemorrhagic cystitis and simultaneous CMV reactivation with cidofovir. *Bone Marrow Transpl.* 26:347–350.

242. Bray, M., M. Martinez, D. Kefauver, M. West, and C. Roy. 2002. Treatment of aerosolized cowpox virus infection in mice with aerosolized cidofovir. *Antiviral Res.* 54:129–142.

243. Smee, D. F., K. W. Bailey, and R. W. Sidwell. 2000. Treatment of cowpox virus respiratory infections in mice with ribavirin as a single agent or followed sequentially by cidofovir. *Antiviral Res.* 11:303–309.

244. Smee, D. F., K. W. Bailey, and R. W. Sidwell. 2002. Treatment of lethal cowpox virus respiratory infections in mice with 2-amino-7-[(1,3-dihydroxyy-2-propoxy)methyl]purine and its orally active diacetate ester prodrug. *Antiviral Res.* 54:113–120.

245. Zedtwitz-Liebenstein, K., E. Presterl, E. Deviatko, and W. Graninger. 2001. Acute renal failure in a lung transplant patient after therapy with cidofovir. *Transpl. Int.* 14:445–446.

246. Geerinck, K., G. Lukito, R. Snoeck, R. De Vos, E. DeClercq, Y. Vanrenterghem, H. Degreef, and B. Maes. 2001. A case of human orf in an immunocompromised patient treated successfully with cidofovir cream. *J. Med. Virol.* 64:543–549.

247. Stragier, I., R. Snoeck, E. DeClercq, J. J. Van Den Oord, M. Van Ranst, and H. De Greef. 2002. Local treatment of HPV-induced skin lesions by cidofovir. *J. Med. Virol.* 67:241–245.

248. Martinelli, C., A. Farese, A. Del Mistro, S. Giorgini, and I. Ruffino. 2001. Resolution of recurrent perianal condylomata acuminata by topical cidofovir in patients with HIV infection. *J. Eur. Acad. Dermatol. Venereol.* 15:568.

249. Houston, S., N. Roberts, and L. Mashinter. 2001. Failure of cidofovir therapy in progressive multifocal leukoencephalopathy unrelated to human immunodeficiency virus. *Clin. Inf. Dis.* 32:150–152.

250. Mazzi, R., S. G. Parisi, L. Sarmati, I. Uccella, E. Nicastri, G. Carolo, F. Gatti, E. Concia, and M. Andreoni. 2001. Efficacy of cidofovir on human herpesvirus 8 viraemia and Kaposi's sarcoma progression in two patients with AIDS. *AIDS* 15:2061–2062.

251. Studies of Ocular Complications of AIDS Research Group, in collaboration with the AIDS Clinical Trials Group. 2000. Long-term follow-up of patients with AIDS treated with parenteral cidofovir for cytomegalovirus retinitis: the HPMPC peripheral cytomegalovirus retinitis trial. *AIDS* 14:1571–1581.

252. Heathcote, E. J., L. Jeffers, and T. Wright. 1988. Loss of serum HBV DNA and HBeAg and seroconversion following short-term (12 weeks) adefovir dipivoxil therapy in chronic hepatitis B: two placebo-controlled phase II studies [abstract]. 49th American Association for the Study of Liver Disease, Chicago, IL, 6–10 November 1998, Abstract 620.

253. Heathcote, E., L. Jeffers, R. Perrillo, T. Wright, M. Sherman, H. Namini, S. Xiong, C. James, V. Ho, J. Fry, and C. Brosgart. 2002. Sustained antiviral response and lack of viral resistance with long term adefovir dipivoxil (ADV) therapy in chronic HBV infection [abstract]. 37th Annual Meeting of the European Association for the Study of the Liver. Madrid, Spain, 17–21 April 2002, Abstract 590.

254. Hadziyannis, S., N. Tassopoulos, E. Heathcote, T. T. Chang, G. Kitis, T. Rizzetto, O. Marcellin, S. G. Lim, M. Wulfsohn, M. Wolman, J. Fru, and C. Brosgart. 2002. Adefovir dipivoxil for the treatment of hepatitis B e-antigen-negative chronic hepatitis B. 37th Annual Meeting of the European Association for the Study of the Liver. Madrid, Spain, 17–21 April 2002, Abstract 648.

255. Fisher, E. J., K. Chaloner, D. L. Cohen, L. B. Grant, B. Alston, C. L. Brosgart, B. Schmetter, W. M. El-Sadr, and J. Sampson, for the Terry Beirn Community Programs for Clinical Research on AIDS. 2001. The safety and efficacy of adefovir dipivoxil in patients with advanced HIV disease: a randomized, placebo-controlled trial. *AIDS* 15:1695–1700.

256. Kurreck, J., E. Wyszko, C. Gillen, and V. A Erdmann. 2002. Design of antisense oligonucleotides stabilized by locked nucleic acids. *Nucleic. Acids. Res.* 30:1911–1918.

257. Field, A. K., 1999. Oligonucleotides as inhibitors of human immunodeficiency virus. Curr Opin Mol Ther 1:323–331.

258. Stone, T. W., and G. J. Jaffe. 2000. Reversible bull's-eye maculopathy associated with intravitreal fomivirsen therapy for cytomegalovirus retinitis. *Am. J. Ophthalmol.* 130:242–243.

259. Vitravene, Study Group. 2002. Safety of intravitreous fomivirsen for treatment of cytomegalovirus retinitis in patients with AIDS. *Am. J. Ophthalmo.* 133:484–498.

260. Dunn, J. P. 2001. Immune recovery uveitis. The Hopkins HIV Report, November 2002. www.hopkins-aids.edu/publications/report=nov01_4.html (accessed 7 October 2003).

261. Amin, H. I., E. Ai, H. R. McDonald, and R. N. Johnson. 2000. Retinal toxic effects associated with intravitreal fomivirsen. *Arch. Ophthalmol.* 118:426–427.

262. Freeman, W. R., and W. R. Freedman. 2001. Renal toxic effects associated with intravitreal fomivirsen. *Arch. Ophthalmol.* 119:458.

263. Moore, R. A., J. E. Edwards, J. Hopwood, and D. Hicks. 2001. Imiquimod for the treatment of genital warts: a quantitative systematic review. *BMC Infect. Dis.* 1:3.

264. Martinez, M. I., I. Sanchez-Carpintero, P. E. North, and M. C. Mihm Jr. 2002. Infantile hemangioma: clinical resolution with 5% imiquimod cream. *Arch. Dermatol.* 138:881–883.

265. Tyring, S. K., I. Arany, M. A. Stanley, M. A. Tomai, R. L. Miller, M. H. Smith, D. J. McDermott, and H. B. Slade. 1998. A randomized, controlled, molecular study of condylomata acuminata clearance during treatment with imiquimod. *J. Infect. Dis.* 178:551–555.

266. Miller, R. L., J. F. Gerster, M. L. Owens, H. B. Slade, and M. A. Tomai. 1999. Imiquimod applied topically: a novel immune response modifier and new class of drug. *Int. J. Immunopharmacol.* 21:1–14.

267. Edwards, L., A. Ferenczy, L. Eron, D. Baker, M. L. Owens, T. L. Fox, A. J. Hougham, and K. A. Schmitt. 1998. Self-administered topical 5% imiquimod cream for external anogenital warts. HPV Study Group. Human Papilloma Virus. *Arch. Dermatol.* 134:25–30.

268. Beutner, K. R., S. L. Spruance, A. J. Hougham, T. L. Fox, M. L. Owens, and J. M. Douglas Jr. 1998. Treatment of genital warts with an immune-response modifier (imiquimod). *J. Am. Acad. Dermatol.* 38:230–239.

269. Hengge, U. R., S. Esser, T. Schultewolter, C. Behrendt, T. Meyer, E. Stockfleth, and M. Goos. 2000. Self-administered topical 5% imiquimod for the treatment of common warts and molluscum contagiosum. *Brit. J. Dermatol* 143:1026–1031.

270. Buck, H. W., M. Fortier, J. Knudsen, and J. Paavonen. 2002. Imiquimod 5% cream in the treatment of anogenital warts in female patients. *Int. J. Gynaecol. Obstet.* 77:231–238.

271. Gilbert, J., M. M. Drehs, and J. M. Weinberg. 2001. Topical imiquimod for acyclovir-unresponsive herpes simplex virus 2 infection. *Arch. Dermatol.* 137:1015–1017.

272. Slade, H. B., T. Schacker, M. Conant, and C. Thoming. 2002. Imiquimod and genital herpes. *Arch. Dermatol.* 138:534.

273. Harrison, C. J., R. L. Miller, and D. I. Bernstein. 2001. Reduction of recurrent HSV disease using imiquimod alone or combined with a glycoprotein vaccine. *Vaccine* 19:1820–1826.

274. Kaidbey, K., M. Owens, M. Liberda, and M. Smith. 2002. Safety studies of topical imiquimod 5% cream on normal skin exposed to ultraviolet radiation. *Toxicology* 178:175–182.

275. Diakomanolis, E., D. Haidopoulos, and K. Stefanidis. 2002. Treatment of high-grade vaginal intraepithelial neoplasia with imiquimod cream. *N. Engl. J. Med.* 347:374.

276. Saiag, P., I. Bourgault-Villada, M. Pavlovic, and C. Roudier-Pujol. 2002. Efficacy of imiquimod on external anogenital warts in HIV-infected patients previously treated by highly active antiretroviral therapy. *AIDS* 16:1438–1440.

277. Diaz-Arrastia, C., I. Arany, S. C. Robazetti, T. V. Dinh, Z. Gatalica, S. K. Tyring, and E. Hannigan. 2001. Clinical and molecular responses in high-grade intraepithelial neoplasia treated with topical imiquimod 5%. *Clin. Cancer Res.* 7: 3031–3033.

278. Gollnick, H., R. Barasso, U. Jappe, K. Ward, A. Eul, M. Carey-Yard, and K. Milde. 2001. Safety and efficacy of imiquimod 5% cream in the treatment of penile genital warts in uncircumcised men when applied three times weekly or once per day. *Int. J. STD AIDS* 12:22–28.

279. Petrow, W., R. Gerdsen, M. Uerlich, O. Richter, and T. Bieber. 2001. Successful topical immunotherapy of bowenoid papulosis with imiquimod. *Brit. J. Dermatol* 145:1022–1023.

280. Weinberg, J. M., A. Stewart, and J. O. Stern. 2001. Successful treatment of extensive condyloma acuminata of the inguinal area and thigh with topical imiquimod cream. *Acta Derm. Venerol.* 81:76–77.

281. Gilbert, J., M. M. Drehs, and J. M. Weinberg. 2001. Topical imiquimod treatment of human papillomavirus in a patient with human immunodeficiency virus. *Acta Derm Venereol.* 81:301–302.

282. Moresi, J. M., C. R. Herbert, and B. A. Cohen. 2001. Treatment of anogenital warts in children with topical 0.05% podofilox gel and 5% imiquimod cream. *Pediatr. Dermatol.* 18:448–450.

283. Adam, M., and M. Stiller. 2001. Direct medical costs for surgical and medical treatment of condylomata acuminata. *Arch. Dermatol.* 137:337–341.

284. Fried, M. W., M. L. Shiffman, R. K. Reddy, C. Smith, G. Marino, F. Goncales, D. Haeussinger, M. Diago, G. Carosi, J.-P. Zarski, J. Hoffman, and J. Yu. 2001. Pegylated (40 kDA) interferon alfa-2a (Pegasys®) in combination with ribavirin: efficacy and safety results from a phase III, randomized, actively-controlled, multicenter study. *Gastroenterology* 120:A55.

285. Freidman-Kien, A. E., L. J. Eron, M. Conant, W. Growdon, H. Badiak, P. W. Bradstreet, D. Fedorczyk, J. R. Trout, and T. F. Plasse. 1998. Natural interferon alfa for treatment of condylomata acuminata. *J. Am. Med. Assoc.* 259:533–538.

286. Vance, J. C., B. J. Bart, R. C. Hansen, R. C. Reichman, C. McEwen, K. D. Hatch, B. Berman, and D. J. Tanner. 1986. Intralesional recombinant alpha-2 interferon for the treatment of patients with condyloma acuminatum or verruca plantaris. *Arch. Dermatol.* 122:272–277.

287. Woo, M. H., and T. G. Burnakis. 1997. Interferon alpha in the treatment of chronic viral hepatitis B and C. *Ann. Pharmacother.* 31:330–337.

288. Jaeckel, E., M. Cornberg, H. Wedemeyer, T. Santantonio, J. Mayer, M. Zankel, G. Pastore, M. Dietrich, C. Trautwein, and M. P. Manns. 2001. German Acute Hepatitis C. Therapy Group. Treatment of acute hepatitis C with interferon alfa-2b. *N. Engl. J. Med.* 345:1452–1457.

289. Causse, X., H. Godinot, M. Chevallier, P. Chossegros, F. Zoulim, D. Ouzan, J. P. Heyraud, T. Fontanges, J. Albrecht, C. Meschievitz, et al. 1991. Comparison of 1 or 3 MU of interferon alfa-2b and placebo in patients with chronic non-A, non-B hepatitis. *Gastroenterology* 101:497–502.

290. Marcellin, P., N. Boyer, E. Giostra, C. Degott, A. M. Courouce, F. Degos, H. Coppere, P. Cales, P. Couzigou, and J. P. Benhamou. 1991. Recombinant human-interferon in patients with chronic non-A, non-B hepatits: A multicenter randomized controlled trial from France. *Hepatology* 13:393–397.

291. Weiland, O., R. Schvarz, R. Wejstal, G. Norkrans, and A. Fryden. 1990. Therapy of chronic post-transfusion non-A, non-B hepatitis with interferon alfa-2b: Swedish experience. *J. Hepatology* 11:S57–S62.

292. Poynard, T., V. Leroy, M. Cohard, T. Thevenot, P. Mathurin, P. Opolon, and J. P. Zarski. 1996. Meta-analysis of interferon randomized trials in the treatment of viral hepatitis C: effects of dose and duration. *Hepatology* 24:778–789.

293. Sheiner, P. A., P. Boros, F. M. Klion, S. N. Thung, L. K. Schluger, J. Y. Lau, E. Mor, C. Bodian, S. R. Guy, M. E. Schwartz, S. Emre, H. C. Bodenheimer Jr., and C. M. Miller. 1998. The efficacy of prophylactic interferon alpha-2b in preventing recurrent hepatitis C after liver transplantation. *Hepatology* 28:831–838.

294. Bini, E. J., and E. H. Weinshel. 1999. Severe exacerbation of asthma: a new side effect of interferon-alpha in patients with asthma and chronic hepatitis C. *Mayo Clin. Proc.* 74:367–370.

295. Wills, R. J., S. Dennis, H. E. Spiegel, D. M. Gibson, and P. I. Nadler. 1984. Interferon kinetics and adverse reaction after intravenous, intramuscular, and subcutaneous infection. *Clin. Pharmacol. Ther.* 35:722–727.

296. Cattelan, A. M., L. Sasset, L. Corti, S. Stiffan, F. Meneghetti, and P. Cadrobbi. 1999. A complete remission of recalcitrant molluscum contagiosum in an AIDS patient following highly active antiretroviral therapy (HAART) [letter]. *J. Infect.* 38:58–60.

297. Nelson, M. R., S. Chard, and S. E. Barton. 1995. Intralesional interferon for the treatment of recalcitrant molluscum contagiosum in HIV antibody positive individuals—a preliminary report. *Int. J. STD AIDS* 6:351–352.

298. Hourihane, J., E. Hodges, J. Smith, M. Keefe, A. Jones, and G. Connett. 1999. Interferon alpha treatment of molluscum contagiosum in immunodeficiency. *Arch. Dis. Child.* 80:77–79.

299. Calista, D., A. Boschini, and G. Landi. 1999. Resolution of disseminated molluscum contagiosum with Highly Active Antiretroviral Therapy (HAART) in patients with AIDS. *Eur. J. Dermatol.* 9:211–213.

300. Horn, C. K., G. R. Scott, and E. C. Benton. 1998. Resolution of severe molluscum contagiosum on effective antiretroviral therapy [letter]. *Br. J. Dermatol.* 138:715–717.

301. Delgado, C., G. E. Francis, and D. Fisher. 1992. The uses and properties of PEG-linked proteins. *Crit. Rev. Ther. Drug Carrier Syst.* 9:249–304.

302. Yamaoka, T., Y. Tabata, and Y. Ikada. 1994. Distribution and tissue uptake of poly(ethylene glycol) with different molecular weights after intravenous administration to mice. *J. Pharm. Sci.* 83:601–606.

303. Reddy, K. R., M. W. Modi, and S. Pedder. 2002. Use of peginterferon alfa-2a (40KD) (Pegasys) for the treatment of hepatitis C. *Adv. Drug Delivery Rev.* 54:571–586.

304. Glue, P., J. W. S. Fang, R. Rouzier-Panis, C. Raffanel, R. Sabo, S. K. Gupta, M. Salfi, and S. Jacobs. 2000. The Hepatitis C. Intervention Therapy Group. Pegylated interferon-alpha2b: pharmacokinetics, pharmacodynamics, safety, and preliminary efficacy data. *Clin. Pharmacol. Ther.* 68:556–567.

305. Reichard, O., G. Norkrans, A. Fryden, J. H. Braconier, A. Sonnerborg, and O. Weiland. 1998. Randomised, double-blind, placebo-controlled trial of interferon alpha-2b with and without ribavirin for chronic hepatitis C. The Swedish Study Group. *Lancet* 351:83–87.

306. Stoia, J. 1998. Hepatitis C: new treatment options. *AIDS Treatment News* 302:5.

307. Davis, G. L., R. Esterban-Mur, V. Rustgi, J. Hoefs, S. C. Gordon, C. Trepo, M. L. Shiffman, S. Zeuzem, A. Craxi, M. H. Ling, and J. Albrecht, for the International Hepatitis Interventional Therapy Group. 1998. Interferon alpha-2b alone or in combination with ribavirin for the treatment of relapse of chronic hepatits C. *N. Engl. J. Med.* 339:1493–1499.

308. Doong, S. L., C. H. Tsai, R. F. Schinazi, D. C. Liotta, and Y. C. Cheng. 1991. Inhibition of the replication of hepatitis B virus in vitro by 2′,3′-dideoxy-3′-thiacytidine and related analogues. *Proc. Natl. Acad. Sci. USA* 88:8495–9499.

309. Ong, J. P., Z. M. Younossi, T. Gramlich, Z. Goodman, J. Mayes, S. Sarbah, and B. Yen-Lieberman. 2001. Interferon alpha 2B and ribavirin in severe recurrent cholestatic hepatitis C. *Transplantation* 71:1486–1487.

310. McHutchinson, J. G. 2002. Hepatitis C advances in antiviral therapy: what is accepted treatment now? *J. Gastroenterol. Hepatol.* 17:431–441.

311. Hoey, J. 2001. Early treatment of acute hepatitis C infection may lead to cure. *CMAJ* 165:1527.

312. Fang, S.-H., M.-Y. Lai, L.-H. Hwang, P.-M. Yang, P.-J. Chen, B.-L. Chiang, and D.-S. Chen. 2001. Ribavirin Enhances Interferon-γ Levels in Patients with Chronic Hepatitis C Treated with Interferon-α. *J. Biomed. Sci.* 8:484–491.

313. Gordon, S. C. 2001. Treatment of viral hepatitis—2001. *Ann. Med.* 33:385–390.

314. Sennfalt, K., O. Reichard, R. Hultkrantz, J. B. Wong, and D. Jonsson. 2001. Cost-effectiveness of interferon alfa-2b with and without ribavirin as therapy for chronic hepatitis C in Sweden. *Scandinavian J. Gastroenterol.* 36:870–876.

315. Bruchfeld, A., L. Stahle, J. Andersson, and R. Schvarcz. 2001. Ribavirin treatment in dialysis patients with chronic hepatitis C virus infection—a pilot study. *J. Viral Hepat.* 8:287–92.

316. Kjaergard, L. L., K. Krogsgaard, and C. Gluud. 2001. Interferon alfa with or without ribavirin for chronic hepatitis C: systematic review of randomised trials. *BMJ* 323:1151–1155.

317. Talal, A. H., K. Weisz, T. Hau, S. Kreiswirth, and D. T. Dieterich. 2001. A preliminary study of erythropoietin for anemia associated with ribavirin and interferon-alpha. *Am. J. Gastroenterol.* 96:2802–2804.

318. Weegink, C. J., R. A. Chamuleau, H. W. Reesink, and D. S. Molenaar. 2001. Development of myasthenia gravis during treatment of chronic hepatitis C with interferon-alpha and ribavirin. *J. Gastroenterol.* 36:723–724.

319. Neuman, M. G., L. M. Blendis, N. H. Shear, I. M. Malkiewicz, A. Ibrahim, G. G. Katz, D. Sapir, Z. Halpern, S. Brill, H. Peretz, S. Magazinik, and F. M. Konikoff. 2001. Cytokine network in nonresponding chronic hepatitis C patients with genotype 1: role of triple therapy with interferon alpha, ribavirin, and ursodeoxycholate. *Clin. Biochem.* 34:183–188.

320. Houck, P., M. Hemphill, S. Lacroix, D. Hirsh, and N. Cox. 1995. Amantadine-resistant influenza A in nursing homes: identification of a resistant virus prior to drug use. *Arch. Intern. Med.* 155:533–537.

321. Ziegler, T., M. L. Hemphill, M. L. Ziegler, G. Perez-Oronoz, A. I. Klimov, A. W. Hampson, H. L. Regnery, and N. J. Cox. 1999. Low incidence of rimantadine resistance in field isolates of influenza A. viruses. *J. Infect. Dis.* 180:935–939.

322. Fritz, R. S., F. G. Hayden, D. P. Calfee, L. M. Cass, A. W. Peng, W. G. Alvord, W. Strober, and S. E. Straus. 1999. Nasal cytokine and chemokine responses in experimental influenza A virus infection: results of a placebo-controlled trial of iv. zanamivir treatment. *J. Infect. Dis.* 180:586–593.

323. Bantia, S., C. D. Parker, S. L. Ananth, L. L. Horn, K. Andries, P. Chand, P. L. Kotian, A. Dehghani, Y. El-Kattan, T. Lin, T. L. Hutchison, J. A. Montgomery, D. L. Kellog, and Y. S. Babu. 2001. Comparison of the anti-influenza virus activity of RWJ-270201 with those of oseltamivir and zanamivir. *Antimicrob. Agents Chemother.* 45:1162–1167.

324. Smith, B. J., J. L. McKimm-Breshkin, M. McDonald, R. T. Fernley, J. N. Varghese, and P. M. Colman. 2002. Structural studies of the resistance of influenza virus neuramindase to inhibitors. *J. Med. Chem.* 45:2207–2212.

325. de los Cobos, J. P., P. Duro, J. Trujols, A. Tejero, F. Batlle, E. Ribalta, and M. Casas. 2001. Methadone tapering plus amantadine to detoxify heroin-dependent inpatients with or without an active cocaine use disorder: two randomised controlled trials. *Drug and Alcohol Dependence* 63: 187–195.

326. Shoptaw, S., P. C. Kintaudi, C. Charuvastra, and W. Ling. 2002. A screening trial of amantadine as a medication for cocaine dependence. *Drug and Alcohol Dependence* 66:217–224.

327. King, B. H., D. M. Wright, M. Snape, and C. T. Dourish. 2001. Case Series: Amantadine open-label treatment of impulsive and aggressive behavior in hospitalized children with developmental disabilities. *J. Am. Child Adolescent Psychiatry* 40:654–657.

328. King, B. H., D. M. Wright, B. L. Handen, L. Sikich, A. W. Zimmerman, W. McMahon, E. Cantwell, P. A. Davanzo, C. T. Dourish, E. M. Dykens, S. R. Hooper, C. A. Jaselskis, B. L. Leventhal, J. Levitt, C. Lord, M. J. Lubetsky, S. M. Myers, S. Ozonoff, B. G. Shah, M. Snape, E. W. Shernoff, K. Williamson, and E. H. Cook Jr. 2001. Double-blind, placebo-controlled study of amantadine hydrochloride in the treatment of children with autistic disorder. *J. Am. Child Adolescent Psychiatry* 40:658–665.

329. Terao, T. 2001. Female sexual dysfunction and antidepressant use. *Am. J. Psychiatry* 158: 326–327.

330. Michelson, D. 2001. Female sexual dysfunction and antidepressant use. *Am. J. Psychiatry* 158:327.

331. Torre, F., and A. Picciotto. 2002. Amantadine: a different approach. *J. Hepatol.* 36:705–709.

332. Bacosi, M., F. Russo, S. D'innocenzo, M. Santolamazza, L. Miglioresi, A. Ursitti, A. De Angelis, F. Patrizi, and G. Ricci. 2002. Amantadine and interferon in the combined treatment of hepatitis C virus in elderly patients. *Hepatol. Res.* 22:231–239.

333. Zeuzem, S., E. Herrmann, J. H. Lee, J. Fricke, A. U. Neumann, M. Modi, G. Colucci, and W. K. Roth. 2001. Viral kinetics in patients with chronic hepatitis C treated with standard or peginterferon alpha2a. *Gastroenterology* 120:1438–1447.

334. Skehel, J. J., A. J. Hay, and J. A. Armstrong. 1978. On the mechanism of inhibition of influenza virus replication by amantadine hydrochloride. *J. Gen. Virol.* 38:97–110.

335. Torre, F., N. Campo, R. Giusto, F. Ansaldi, G. C. Icardi, and A. Picciotto. 2001. Antiviral activity of amantadine inelderly patients with chronic hepatitis C. *Gerontology* 47:330–333.

336. Zapata, L., F. Sanchez-Avila, F. Vargas, and D. Kershenobich. 1997. Presentation. American Gastroenterology Association Digestive Disease Week Meeting. Washington, DC May 1997.

337. Anonymous. 2002. The role of amantadine in combination with interferon in the treatment of chronic hepatitis C. http://hepatitis-c.de/amantad.htm (accessed 6 November 2002).

338. Tabamo R. E., and A. DiRocco. 2002. Alopecia induced by dopamine agonists. *Neurology* 58:829–830.

339. Hornick, R. B., Y. Togo, S. Mahler, and D. Iezzoni. 1969. Evaluation of amantadine hydrochloride in the treatment of A2 influenzal disease. *Bulletin of the WHO* 41:671–676.

340. Kitamoto, O. 1971. Therapeutic effectiveness of amantadine hydrochloride in naturally occurring Hong Kong influenza double-blind studies. *Jap. J. Tuberculosis Chest Diseases* 17:1–7.

341. Published, data only. Knight, V., D. Fedson, J. Baldini, R. G. Douglas, and R. B. Couch. 1969. Amantadine therapy of epidemic

influenza A2 (Hong Kong). Antimicrobial agents chemother. 9:370–371.

342. Younossi, Z. M., K. D. Mullen, W. Zakko, S. Hodnick, E. Brand, D. S. Barnes, W. D. Carey, A. C. McCullough, K. Easley, N. Boparai, and T. Gramlich. 2001. A randomized, double-blind controlled trial of interferon alpha-2b and ribavirin vs. interferon alpha-2b and amantadine for treatment of chronic hepatitis C. non-responder to interferon monotherapy. *J. Hepatol.* 34:128–133.

343. Jefferson, T. O., V. Demicheli, J. J. Deeks, and D. Rivetti. 2002. Amantadine and rimantadine for preventing and treating influenza A in adults. (Cochrane Reviews.) In: The Cochrane Library. Oxford: Update Software, Issue 4, 2002.

344. Dolin, R., R. C. Reichman, H. P. Madore, R. Maynard, P. N. Linton, and J. Webber-Jones. 1982. A controlled trial of amantadine and rimantadine in the prophylaxis of influenza A infection. *N. Engl. J. Med.* 307:580–584.

345. Hayden, F. G., J. M. Gwaltney, R. L. van de Castle, K. F. Adams, and B. Giordani. 1981. Comparative toxicity of amantadine hydrochloride and rimantadine hydrochloride in healthy adults. *Antimicrob. Agents Chemother.* 19:226–233.

346. Kantor, R. J., D. W. Potts, D. Stevens, and G. R. Noble. 1980. Prevention of influenza A/USSR/77 (H1N1): an evaluation of the side effects and efficacy of amantadine in recruits at Fort Sam Houston. *Military Med.* 145:312–315.

347. Muldoon, R. L., E. D. Stanley, and G. G. Jackson. 1976. Use and withdrawal of amantadine chemoprophylaxis during epidemic influenza A. *Am. Rev. Respiratory Disease* 113:487–491.

348. Payler, D. K., and P. A. Purdham. 1984. Influenza A prophylaxis with amantadine in a boarding school. *Lancet* 1:502–504.

349. Hayden, F. G., W. J. Hall, and R. G. Douglas. 1980. Therapeutic effects of aerosolized amantadine in naturally acquired infection due to influenza A virus. *J. Infect. Dis.* 141:535–542.

350. Morris, H. H., and W. F. McCormick. 1980. Neuroleptic malignant syndrome. *Arch. Neurol.* 37:462–465.

351. Ito, T., K. Shibata, A. Watannbe, and J. Akabase. 2001. Neuroleptic malignant syndrome following withdrawal of amantadine

in a patient with influenza A. encephalopathy. *Eur. J. Pediatrics* 160:401.

352. Fredericksen, B. L., B. L. Wei, J. Yao, T. Luo, and J. V. Garcia. 2002. Inhibition of endosomal/lysosomal degradation increases the infectivity of human immunodeficiency virus. *J. Virol.* 76:11440–11446.

353. Hayden, F. G., and R. B. Couch. 1993. Clinical and epidemiological importance of influenza A viruses resistant to amantadine and rimantadine. In: C. Hannoun et al., Eds. *Options for the Control of Influenza* II. Amsterdam: Excerpta Medica, 1993, pp. 333–342.

354. Monto, A. S., S. E. Ohmit, K. Hornbuckle, and C. L. Pearce. 1995. Safety and efficacy of long-term use of rimantadine for prophylaxis of type A influenza in nursing homes. *Antimicrob. Agents Chemother.* 39:2224–2228.

355. Belshe, R. B., M. Hall Smith, C. B. Hall, R. Betts, and A. J. Hay. 1988. Genetic basis of resistance to rimantadine emerging during treatment of influenza virus infection. *J. Virol.* 62:1508–1512.

356. Clover, R. D., S. A. Crawford, T. D. Abell, C. N. Ramsey, W. P. Glezen, and R. B. Couch. 1986. Effectiveness of rimantadine prophylaxis of children within families. *Am. J. Dis. Child.* 140:706–709.

357. Couch, R. B. 2000. Influenza: prospects for control. *Ann. Intern. Med.* 133:992–998.

358. Morris, S. J., H. Smith, and C. Sweet. 2002. Exploitation of the herpes simplex virus translocating protein VP22 to carry influenza virus proteins into cells for studies of apoptosis: direct confirmation that neuraminidase induces apoptosis and indications that other proteins may have a role. *Arch. Virol.* 147:961–979.

359. Burls, A., W. Clark, T. Stewart, C. Preston, S. Bryan, T. Jefferson, and A. Fry-Smith. 2002. Zanamivir for the treatment of influenza in adults: a systematic review and economic evaluation. *Health Technol. Assess* 6:1–87.

360. Hayden, F. G., A. D. Osterhaus, J. J. Treanor, D. M. Fleming, F. Y. Aoki, K. G. Nicholson, A. M. Bohnen, H. M. Hirst, O. Keene,

and K. Wightman, for the GG167 Influenza Study Group. 1997. Efficacy and safety of the neuraminidase inhibitor zanamivir in the treatment of influenzavirus infections. *N. Engl. J. Med.* 337:874–880.

361. Maeda, M., Y. Fukunaga, T. Asano, M. Migita, T. Ueda, and J. Hayakawa. 2002. Zanamivir is an effective treatment for influenza in children undergoing therapy for acute lymphoblastic leukemia. *Scand. J. Infect. Dis.* 34:632–633.

362. Boivin, G., and N. Goyette. 2002. Susceptibility of recent Canadian influenza A and B virus isolates to different neuraminidase inhibitors. *Antiviral Res.* 54:143–147.

363. Hayden, F. G., L. V. Gubareva, A. S. Monto, T. C. Klein, M. J. Elliot, J. M. Hammond, S. J. Sharp, and M. J. Ossi, for the Zanamivir Family Study Group. 2000. Inhaled zanamivir for the prevention of influenza in families. *N. Engl. J. Med.* 343(18):1282–1289.

364. Hayden, F. G., R. Belshe, C. Villanueva, R. Lanno, C. Hughes, I. Small, R. Dutkowski, P. Ward, and J. Carr. 2004. Management of influenza in households: a prospective, randomized comparison of oseltamivir treatment with or without postexposure prophylaxis. *J. Infect. Dis.* 189:440–449.

365. Anonymous. 2003. Oseltamivir: new prevention; an antiviral agent with little impact on influenza. *Prescrire Int.* 12:85–88.

366. McClellan, K., and C. M. Perry. 2001. Oseltamivir: a review of its use in influenza. Drugs 61:263–283.

367. Bowles, S. K., W. Lee, A. E. Simor, M. Vearncombe, M. Loeb, S. Tamblyn, M. Fearon, Y. Li, and A. McGeer, for the Oseltamivir Compassionate Use Program Group. 2002. Use of Oseltamivir during influenza outbreaks in Ontario nursing homes, 1999–2000. *JAGS* 50:608–616.

368. Gillissen, A., and G. Hoffken. 2002. Early therapy with the neuraminidase inhibitor oseltamivir maximizes its efficacy in influenza treatment. *Med. Microbiol. Immunol.* 191:165–168.

369. Nicholson, K. G., F. Y. Aoki, A. D. Osterhaus, S. Trottier, O. Carewicz, C. H. Mercier, A. Rode, N. Kinnersley, and P. Ward. 2000. Efficacy and safety of oseltamivir in treatment of acute

influenza: a randomized controlled trial. Neuraminidase Inhibitor Flu Treatment Investigator Group. *Lancet* 356:1856.

370. Doucette, K. E., and F. Y. Aoki. 2001. Oseltamivir: a clinical and pharmacological perspective. *Expert Opin. Pharmacother.* 2:1671–1683.

371. Bardsley-Elliot, A., and S. Noble. 1999. Oseltamivir. *Drugs* 58:851–860.

372. Welliver, R., A. S. Monto, O. Carewicz, E. Schatteman, M. Hassman, J. Hedrick, H. C. Jackson, L. Huson, P. Ward, J. S. Oxford, et al. 2001. Effectiveness of oseltamivir in preventing influenza in household contacts. *J. Am. Med. Assoc.* 285:748–754.

373. Li, L., B. Cai, M. Wang, and Y. Zhu. 2003. A double-blind, randomized, placebo-controlled multicenter study of oseltamivir phosphate for treatment of influenza infection in China. *Chin. Med. J.* 116:44–48.

374. Peters, P. H., Jr., S. Gravenstein, P. Norwood, V. De Bock, A. Van Couter, M. Gibbens, T. A. von Planta, and P. Ward. 2001. Long-term use of oseltamivir for the prophylaxis of influenza in a vaccinated frail older population. *J. Am. Geriatr. Soc.* 49:1025–31.

375. Treanor, J. J., F. G. Hayden, P. S. Vrooman, R. Barbarash, R. Bettis, D. Riff, S. Singh, N. Kinnersley, P. Ward, and R. G. Mills, for the US Oral Neuraminidase Study Group. 2000. Efficacy and safety of the oral neuraminidase inhibitor oseltamivir in treating acute influenza: a randomized controlled trial. *J. Am. Med. Assoc.* 283:1016–1024.

376. Snell, P., C. Oo, A. Dorr, and J. Barrett. 2002. Lack of pharmacokinetic interaction between the oral anti-influenza neuraminidase inhibitor prodrug oseltamivir and antacids. *Br. J. Clin. Pharmacol.* 54:372–377.

377. Hill, G., T. Cihlar, C. Oo, E. S. Ho, K. Prior, H. Wiltshire, J. Barrett, B. Liu, and P. Ward. 2002. The anti-influenza drug oseltamivir exhibits low potential to induce pharmacokinetic drug interactions via renal secretion—correlation of in vivo and in vitro studies. *Drug Metabolism and Disposition* 30:13–19.

378. Oo, C., J. Barrett, G. Hill, J. Mann, A. Dorr, R. Dutkowski, and P. Ward. 2001. Pharmacokinetics and dosage recommendations

for an oseltamivir oral suspension for the treatment of influenza in children. *Paediatr. Drugs* 3:229–236.

379. Whitley, R. J., F. G. Hayden, K. S. Reisinger, N. Young, R. Dutkowski, D. Ipe, R. G. Mills, and P. Ward. 2001. Oral oseltamivir treatment of influenza in children. *Pediatr. Infect. Dis. J.* 20:127–133.

380. Birch, C. J., D. P. Tyssen, G. Tachedjian, R. Doherty, K. Hayes, A. Mijch, and C. R. Lucas. 1992. Clinical effects and in vitro studies of trifluorothymidine combined with interferon-alpha for treatment of drug-resistant and -sensitive herpes simplex virus infection. *J. Infect. Dis.* 166:108–112.

381. Spector, A., S. A. M. Tyndall, and E. Kelley. 1983. Inhibition of human cytomegalovirus by trifluorothymidine. *Antimicrob. Agents Chemother.* 23:113–118.

382. Kessler, H., A. Hurwitz, C. Farthing, C. A. Benson, J. Feinberg, D. R. Kuritzkes, T. C. Bailey, S. Safrin, R. T. Steigbigel, S. H. Cheeseman, G. F. McKinley, B. Wettlaufer, S. Owens, T. Nevin, and J. A. Korvick. 1996. Pilot study of topical trifluridine for the treatment of acyclovir-resistant mucocutaneous herpes simplex disease in patients with AIDS (ACTG 172). AIDS Clinical Trials Group. *J. Acquir. Immune Defic. Syndr. Hum. Retrovirol.* 12:147–152.

383. Murphy, M., A. Morley, R. P. Eglin, and E. Monteiro. 1992. Topical trifluridine for mucocutaneous acyclovir-resistant herpes simplex II in AIDS patient. *Lancet* 340:1040.

384. Vastag, B. 2003. Experts weigh prevention, therapy for ocular vaccinia in smallpox vaccinees. *JAMA* 289:2198–2199.

385. Semba, R. D. 2003. The ocular complications of smallpox and smallpox immunization. *Arch. Ophthalmol.* 121:715–719.

386. Smallpox vaccine adverse events among civilians—United States, February 25–March 3, 2003. *Arch. Derm.* 139:683–684.

387. Smallpox vaccine adverse events among civilians—United States, February 25–March 3, 2003. *MMWR* 52:180–181; 191, 2003.

388. Whitley, R. J. 2003. Other antiviral agents. In: R. G. Finch, D. Greenwood, S. R. Norrby, and R. J. Whitley, Eds. *Antibiotic and Chemotherapy*, 8th ed. New York: Livingston, 2003, pp. 505.

389. Smith, K. J., C. Kahlter, D. C. Davis, W. D. James, H. G. Skelton, and P. Angritt. 1991. Acyclovir-resistant varicella zoster responsive to foscarnet. *Arch. Dermatol.* 127:1069–1071.

390. Oberg, B. 1989. Antiviral effects of phosphonoformate (PFA, foscarnet sodium). *Pharmacol. Ther.* 40:213–285.

391. Safrin, S., T. Assaykeen, S. Follansbee, and J. Mills. 1990. Foscarnet therapy for acyclovir-resistant mucocutaneous herpes simplex virus infection in 26 AIDS patients: preliminary data. *J. Infect. Dis.* 161:1078–1084.

392. Balfour, H. H. Jr. 1999. Antiviral Drugs. *N. Engl. J. Med.* 340: 1255–1268.

393. Devianne-Garrigue, I., I. Pellegrin, R. Denisi, M. Dupon, J. M. Ragnaud, P. Barbeau, D. Breilh, B. Leng, H. J. Fleury, and J. L. Pellegrin. 1998. Foscarnet decreases HIV-1 plasma load. *J. Acquir. Immune Defic. Syndr. Hum. Retrovirol.* 18:46–50.

394. Løkke Jensen, B., K. Weismann, L. Mathiesen, and H. Klem Thomsen. 1993. Atypical varicella-zoster infection in AIDS. *Acta Derm. Venereol.* 73:123–125.

395. Paar, D. P., and S. E. Straus. 1991. Treatment of acyclovir (ACV)-resistant zoster with foscarnet in a man with AIDS [abstract no. 206]. *Antivir. Res.* 15(Suppl 1):153.

396. Safrin, S., T. G. Berger, I. Gilson, P. R. Wolfe, C. B. Wofsy, J. Mills, and K. K. Biron. 1991. Foscarnet therapy in five patients with AIDS and acyclovir-resistant varicella-zoster virus infection. *Ann. Intern. Med.* 115:19–21.

397. Javaly, K., M. Wohlfeiler, R. Kalayjian, T. Klein, Y. Bryson, and K. Grafford. 1999. Treatment of mucocutaneous herpes simplex virus infections unresponsive to acyclovir with topical foscarnet cream in AIDS patients: a phase I/II study. *J. Acquire. Immune Defic. Syndr.* 21:301–306.

398. Boulanger, E. 1999. Human herpesvirus 8: Pathogenic role and sensitivity to antiviral drugs. *Ann. Biol. Clin. (Paris)* 57:19–28.

399. Boivin, G., A. Gaudreau, E. Toma, R. Lalonde, J. P. Routy, G. Murray, J. Handfield, and M. G. Bergeron. 1999. Human herpesvirus 8 DNA load in leukocytes of human immunodeficiency virus-infected subjects: correlation with the presence of

Kaposi's sarcoma and response to anti-cytomegalovirus therapy. *Antimicrob. Agents Chemother.* 43:377–380.

400. Glesby, M. J., D. R. Hoover, S. Weng, N. M. Graham, J. P. Phair, R. Detels, M. Ho, and A. J. Saah. 1996. Use of antiherpes drugs and the risk of Kaposi's sarcoma: data from the Multicenter AIDS Cohort Study. *J. Infect. Dis.* 173:1477–1480.

401. Mocroft, A., M. Youle, B. Gazzard, J. Morcinek, R. Halai, and A. N. Phillips. 1996. Anti-herpesvirus treatment and risk of Kaposi's sarcoma in HIV infection. Royal Free/Chelsea and Westminster Hospitals Collaborative Group. *AIDS* 10:1101–1105.

402. Morfeldt, L., and J. Torrsander. 1994. Long-term remission of Kaposi's sarcoma following foscarnet treatment in HIV-infected patients. *Scand. J. Infect. Dis.* 26:749–752.

403. Gilbert, C., M. H. LeBlanc, and G. Boivin. 2001. Case study: rapid emergence of a cytomegalovirus UL97 mutant in a heart-transplant receipient on pre-emptive ganciclovir therapy. *Herpes* 8:80–82.

404. DeClercq, E., L. Naesens, L. De Bolle, D. Schols, Y. Zhang, and J. Neyts. 2001. Antiviral agents active against human herpesviruses HHV-6, HHV-7 and HHV-8. *Rev. Med. Virol.* 11: 381–395.

405. Ohta, H., Y. Matsuda, S. Tokimasa, A. Sawada, J. Y. Kim, J. Sashihara, K. Amo, H. Miyagawa, K. Tanaka-Taya, S. Yamamoto, Y. Tano, T. Aono, K. Yamanishi, S. Okada, and J. Hara. 2001. Foscarnet therapy for ganciclovir-resistant cytomegalovirus retinitis after stem cell transplantation: effective monitoring of CMV infection by quantitative analysis of CMV mRNA. *Bone Marrow Transplant* 27:1141–1145.

406. Pelosi, E., K. A. Hicks, S. L. Sacks, and D. M. Coen. 1992. Heterogeneity of a herpes simplex virus clinical isolate exhibiting resistance to acyclovir and foscarnet. *Adv. Exp. Med. Biol.* 312:151–158.

407. Pope, L. E., J. F. Marcelletti, L. R. Katz, J. Y. Lin, D. H. Katz, M. L. Parish, and P. G. Spear. 1998. The anti-herpes simplex virus activity of n-docosanol includes inhibition of the viral entry process. *Antiviral Res.* 40:85–94.

408. Spruance, S. L. 2000. N-docosanol (Abreva) for herpes labialis: problems and questions. *J. Am. Acad. Dermatol.* 47:457–458.

409. Katz, D. H., J. F. Marcelletti, M. H. Khalil, L. E. Pope, and L. R. Katz. 1991. Antiviral acitivity of 1-docosanol, an inhibitor of lipid-enveloped viruses including herpes simplex. *Proc. Natl. Acad. Sci. USA* 88:10825–10829.

410. Habbema, L., K. De boulle, G. A. Roders, and D. H. Katz. 1996. n-Docosanol 10% cream in the treatment of recurrent herpes labialis: a randomized, double-blind, placebo-controlled study. *Acta Dermatol. Venerol.* 76:479–481.

411. Spruance, S. L., and M. B. McKeough. 2000. Combination treatment with famciclovir and a topical corticosteroid gel versus famciclovir alone for experimental ultraviolet radiation-induced herpes simplex labialis: a pilot study. *J. Infect. Dis.* 181: 1906–1910.

Chapter 4

Vaccines and Immunotherapies

INTRODUCTION

Patients are inoculated with one of two intents: prevention of a disease through the immune response (vaccination) and prophylaxis to protect those already exposed to a disease and for whom regular vaccination would not be effective. If humans could control virus transmittal in nonhuman reservoirs, eliminate vectors, and improve sanitation, then vaccines and other immunomodulators would be less necessary. Instead, many human activities may promote opportunities for virus transmittal and improper sanitation, particularly in third-world countries when new agricultural crops or production methods are introduced; populations become concentrated in an area with new economic development and no sanitary infrastructure; or in populations that move into vector habitats that were previously undisturbed. Nonhuman animal reservoirs can be controlled through vaccination, removal of stray or wild animals, and quarantine. Vector control usually involves draining swamps, spraying insecticides, using insect repellent and long-sleeved or -legged clothes, screening, etc. Improving sanitation involves breaking the fecal-oral transmission cycle, which includes drinking water chlorination and proper treatment of wastewater. The use of vaccines is only one aspect of controlling the spread of viruses and should be used along with other public health measures.

The global eradication of poliomyelitis is currently underway, with an unmet target goal of 2000 (1). A number of other virus vaccines have led to notable decreases in infections and complications. In 2002, an all-time low of 37 cases of measles was recorded in the United States. Worldwide eradication for measles is targeted for 2005–2010. Currently available vaccines provide a basic framework of knowledge and experience with which other virus vaccines can be developed. The incidence of many viral infections, such as herpes simplex viruses, human papillomaviruses, and HIV, as well as newly emerging viruses, such as Ebola and West Nile viruses, means that no let up in vaccine development is in sight (Fig. 4.1).

By administering antibodies from another host, usually in an antibody-containing gamma globulin preparation, into a susceptible individual, some form of temporary immunity either protects the individual from getting the disease or reduces the effects of the disease. Active prophylaxis, delivered as a vaccine, stimulates an antibody response via T lymphocytes. The vaccine efficacy is measured in the length of immunity (over time) and the proportion of persons vaccinated who demonstrate immunity. While immunity diminishes over time, recent studies indicate

————————————————————————————▶

Fig. 4.1 Occurrence of Emerging Viral Diseases and Vaccine Development (1950–2003). Vaccines with the most impact are those designed to eradicate viral diseases of childhood. For some diseases, vaccines are available but are not routinely administered to anyone other than animal care workers, foresters, or health-care workers due to limited availability, adverse events, or incidental exposure. A 100% vaccination rate is usually not achieved. Some diseases, such as yellow fever, depend upon vector control and have reemerged as agricultural practices and vector-control policy have changed. In summary, progress is being made, but the viruses are emerging faster than they are being eradicated or controlled.

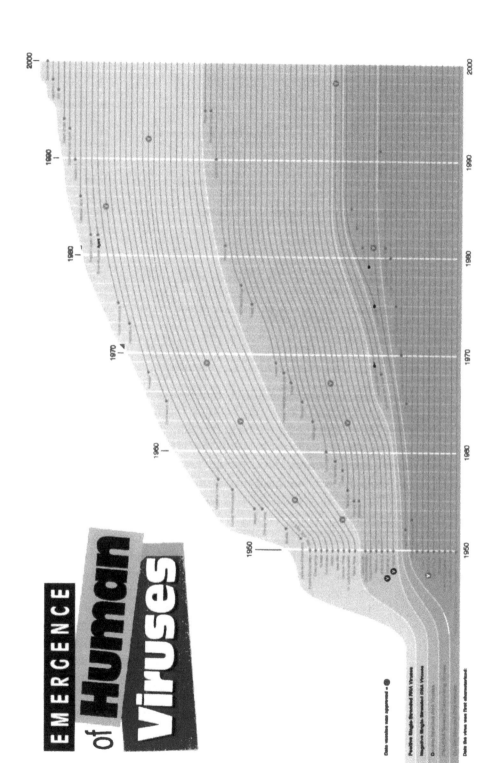

EMERGENCE of **Human Viruses**

Table 4.1 Vaccines Approved for Viruses (USA) 2003

Virus Vaccine	Type of Vaccine	Year Released
Adenovirus	Live oral, type 4	1971
Adenovirus	Live oral, type 7	1971
Hepatitis A	Inactivated	1995
Hepatitis B	Recombinant	1986
Influenza	Inactivated	1945
Japanese Encephalitis	Inactivated	1992
Measles	Live	1963
Mumps	Live	1967
Rubella	Live	1969
Poliovirus	Inactivated	1955
Poliovirus	Live oral	1963
Rabies	Inactivated	1885
Smallpox	Live	1796
Varicella	Live	1995
Yellow Fever	Live	1953

that those vaccinated against smallpox over 30 years ago continue to demonstrate some level of immunity to the smallpox virus. Many vaccines have been developed since the original cowpox (smallpox) vaccine in 1796. As viruses have become more prominent and vaccine technology has changed, vaccines of various etiologies are being approved on a regular basis (Table 4.1).

Currently, vaccines are derived from three different mechanisms:

Attenuated live viral vaccine. A live vaccine containing a virus that has been manipulated in the laboratory. These special viruses can infect and replicate in the vaccine to produce an immune response without causing illness. There is always the danger that the virus will mutate to a more pathogenic form. Fortunately, current in vitro, in vivo, and clinical tests must assess and report this risk before the vaccine is licensed for use in the general population. New recombinant DNA strains have had genetic regions deleted that are most likely to mutate to pathogenic strains. Most of the vaccines developed prior to 1960 were attenuated live vaccines. Varicella, yellow fever, measles, mumps, rubella, oral polio vaccine, and some adenovirus vaccines are examples of attenuated live viral vaccines.

Killed viral vaccines (inactivated). Whole virus particles or some component of the virus, either of which has been deactivated chemically or physically. These vaccines do not cause infection but stimulate an immune reaction. Usually, repeated doses are required as one dose does not confer lifelong immunity. Large quantities of viral antigens per dose are necessary to produce an adequate response. Influenza, Salk polio, rabies, and Japanese encephalitis vaccines are of this type.

Recombinant antigens. Tend to be newer versions of earlier vaccines and furnish better protection with less risk and fewer side effects. Specific components that elicit production of protective antibodies are cloned. These express the gene that encodes that protein or protein complex. The new hepatitis B vaccine is this type.

The different types of vaccines that produce immune responses in a variety of cell types are shown in Table 4.2. Vaccine-induced immunity is a relative science. Selecting the correct dosage(s), timing of dosages, and determining the long-term efficacy are trials facing vaccine development. Normally, B cells, CD8$^+$ T cells and CD4$^+$ T cells mediate immune functions. B-cell functions may involve secretion of IgG antibodies or secretory IgA antibodies. CD4$^+$ and CD8$^+$ T cells provide support for B cells and CD8$^+$ T cells assist in killing human leukocyte antigen (HLA)-matched infected cells. B cells, when mediated by T-helper cells, are thought to provide long-lasting immunity despite negative antibody test results (2).

Table 4.2 Roles of Different Cell Types in Vaccine-Induced Immune System Development

B-cells	Live-attenuated virus vaccines, inactivated virus vaccines, protein antigens, capsular polysaccharides with or without carrier.
CD8$^+$ T cells	Live-attenuated virus vaccines.
CD4$^+$ T cells	Live-attenuated virus vaccines, inactivated virus vaccines, protein antigens, and capsular polysaccharides only with a protein carrier.

The development of vaccines may take decades to characterize, develop genetic-splicing methods to improve safety and efficacy, and complete appropriate testing. Still, even after vaccines are developed, many persons choose for a variety of reasons not to be vaccinated. Therefore antivirals, prophylaxis therapies, vaccines, and other immunomodulators all have a role to play in disease eradication and cure.

SMALLPOX AND OTHER POXVIRUSES

Smallpox

In 1796, Edward Jenner first demonstrated that inoculation of cowpox virus into human skin could lead to protection from subsequent smallpox infection (3). He named the inoculation substance *vaccine,* based on the Latin word, *vacca*, meaning cow. The more effective vaccines used for smallpox vaccination are derived from the vaccinia virus that is similar to cowpox. Several strains of the live attenuated virus vaccine were employed in eradication of the disease. The smallpox vaccine has been the prototype of success of a viral vaccine. Prior to immunization, smallpox infection relentlessly killed hundreds of millions of persons and left many badly scarred and/or blind. The mortality rate ranged between 20–30%. The worldwide eradication of this disease in 1977 is considered the greatest success story in medical history. The recent accidental introduction of monkeypox into the United States via the Gambian pouched rat illustrates the need for better vaccines and perhaps vaccines with a broader range of targets. Immunity provided by the current smallpox vaccination reduces the effects of monkeypox virus on humans by 85%.

Vaccine production ended two decades ago and most Americans under the age of 35 have not been vaccinated. Smallpox eradication occurred because every child was immunized before attending public school, thus reducing the exposure of infected children to nonimmunized children and their families (4). Approximately 60 million vaccine doses remain worldwide and more vaccine is bring produced (5). Immunologic status of the older population is questionable but there are some reports of lingering immunity (6–8). At least 119,000,000 people in the United States have never been immunized (9). There are some indications from recent revaccinations of older persons that some degree of immunity still exists, albeit variable among the population. The destruction of the two remaining smallpox virus reserves in Atlanta and near Moscow has been a source of ongoing debate. Opponents of destruction contend that the virus stocks would be helpful for future research, such as smallpox pathogenesis and the production of new antiviral agents (10,11). Fear of undisclosed reserves is also a concern. Proponents argue that the virus genome has already been cloned and sequenced and is unnecessary for research (12).

Destruction of the virus reserves will likely be halted as concerns for bioterrorism increase. Of concern since the collapse of the Soviet Union is that existing stocks of virus, combined with the technology for maintaining and activating the stocks, may have passed into non-Russian hands (13). Should these undocumented virus stocks fall into the domain of terrorists, strategic outbreaks among the unvaccinated or underimmunized could begin an epidemic that would be difficult to contain. Smallpox is considered to be an ideal bioterroist avenue as it is easily transmitted, has a high mortality rate, requires specific action for public health response, and could cause social and community disarray (14). Models based on the assumption that 100 persons are initially infected and each infects three more predict that quarantine could stop or eradicate such an outbreak if 50% of those with overt symptoms were quarantined. At risk would be family members (50% risk to the unvaccinated), school children, health-care workers, etc. Vaccination alone would only stop the transmission within a year if the disease transmittal rate were reduced to ≤ 0.85 persons infected per initially infected person. Therefore, a combination vaccination-quarantine program is necessary (25% daily quarantine and a vaccination reduction of smallpox transmission by $\geq 33\%$). Given the scenario, approximately 4,200 cases would occur over the period of a year. Approximately 215,500 vaccine doses would need to be administered to stop the outbreak (15). Vaccination distribution using two distinct models predicts that mass vaccination (MV) is superior over traced vaccination (TV). TV involves contact tracing with susceptible and exposed individuals being administered the vaccine, whereas MV occurs when everyone is vaccinated simultaneously according to a schedule. In these models, MV results in both fewer deaths and more rapid resolution of an epidemic (16). Vaccine production remains limited although numbers of available vaccine stock are increasing. Plans are to voluntarily vaccinate smallpox response teams, public health authorities and staff, and some law enforcement staff. The military were the first to be vaccinated (17).

Smallpox transmission occurs via droplets or as an aerosol from the respiratory tract or by fomite exposure to bedding or clothing. An incubation period of 7–17 days (average of 12 days) is followed by a fever for 2–4 days. A rash ensues that lasts for weeks as papules become vesicles, followed by pustules and scabs. A characteristic of smallpox that separates it from the initial chickenpox diagnosis is that all skin eruptions in a localized area are in the same stage at any given point in time. Chickenpox lesions are more superficial than the hard, deep-seated lesions of smallpox. Localized eruptions of HSV-2 may mimic smallpox (18). Disease transmission may occur as the fever (prodrome) phase ends and during the rash phase. As the lesions scab over, transmission decreases (19).

The smallpox vaccination is a suspended live vaccine derived from vaccinia. To prevent bacterial contamination of the lyophilized vaccine, polymyxin B, dihydrostreptomycin, chlortetracycline, and neomycin are included in the preparation. Other preparations under study include a calf-derived vaccine and a vaccinia virus grown in monkey kidney and human fibroblast cells.

Adverse Effects

Live vaccine can cause many adverse effects. (20,21). In a mass smallpox vaccination plan, to immunize 75% of the population (aged 1–65), 4600 serious adverse events and 285 deaths will occur (22).

Pustule formation. One of the negative impacts of the current smallpox vaccine program has been the realization that smallpox vaccine causes a noticeable pustule when immunization occurs. Many people currently being vaccinated have no prior experience with this type of vaccine. We have become accustomed to viral vaccines that are administered as a "shot"—i.e., influenza, hepatitis, MMR (measles, mumps and rubella), and VZV (chickenpox)—where an adverse effect consists of a little erythema and edema surrounding the injection sites. An open wound, improperly cared for, can become infected or can cause variolation on other body parts. The eyes are particularly sensitive to keratitis from fomite transmittal.

Allergy to vaccine components or residual immunity. Presence of a rapidly-forming erythema without development of the vesicle or pustule may indicate past vaccination immunity and/or allergy to vaccine compounds.

Death. Approximately one death per million vaccinations occurs. These usually occur among infants.

Local reactions. Most brief symptomatic reactions include fever, muscle aches, headache, nausea, and/or fatigue.

Eczema vaccinatum. Where active (or even healed) eczema/atopic dermatitis occurs, eczema vaccinatum can occur.

Immunocompromised. Progressive vaccinia may occur in patients with depressed cell-mediated immunity with increased numbers of HIV-positive patients and widespread use of immunosuppressive drugs.

Neurologic implications. Post vaccinal encephalomyelitis (PVEM) may occur even if there is no contraindication for vaccination (23). There are few signs of viral dissemination on the vaccine skin site, but neurologic symptoms may begin in 2–30 days after rash onset. Initial complaints are very similar to local reactions reported by others except that high fevers and other neurologic signs occur. Seizures are most frequent in children. Rates of PVEM differ and this is attributed to: 1) strain of vaccinia virus; 2) vaccine preparation; 3) viability of vaccinia virus used; 4) method of vaccine delivery; and 5) level of post vaccine surveillance (23).

Special Considerations

> **Vaccination of pregnant women.** There are reported cases of fetal vaccinia occuring after vaccination during pregnancy.
>
> **Coadministration of vaccine immune globin (VIG) with smallpox vaccine.** VIG may prevent or decrease the severity of smallpox. Post-exposure vaccination may also be effective if it is administered with in 4 days of known exposure.
>
> **Exposed persons with vaccine contraindications.** Administration of smallpox vaccine and VIG simultaneously can reduce side effects for those with vaccine contraindications who are exposed to an infected person (24).

New Vaccines for Poxviruses Currently under Investigation

Cell culture and recombinant vaccines may produce solid immunity with fewer complications. Should monkeypox continue to be transmitted from animal reservoirs to humans, there may be some effort to develop a vaccine. Fortunately, some immunity to many of the poxviruses is provided by the smallpox vaccination. One of the positions against destroying the remaining smallpox cultures is that the smallpox virus, itself, may become the backbone for a multiple-pox virus that would extend protection against orf, molluscum contagiosum, vaccinia, and other poxviruses. Others respond that the manipulated poxvirus strains are now the most important as they can confer immunity and do not cause disease. Obviously, the threat of poxviruses being used for terrorism is factored into the decision-making process.

MEASLES, MUMPS, AND RUBELLA VACCINES

Measles, mumps, and rubella are described in Chapter 3. Each of these viruses has its own vaccine to be described later. The vaccination for these three classic childhood diseases is typically given as a combination MMR vaccine (Table 4.3). Combination vaccines tend to require fewer total immunizations to achieve a satisfactory efficacy rate, are usually less expensive, and provide a greater opportunity to inoculate masses of people in a short period of time (25).

Table 4.3   Immunization Schedules

Footnotes for
Recommended Adult Immunization Schedule
by Age Group and Medical Conditions, United States, 2003–2004

1. **Tetanus and diphtheria (Td)**—Adults including pregnant women with uncertain histories of a complete primary vaccination series should receive a primary series of Td. A primary series for adults is 3 doses: the first 2 doses given at least 4 weeks apart and the 3rd dose, 6–12 months after the second. Administer 1 dose if the person had received the primary series and the last vaccination was 10 years ago or longer. Consult *MMWR* 1991; 40 (RR-10): 1–21 for administering Td as prophylaxis in wound management. The ACP Task Force on Adult Immunization supports a second option for Td use in adults: a single Td booster at age 50 years for persons who have completed the full pediatric series, including the teenage/young adult booster. *Guide for Adult Immunization*. 3rd ed. ACP 1994:20.

2. **Influenza vaccination**—Medical indications: chronic disorders of the cardiovascular or pulmonary systems including asthma; chronic metabolic diseases including diabetes mellitus, renal dysfunction, hemoglobinopathies, or immunosuppression (including Immunosuppression caused by medications or by human immunodefidency virus [HIV]), requiring regular medical follow-up or hospitalization during the preceding year; women who will be in the second or third trimester of pregnancy during the influenza season. Occupational indications: health-care workers. Other indications: residents of nursing homes and other long-term care facilities; persons likely to transmit influenza to persons at high-risk (in-home care givers to persons with medical indications, household contacts and out-of-home caregivers of children birth to 23 months of age, or children with asthma or other indicator conditions for influenza vaccination, household members and care givers of elderly and adults with high-risk conditions); and anyone who wishes to be vaccinated. For healthy persons aged 5–49 years without high risk conditions, either the inactivated vaccine or the intranasally administered influenza vaccine (Flumist) may be given. *MMWR* 2003; 52 (RR-B):1–36; *MMWR* 2003; 53 (RR-13):1–8.

3. **Pneumococcal polysaccharide vaccination**—Medical indications: chronic disorders of the pulmonary system (excluding asthma), cardiovascular diseases, diabetes mellitus, chronic liver diseases including liver disease as a result of alcohol abuse (e.g., cirrhosis), chronic renal failure or nephrotic syndrome, functional or an atomic asplenia (e.g., sickle cell disease or splenectomy), immunosuppressive conditions (e.g., congenital immunodeficiency, HIV infection, leukemia, lymphoma, multiple myeloma, Hodgkins disease, generalized malignancy, organ or bone marrow transplantation), chemotherapy with alkylating agents, antimetabolites, or long-term systemic corticosteroids. Geographic/other indications: Alaskan Natives and certain American Indian populations. Other indications: residents of nursing homes and other long-term care facilities. *MMWR* 1997; 45(RR-8):1–24.

4. **Revaccination with pneumococcal polysaccharide vaccine**—One time revaccination after 5 years for persons with chronic renal failure or nephrotic syndrome, functional or anatomic asplenia (e.g., sickle cell disease or splenectomy), immunosuppressive conditions (e.g., congenital immunodeficiency, HIV infection, leukemia, lymphoma, multiple myeloma, Hodgkins disease, generalized malignancy, organ or bone marrow transplantation), chemotherapy with alkylating agents, antimetabolites, or long-term systemic corticosteroids. For persons 65 and older, one-time revaccination if they were vaccinated 5 or more years previously and were aged less than 65 years at the time of primary vaccination. *MMWR* 1997; 46(RR-8):1–24.

5. **Hepatitis B vaccination**—Medical indications: hemodialysis patients, patients who receive dotting-factor concentrates. Occupational indications: health-care workers and public-safety workers who have exposure to blood in the workplace, persons in training in schools of medicine, dentistry, nursing, laboratory technology, and other allied health professions. Behavioral indications: injecting drug users, persons with more than one sex partner in the previous 6 months, persons with a recently acquired sexually-transmitted disease (STD), all clients in STD clinics, men who have sex with men. Other indications: household contacts and sex partners of persons with chronic HBV infection, clients and staff of institutions for the developmentally disabled, international travelers who will be in countries with high or intermediate prevalence of chronic HBV infection for more than 6 months, inmates of correctional facilities. *MMWR* 1991; 40 (RR-13):1–19.
(www.cdc.gov/travel/diseases/hby.htm)

6. **Hepatitis A vaccination**—For the combined HepA-HepB vaccine use 3 doses at 0, 1, 6 months). Medical indications: persons with dotting-factor disorders or chronic liver disease. Behavioral indications: men who have sex with

(continued)

Table 4.3 (Continued)

Footnotes for
Recommended Adult Immunization Schedule
by Age Group and Medical Conditions, United States, 2003–2004

men, users of injecting and noninjecting illegal drugs. Occupational indications: persons working with HAV-infected primates or with HAV in a research laboratory setting. Other indications: persons traveling to or working in countries that have high or intermediate endemicity of hepatitis A.
MMWR 1999; 48 (RR-12):1–37, (www.cdc.gov/travel/diseases/hav.htm)

7. **Measles, Mumps, Rubella vaccination (MMR)**—Measles component: Adults born before 1957 may be considered immune to measles. Adults born in or after 1957 should receive at least one dose of MMR unless they have a medical contraindication, documentation of at least one dose or other acceptable evidence of immunity. A second dose of MMR is recommended for adults who:

- are recently exposed to measles or in an outbreak setting
- were previously vaccinated with killed measles vaccine
- were vaccinated with an unknown vaccine between 1963 and 1967
- are students in post-secondary educational institutions
- work in health care facilities
- plan to travel internationally

Mumps component: 1 dose of MMR should be adequate for protection. Rubella component: Give 1 dose of MMR to women whose rubella vaccination history is unreliable and counsel women to avoid becoming pregnant for 4 weeks after vaccination. For women of child-bearing age, regardless of birth year, routinely determine rubella immunity and counsel women regarding congenital rubella syndrome. Do not vaccinate pregnant women or those planning to become pregnant in the next 4 weeks. If pregnant and susceptible, vaccinate as early in postpartum period as possible.
MMWR 1998; 47 (RR-8):1–57; *MMWR* 2001; 50:1117.

8. **Varicella vaccination**—Recommended for all persons who do not have reliable clinical history of varicella infection, or serological evidence of varicella zoster virus (VZV) infection who may be at high risk for exposure or transmission.

This includes, health-care workers and family contacts or immunocompromised persons, those who live or work in environments where transmission is likely (e.g., teachers of young children, day care employees, and residents and staff members in institutional settings), persons who live or work in environments where VZV transmission can occur (e.g., college students, inmates and staff members of correctional institutions, and military personnel), adolescents and adults living in households with children, women who are not pregnant but who may become pregnant in the future, international travelers who are not immune to infection.
Note: Greater than 95% of U.S. born adults are immune to VZV. Do not vaccinate pregnant women or those planning to become pregnant in the next 4 weeks. If pregnant and susceptible, vaccinate as early in postpartum period as possible.
MMWR 1996; 45 (RR-11):1–36; *MMWR* 1999; 48 (RR-6):1–5.

9. **Meningococcal vaccine (quadrivalent polysaccharide for serogroups A, C, Y, and W-135)**—Consider vaccination for persons with medical indications: adults with terminal complement component deficiencies, with anatomic or functional asplenia. Other indications: travelers to countries in which disease is hyperendemic or epidemic (*meningitis belt* of sub-Saharan Africa, Mecca, Saudi Arabia for Hajj). Revaccination at 3–5 years may be indicated for persons at high risk for infection (e.g., persons residing in areas in which disease is epidemic). Counsel college freshmen, especially those who live in dormitories, regarding meningococcal disease and the vaccine so that they can make an educated decision about receiving the vaccination. *MMWR* 2000; 49 (RR-7):1–20.
Note: The AAFP recommends that colleges should take the lead on providing education on meningococcal infection and vaccination and offer it to those who are interested. Physicians need not initiate discussion of the meningococcal quadravalent polysaccharide vaccine as part of routine medical care.

(continued)

Table 4.3 *(Continued)*

Recommended Adult Immunization Schedule by Age Group and Medical Conditions United States, 2003–2004

Summary of Recommendations Published by

The Advisory Committee on Immunization Practices

 Department of Health and Human Services
Centers for Disease Control and Prevention

(continued)

Table 4.3 *(Continued)*

Recommended Childhood and Adolescent Immunization Schedule – United States, January – June 2004

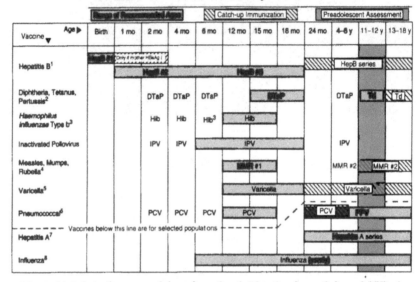

This schedule indicates the recommended ages for routine administration of currently licensed childhood vaccines, as of December 1, 2003, for children through age 18 years. Any dose not given at the recommended age should be given at any subsequent visit when indicated and feasible. ▨ Indicates age groups that warrant special effort to administer those vaccines not previously given. Additional vaccines may be licensed and recommended during the year. Licensed combination vaccines may be used whenever any components of the combination are indicated and the vaccine's other components are not contraindicated. Providers should consult the manufacturers' package inserts for detailed recommendations. Clinically significant adverse events that follow immunization should be reported to the Vaccine Adverse Event Reporting System (VAERS). Guidance about how to obtain and complete a VAERS form can be found on the internet: http://www.vaers.org/ or by calling 1-800-822-7967.

1. Hepatitis B (HepB) vaccine. All infants should receive the first dose of hepatitis B vaccine soon after birth and before hospital discharge; the first dose may also be given by age 2 months if the infant's mother is hepatitis B surface antigen (HBsAg) negative. Only monovalent HepB can be used for the birth dose. Monovalent or combination vaccine containing HepB may be used to complete the series. Four doses of vaccine may be administered when a birth dose is given. The second dose should be given at least 4 weeks after the first dose, except for combination vaccines which cannot be administered before age 6 weeks. The third dose should be given at least 16 weeks after the first dose and at least 8 weeks after the second dose. The last dose in the vaccination series (third or fourth dose) should not be administered before age 24 weeks.

Infants born to HBsAg-positive mothers should receive HepB and 0.5 mL of Hepatitis B Immune Globulin (HBIG) within 12 hours of birth at separate sites. The second dose is recommended at age 1 to 2 months. The last dose in the immunization series should not be administered before age 24 weeks. These infants should be tested for HBsAg and antibody to HBsAg (anti-HBs) at age 9 to 15 months.

Infants born to mothers whose HBsAg status is unknown should receive the first dose of the HepB series within 12 hours of birth. Maternal blood should be drawn as soon as possible to determine the mother's HBsAg status; if the HBsAg test is positive, the infant should receive HBIG as soon as possible (no later than age 1 week). The second dose is recommended at age 1 to 2 months. The last dose in the immunization series should not be administered before age 24 weeks.

(continued)

Table 4.3 (Continued)

2. **Diphtheria and tetanus toxoids and acellular pertussis (DTaP) vaccine.** The fourth dose of DTaP may be administered as early as age 12 months, provided 6 months have elapsed since the third dose and the child is unlikely to return at age 15 to 18 months. The final dose in the series should be given at age ≥4 years. Tetanus and diphtheria toxoids (Td) is recommended at age 11 to 12 years if at last 5 years have elapsed since the last dose of tetanus and diphtheria toxoid-containing vaccine. Subsequent routine Td boosters are recommended every 10 years.

3. *Haemophilus Influenzae* **type b (Hib) conjugate vaccine.** Three Hib conjugate vaccines are licensed for infant use. If PRP-OMP (PedvaxHIB or ComVax [Merck] is administered at ages 2 and 4 months, a dose at age 6 months is not reqeired. DTaP/Hib combination products should not be used for primary immunization in infants at ages 2, 4 or 6 months but can be used as boosters following any Hib vaccine. The find dose in the series should be given at age ≥12 months.

4. **Measles, mumps, and rubella vaccine (MMR).** The second dose of MMR is recommended routinely at age 4 to 6 years but may be administered during any visit, provided at least 4 weeks have elapsed since the first dose and both doses are administered beginning at or after age 12 months. Those who have not previously received the second dose should complete the schedule by the 11- to 12-year-old visit.

5. **Varicella vaccine.** Varicella vaccine is recommended at any visit at or after age 12 months for susceptible children (i.e., those who lack a reliable history of chickenpox). Susceptible persons age ≥13 years should receive 2 doses, given at least 4 weeks apart.

6. **Pneumococcal vaccine.** The heptavalent pneumococcal conjugate vaccine (PCV) is recommended for all children age 2 to 23 months. It is also recommended for certain children age 24 to 59 months. The final dose in the series should be given at age ≥12 months. Pneumococcal polysaccharide vaccine (PPV) is recommended in addition to PCV for certain high-risk groups. See *MMWR* 2000;49(RR-9):1–38.

7. **Hepatitis A vaccine.** Hepatitis A vaccine is recommended for children and adolescents is selected states and regions and for certain high-risk groups; consult your local public health authority. Children and adolescents in these states, regions, and high-risk groups who have not been immunized against hepatitis A can begin the hepatitis A immunization series during any visit. The 2 doses in the series should be administered at least 6 months apart. See *MMWR* 1999;48(RR-12):1–37.

8. **Influenza vaccine.** Influenza vaccine is recommended annually for children age ≥6 months with certain risk factors (including but not limited to children with asthma, cardiac disease, sickle cell disease, human immunodeficiency virus infection, and diabetes; and household members of persons in high-risk groups [see *MMWR* 2003;52 (RR-8):1–36]) and can be administered to all others wishing to obtain immunity. In addition, healthy children age 6 to 23 months are encouraged to receive influenza vaccine if feasible, because children in this age group are at substantially increased risk of influenza-related hospitalizations. For healthy persons age 5 to 49 years, the intranasally administered live-attenuated influenza vaccine (LAIV) is an acceptable alternative to the intramuscular trivalent inactivated influenza vaccine (TIV). See *MMWR* 2003;52(RR-13):1–8. Children receiving TIV should be administered a dosage appropriate for their age (0.25 mL if age 6 to 35 months or 0.5 mL if age ≥3 years). Children age ≤ 8 years who are receiving influenza vaccine for the first time should receive 2 doses (separated by at least 4 weeks for TIV and at least 6 weeks for LAIV).

For additional information about vaccines, including precautions and contraindications for immunization and vaccine shortages, please visit the National Immunization Program Web site at www.cdc.gov/nip/ or call the National Immunization Information Hotline at 800-232-2522 (English) or 800-232-0233 (Spanish)

Approved by the Advisory Committee on Immunization Practices (www.cdc.gov/nip/acip), the American Academy of pediatrics (www.aap.org), and the American Academy of Family Physicians (www.aafp.org).

(continued)

Table 4.3 (Continued)

For Children and Adolescents Who Start Late or Who Are >1 Month Behind

The tables below give catch-up schedules and minimum intervals between doses for children who have delayed immunizations. There is no need to restart a vaccine series regardless of the time that has elapsed between doses. Use the chart appropriate for the child's age.

Catch-up schedule for children age 4 months through 6 years

Dose 1 (Minimum Age)	Minimum Interval Between Doses			
	Dose 1 to Dose 2	Dose 2 to Dose 3	Dose 3 to Dose 4	Dose 4 to Dose 5
DTaP (6 wk)	4 wk	4 wk	6 mo	6 mo[1]
IPV (6 wk)	4 wk	4 wk	4 wk[2]	
HepB[3] (birth)	4 wk	8 wk (and 16 wk after first dose)		
MMR (12 mo)	4 wk[4]			
Varicella (12 mo)				
Hib[5] (6 wk)	4 wk: If first dose given at age <12 mo. 8 wk (as final dose): If first dose given at age 12–14 mo. No further doses needed: If first dose given at age ≥ 15 mo	4 wk[6]: If current age <12 mo. 8 wk (as final dose)[6]: If current age ≥12 mo and second dose given at age <15 mo. No further doses needed: If previous dose given at age ≥15 mo	8 wk (as final dose): this dose only necessary for children age 12 mo–5 y who received 3 doses before age 12 mo	
PCV[7] (6 wk)	4 wk: If first dose given at age <12 mo and current age <24 mo. 8 wk (as final dose): If first dose given at age ≥12 mo or current age 24–59 mo. No further doses needed: for healthy children if first dose given at age ≥24 mo	4 wk: If current age <12 mo. 8 wk (as final dose): If current age ≥12 mo. No further doses needed: for healthy children if previous dose given at age ≥24 mo	8 wk (as final dose): this dose only necessary for children age 12 mo–5 y who received 3 doses before age 12 mo	

(continued)

Table 4.3 *(Continued)*

For Children and Adolescents Who Start Late or Who Are >1 Month Behind

The tables below give catch-up schedules and minimum intervals between doses for children who have delayed immunizations. There is no need to restart a vaccine series regardless of the time that has elapsed between doses. Use the chart appropriate for the child's age.

Catch-up schedule for children age 7 through 18 years

	Minimum Interval Between Doses		
	Dose 1 to Dose 2	Dose 2 to Dose 3	Dose 3 to Booster Dose
TD:	4 wk	TD: 6 mo	TD[8]: 6 mo: If first dose given at age <12 mo and current age <11 y 5 y: If first dose given at age ≥12 mo and third dose given at age <7 y and current age ≥ 11 y 10 y: If third dose given at age ≥ 7 y
IVP[9]:	4 wk	IPV[9]: 4 wk	IPV[2,9]
HepB:	4 wk	HepB: 8 wk (and 16 wk after first dose)	
MMR:	4 wk		
Varicella[10]:	4 wk		

(continued)

Table 4.3 (Continued)

1. **DTaP:** The fifth dose is not necessary if the fourth dose was given after the fourth birthday.

2. **IPV:** For children who received an all-IPV or all-oral poliovirus (OPV) series, a fourth dose is not necessary if third dose was given at age ≥4 years. If both OPV and IPV were given as part of a series, a total of 4 doses should be given, regardless of the child's current age.

3. **HepB:** All Children and adolescents who have not been immunized against hepatitis B should begin the HepB immunization series during any visit. Providers should make special efforts to immunize children who were born in, or whose parents were born in, areas of the world where hepatitis B virus infection is moderately or highly endemic.

4. **MMR:** The second dose of MMR is recommended routinely at age 4 to 6 years but may be given earlier if desired.

5. **Hib:** Vaccine is not generally recommended for children age ≥5 years.

6. **Hib:** If current age <12 months and the first 2 doses were PRP-OMP (PedvaxHIB or ComVax [Merck]), the third (and final) dose should be given at age 12 to 15 months and at least 8 weeks after the second dose.

7. **PCV:** Vaccine is not generally recommended for children age ≥5 years.

8. **Td:** For children age 7 to 10 years, the interval between the third and booster dose is determined by the age when the first dose was given. For adolescents age 11 to 18 years, the interval is determined by the age when the third dose was given.

9. **IPV:** Vaccine is not generally recommended for persons age ≥18 years.

10. **Varicella:** Give 2-dose series to all susceptible adolescents age ≥13 years.

Reporting Adverse Reactions
Report adverse reactions to vaccines through the federal Vaccine Adverse Event Reporting System. For information on reporting reactions following immunization, please visit www.vaers.org or call the 24-hour national toll-free information line (800)822-7967.

Disease Reporting
Report suspected cases of vaccine-preventable diseases to your state or local health department.

For additional information about vaccines, including precautions and contraindications for immunization and vaccine shortages, please visit the National Immunization Program Web site at www.cdc.gov/nip or call the National Immunization Information Hotline at 800-232-2522 (English) or 800-232-0233 (Spanish).

(continued)

Table 4.3 (*Continued*)

Recommended Adult Immunization Schedule, United States, 2003–2004
by Age Group

Age Group ▶ Vaccine ▼	19–49 Years	50–64 Years	65 Years and older
Tetanus, Diphtheria (Td)*	1 does booster every 10 years[1]		
Influenza	1 dose annually[2]	1 dose annually[2]	
Pneumococcal (polysaccharide)	1 dose[3,4]		1 dose[3,4]
Hepatitis B*	3 doses (0, 1–2, 4–6 months)[5]		
Hepatitis A	2 doses (0, 6–12 months)[6]		
Measles, Mumps, Rubella (MMR)*	1 dose if measles, mumps, or rubella vaccination history is unreliable; 2 doses for persons with occupassional or other indications[7]		
Varicella*	2 doses (0, 4–8 weeks) for persons who are susceptible[8]		
Meningococcal (polysaccharide)	1 dose[9]		

See Footnotes for Recommended Adult Immunization Schedule, by Age Group and Medical Conditions United States, 2003–2004 on back cover

☐ For all persons in this group   ◩ Catch-up on childhood vaccinations   ▨ For persons with medical/ exposure indications

* Covered by the Vaccine injury Compensation Program For Information on how to file a claim call 800-338-2382. Please also disit www.hrq.gov/otp/vicp. To file a claim for vaccine injury contact: U.S. Court of Federal Claims, 717 Madison Place, H.W., Washington D.C. 20005, 202-219-9657.

This schedule indicates the recommended age groups for routine administration of currently licensed vaccines for persons 19 years of age and older. Licensed combination vaccines may be used whenever any components of the combination are indicated and the vaccines other components are not contraindicated Providers should consult the manufactures' package inserts for detailed recommendations.

Report all clinically significant post-vaccination reactions to the Vaccine Adverse Event Reporting System (VAERS). Reporting forms and instructions on filing a VAERS report are available by calling 800-822-7967 or from the VAERS website at www.vaers.org.

For additional information about the vaccines listed above and contraindications for immunization, visit the National Immunization Program Website at www.cdc.gov/nip/ or call the National Immunization Hotline at 800-232-2522 (English) or 800-232-0233 (Spanish).

Approved by the Advisory Committee on Immunization Practices (ACIP), and accepted by the American College of Obstetridans and Gynecologists (ACOG) and the American of Family Physicians (AAFP)

(*continued*)

Table 4.3   *(Continued)*

Recommended Adult Immunization Schedule, United States, 2003–2004 by Medical Conditions

Medical Conditions ▼ \ Vaccine ▶	Tetanus-Diphtheria (Td)[a,1]	Influenza[2]	Pneumo-coccal (polysacch-aride) [3,4]	Hepatitis B[a,5]	Hepatitis A[6]	Measles, Mumps, Rubelia (MME)[a,7]	Varicalla[a,8]
Pregnancy		A					
Diabetes, heart disease, chronic pulmonary disease, chronic liver disease, including chronic alcoholism		B	C		D		
Congenital immunodeficiency, leukemia, lymphoma, generalized malignancy, therapy with alkylating agents, antimetabolites, radiation or large amounts of corticosteroids			E				F
Renal failure / and stage renal disease, recipients of hemodialysis or clotting factor concentrates			E	G			
Asplenia including elective splenectomy and terminal complement component deficiencies		H	E,I,J				
HIV infection			E,K			L	

See Special Notes for Medical Conditions below—also see Footnotes for Recommended Adult Immunization Schedule, by Age Group and Medical Conditions United States, 2003-2004 on back cover

▪ For all persons in this group   ◩ Catch-up on childhood vaccinations   ▨ For persons with medical/ exposure indications   ▫ Contraindicated

Special Notes for Medical Conditions

A. For women without chronic diseases/conditions, vaccinate If pregnancy will be at 2nd or 3rd trimester during influenza season. For women with chronic deseases/conditions, vaccinate at any time during the pregnancy.

B. Although chronic liver disease and alcoholism are not indicator conditions for influenza vaccination, give 1 dose annually if the patent is ≥50 years, has other indications for influenza vaccine, or if the patient requests vaccination.

C. Asthma a is an indication condition for influenza but not for pneumococcal vaccination.

D. For all persons with chornic liver disease.

E. For persons < 65 years revaccinate once after 5 years or more have elapsed since initial vaccination.

F. Persons with impaired humoral immunity but intact cellular immunity may be vaccinated, *MMWR* 1999;48 (RR-06):1–5.

G. Hemodialysis patients: Use special formulation of vaccine (40 ug/mL) or two 1.0 ml 20 ug doses given at one site. Vaccinate early in the course of renal disease. Assess antibody iters to hep B surface antigen (anti-HBs) levels annually. Administer additional doses if anti-HBs levels decline to < 10 milliinternational units (mlUl/mL.

H. There are no data specially on risk of severe or complicated influenza infections among persons with asplenia. However, Influenza is a risk factor for secondary bacterial infections that may cause severe disease in asplenics.

I. Administer meningococcal vaccine and consider Hib vaccine.

J. Elective splenectomy: vaccinate at least 2 weeks before surgery.

K. Vaccinate as close to diagnosis as possible when CD4 cell counts are highest.

L. Withhold MMR or other measles containing vaccines from HIV-infected persons with evidence of severe immunosuppression. *MMWR* 1998;47 (RR-8):21–22; *MMWR* 2002:51 (RR-02);22–24.

Live virus vaccines for measles, mumps, rubella were introduced in the 1960s and, after widespread implementation in the United States, annual reported cases of these infections declined by more than 98% (26). The most recent recommendations by the Centers for Disease Control and Prevention (CDC) suggest vaccination with the first MMR dose at 12–15 months and the second dose at 4–6 years of age (27). Two doses confer 92% immunity, which is sufficient to prevent epidemics.

Special Considerations

Pregnancy. Because these vaccines consist of live attenuated viruses, they should not be administered to pregnant women or those planning to become pregnant in the next 3 months. The theoretical risk of congenital rubella syndrome after immunization has been the primary concern. However, a study of 321 women who had received the rubella vaccine 3 months before or after conception revealed no congenital malformations compatible with congenital rubella infection (27).

Immunosuppressed. Immunization is also contraindicated in immunosuppressed patients, although it can be administered to individuals with asymptomatic HIV infection as well as persons with mild immunosuppression.

Healthy individuals. In healthy individuals, minor illnesses with or without fever are not a contraindication to vaccination.

Patients with a history of anaphylactic hypersensitivity to neomycin. These persons should not receive the MMR vaccine.

Egg allergy. The vaccine can be administered to patients with an allergy to eggs, since the risk for severe anaphylactic reactions is exceedingly low (28,29). It is recommended that these patients be observed for 90 minutes after immunization (29). Khahoo and Loch (28) report that most severe cardiorespiratory allergic reactions were reported in children who were most likely allergic to the gelatin or neomycin in the vaccine rather than ovalbumin.

Measles

Measles virus has been noted to be the most infectious disease of humankind, in terms of the minimal number of virions necessary to produce infection (30). An estimated 75% of susceptible family contacts who are exposed to a case of measles develop the disease (31). Because humans are the only reservoir for measles virus, global eradication is technically feasible. A meeting cosponsored by the World Health Organization, CDC, and the Pan American Health Organization convened in 1996 and adopted the goal of global eradication by a target date during 2005–2010 (32). Due to universal childhood immunization in the United States, measles is no longer considered an indigenous disease in this country. In 2001, a total of 116 confirmed measles cases were reported—54 internationally imported and 62 indigenous (37 import linked and 25 unknown sources). In 2002, a total of only 37 cases of measles were confirmed, which represents a record low number of reported cases. It is important, however, to guard against complacency with these encouraging figures. In 2003, 39 cases had been confirmed by August, which should serve as a reminder of the continuing need for vaccination (33).

Lack of compliance with routine MMR vaccination in the past led to a resurgence of measles infection in the United States from 1989–1991, with some deaths reported (32). Moreover, greater than 1 million children die of measles each year in Third World countries (34). The current measles vaccine is a further attenuated version of the live preparations previously available, resulting in fewer adverse reactions in recipients. It is produced by culturing the Moraten virus strain in chick embryo cells. Measles vaccination produces a mild or inapparent infection which is noncommunicable. Both humoral and cellular immune responses develop as a result (35). After receiving two doses of vaccine, 95–99% of recipients develop serologic evidence of immunity to measles (36,37). Immunity is thought to be life-long, similar to that acquired after infection with the wild-type virus (38). Measles infection has rarely been reported in patients with previously documented postimmunization seroconversion (39,40). In a recent measles outbreak in

Campania, Italy, low vaccination rates (76%) were cited as the main cause (41).

Adverse Effects

Adverse effects after measles vaccination are typically mild.

> **Fever.** Five to 15 percent of recipients develop a fever of at least 103°F for 1–2 days, generally between 5–12 days after immunization (42). These individuals are largely asymptomatic, but some may develop a transient viral exanthem (26).
>
> **Encephalitis.** An associated encephalitis or encephalopathy has rarely been reported after immunization, and occurs in less than 1 per 1 million vaccinees (43).
>
> **Subacute sclerosing panencephalitis.** There have been early concerns about the association of measles vaccination and subacute sclerosing pancencephalitis (SSPE), since this complication may occur with natural infection. A small number of reports have described the occurrence of SSPE in persons with a history of vaccination but no known history of infection (44–46). More recent evidence indicates that at least some of those cases had unrecognized natural measles infection prior to vaccination, and the SSPE was directly related to the infection (27). Widespread measles immunization has nearly eliminated SSPE in the United States, and the live measles vaccine does not increase the risk for this complication (27).

More recently, the measles vaccine has been administered as an aerosolized vaccine. Aerosol administration has fewer side effects than injection inoculation. Immunogenicity is superior in the aerosol administration when compared with traditional injections. Thus the potential efficacy and cost warrant further studies of aerosol measles immunizations (47).

Mumps

The live attenuated mumps vaccine (Jeryl-Lynn strain) is prepared in chick embryo cell culture. Immunization produces a mild subclinical infection that is noncommunicable. Early clinical studies have shown that 97% of children and 93% of adults develop serological evidence of immunity after vaccination (48–50). Outbreak-based studies, however, have reported lower efficacy rates, ranging from 75–95% protection from infection (51–54). Although the duration of immunity in vaccine recipients is not completely known, serologic and epidemiologic evidence suggests that immunity persists for at least 30 years (55–58).

Adverse Effents

Adverse reactions are generally mild and uncommon after mumps vaccination.

> **Fever, parotitis, and exanthem.** Low-grade fever, mild parotitis, and a viral exanthem have been reported.
>
> **Neurological effects.** Serious reactions such as adverse neurological effects are extremely rare and have not been causally associated with the mumps vaccine (59).

Rubella

Three different live attenuated rubella vaccine strains were initially developed and licensed in the United States. These were all replaced in 1979 by the RA 27/3 (rubella abortus 27, explant 3) vaccine which is grown in human diploid fibroblast cell culture. This vaccine produces nasal antibodies as well as higher and more persistent antibody titers, which better mimic the immune protection developed after natural infection (60,61).

Vaccination induces an antibody response in more than 97% of recipients (49,62). Immunity in vaccine recipients is thought to be lifelong, and has been shown to persist for at least 16 years (63,64).

Adverse Effects

Adverse effects after rubella vaccination are typically mild.

> **Fever, lymphoadenopathy, or exanthem.** 5–15% of vaccinated children develop fever, lymphadenopathy,

or a viral exanthem, typically between 5–12 days after vaccination (50,65).

Arthralgia/arthritis. Arthralgias and arthritis are a frequent complication in adult vaccinees, particularly women, and may develop in 25–40% of this population group (66–68). Occurrences in children are rare (0.5%) (66). These joint symptoms typically begin within the first 3 weeks after vaccination and remit within 11 days. The knees and the fingers are most frequently involved, but any joint may be affected (67).

Special Considerations

Pregnancy and vaccination rates. Failure to achieve 50–60% immunity to rubella by vaccination leaves women of childbearing age susceptible to developing rubella infection during pregnancy. This often causes congenital rubella in children born of mothers who contract rubella during early pregnancy. For example, rubella immunization in Greece was classed as "optional," but less than 50% of the children were vaccinated. An epidemic in Greece in 1993 affected more women of childbearing age than ever before. This, in turn, was followed by the births of the largest number of babies with congenital rubella ever recorded in Greece (69).

VARICELLA-ZOSTER VIRUS VACCINE

Prior to the widespread availability of varicella vaccine, yearly U.S. figures for varicella disease included approximately 4 million cases, 11,000 hospitalizations, and 100 deaths (70). The currently available varicella vaccine in the United States is a live-attenuated Oka strain vaccine approved in 1995. The vaccine is very safe and effective (71–73). Clinical trials began over 20 years earlier in Japan after the vaccine was developed by attenuation of virus isolated from the vesicular fluid of a healthy boy (with the surname Oka) with natural varicella infection (74). These initial studies showed a 90% seroconversion rate 4 weeks after vaccination with few clinical reactions (75). Follow-up studies showed that the vaccine protected against chickenpox for at least 17–19 years, and all of the subjects had persistent antibodies and delayed-type skin reactions to the varicella-zoster antigen (76). In the United States, a double-blind, placebo-controlled study of the Oka vaccine in 914 children revealed an efficacy of 100% at 9 months (77). After a seven-year follow-up, 95% of the subjects remained free of clinical disease with chickenpox (78). Compared with the disease rates of unvaccinated children in the United States, it appears that the Oka vaccine reduces the rate of varicella in children participating in the clinical trials by 65–90% (74). Additional studies in the United States have shown that the Oka vaccine induces humoral and cell-mediated immunity in healthy children (79–81), both of which have been demonstrated to persist for at least 8 years (82). Delayed-type hypersensitivity skin reactions to varicella-zoster virus antigens have also been shown to occur for at least 10 years after vaccination (83).

Studies of adolescents and adults have demonstrated that 2 doses 4–8 weeks apart were necessary to produce seroconversion rates and antibody responses similar to those obtained in healthy children (84). Vaccination is recommended for susceptible adults, particularly those in high-risk situations (health-care personnel, etc.). The vaccine is recommended for all children who have no history of chickenpox and is required to attend school in most states. Clinical studies have also evaluated the use of vaccination in immunosuppressed children and adolescents, particularly in those with acute lymphocytic leukemia (85–87). Results indicated that vaccination is safe for those who are at least 1 year away from induction chemotherapy if the current chemotherapy is halted around the time of vaccination and the patient's lymphocyte counts are >700/mm^3. The immune response in these individuals is lower than that of healthy recipients, thus requiring 2 doses separated by 3 months. Transmission of varicella from these vaccinees may occur if a vaccine-associated rash develops, although the risk of transmission is about one-fourth that of natural varicella (20–25% vs 87%) (88). The Oka vaccine should be given as a single dose to children 12 months to 12 years of age. Individuals over the age of 13 should receive 2 doses, 4–8 weeks apart. The duration of protection is unknown at this time, and the need for a booster immunization is uncertain. It has been observed that vaccinees who are exposed to natural varicella have a boost in antibody levels. However, it is postulated that in a highly vaccinated population, a lack of exposure to natural varicella may result in waning immunity for some.

Adverse Effects

Modified varicella-like syndrome. Multiple studies have reported a modified varicella-like syndrome (MVLS) in some vaccinated children after exposure to the natural wild-type varicella virus (78,89,90). The average rate of MVLS varies from 0.00–2.72% of vaccinated children each year after vaccination with the U.S. licensed Oka strain vaccine. These children typically develop a milder form of disease with less than 50 lesions. Most children do not have associated fever, and only 50% of them develop vesicular lesions (91). None of the cases have been associated with systemic or serious disease. It has been noted that more complete and long-lasting protection from varicella is associated with a stronger antibody response to vaccination (89).

Latent infection. Herpes zoster can later develop either from the Oka strain vaccine-type virus or from natural wild-type varicella-zoster virus (92,93). There have been several reports of mild herpes zoster in healthy children who had previously received the varicella vaccine. The incidence is less than that seen in children with prior chickenpox (94), such that vaccinated persons may have a decreased risk for herpes zoster.

Tenderness, erythema, or induration at the injection site. This most common side effect occurs in 19.3–24.4% of injection sites.

Fever. Fever occurred in 10.2–14.7% of clinical trial subjects and a generalized varicella-like rash developed in 3.8–5.5% of subjects.

Rash. A generalized varicella-like rash developed in 3.8–5.5% of cases. A localized varicella-like rash at the injection site may also occur.

Special Considerations

Exposure to high-risk patients. The likelihood of transmission of the vaccine virus from a healthy vaccinee is low, but may be more likely if a rash develops after vaccination. One case of transmission from a vaccinated child to a susceptible mother has been reported in the United States, but it is suspected that the child may have been concurrently infected with natural wild-type varicella. Individuals receiving vaccination should avoid close association with susceptible high-risk individuals for up to 6 weeks, if possible.

Pregnancy. This vaccination is also contraindicated in pregnancy or any women planning to become pregnant within 3 months, since this is a live attenuated virus and natural varicella is known to cause fetal harm.

Susceptible contact exposure. Recent data indicates that the varicella vaccine is highly effective in preventing disease in susceptible contacts when given within 36 hours of exposure (95).

INFLUENZA VIRUS VACCINE

Influenza types A and B are discussed in Chapter 3.

Every year, immunologists and epidemiologists prepare a vaccine combination based on an educated guess. The new vaccine must be developed and produced rapidly to meet expected needs. Pandemics, such as those in 1917–1919, 1957, 1968, 1977, and 1997, present even more challenges, particularly with the need for safety, quality, and efficacy of the vaccine. Most influenza vaccines are influenza virus grown in embryonated hen's eggs, purified and inactivated. Concerns of this type of vaccine are that it takes 7–8 months of lead time to produce the vaccine. Often a single 15 μg heamagglutinin dose may not confer sufficient immunity. On the other hand, whole virus vaccines are more immunogenic than split or sub-unit vaccines. H5 vaccines may need an adjuvant (96). Soluble, recombinant forms of influenza A virus have been suggested (97). Other suggestions for improved vaccines are better vaccine production technologies, reverse genetics technology, and novel adjuvants to improve immunogenicity (98). Currently, the trivalent inactivated vaccines are available as subvirion (split), purified surface antigen (subunit), and whole virus preparations.

Those who are most at risk for influenza complications are the very young and the very elderly. More than 80% of children and young adults who received influenza vaccination developed high levels of antibody titers (99). Whole-virus influenza vaccines should not be given to children ≤12 years old, due to increased potential for febrile reactions (100). Therefore, for children 1–16 years old, the inactivated trivalent influenza vaccines are well tolerated and provided 91.4% efficacy for influenza A H1N1 and 77.3% efficacy for influenza A H3N2 (101).

Vaccination in the elderly has been shown to lessen the risk of complications, hospitalization and death (102,103). In children and young adults, the influenza vaccine has been 70–90% effective in preventing influenza during controlled trials with a good match between the vaccine and circulating influenza strains (104,106). In the elderly, inactivated virus vaccines have less efficacy due to the declining integrity of elderly immune systems. Only 17% of persons over 65 years are expected to increase antibody titers to all three vaccines components and 46% fail to respond to any of them. Perhaps a prophylactic treatment, such as neuraminidase inhibitors can be used to boost immunogenicity (107). A study of vaccination in low-risk elderly persons demonstrated a 58% efficacy in preventing laboratory-confirmed influenza (108). When studied in elderly nursing home residents, influenza vaccine is 30–40% effective in preventing influenza illness, but is also 50–60% effective in preventing pneumonia or hospitalization and 80% effective in preventing death (109,110). Immunity following influenza vaccination begins within 1–2 weeks and rarely persists beyond 1 year (111). Protective antibody levels may only last 4 months or less in certain elderly patients (112). In addition, the strains of influenza may differ significantly from one season to the next, thus increasing the need for annual vaccinations.

Influenza immunization is indicated for anyone aged ≥6 months who is at increased risk for complications of influenza or is in contact with those individuals (i.e. caregivers, medical personnel). The at-risk population includes persons ≥65 years of age, residents of nursing homes, those with chronic pulmonary or cardiovascular disorders, and persons with HIV. Vaccination is also indicated for individuals who desire to decrease their risk for influenza infection. The immunization regimen consists of one dose given each year, from September through mid-November, to prepare for the winter's influenza activity. Administration of the vaccine is still recommended after mid-November if influenza activity has not peaked in the community. Previously unvaccinated children <9 years of age should receive 2 vaccine doses at least 1 month apart to develop sufficient antibody levels (100).

Adverse Effects

These symptoms typically begin within 6–12 hours and persist for 1–2 days. In one clinical trial, the incidence of adverse effects did not differ between the vaccinated group and placebo (113).

Fever.
Malaise.
Headache.
Arthralgia.
Myalgia.
Guillain-Barré syndrome (GBS). A significantly increased frequency of GBS was found with the 1976 swine influenza vaccine (114), but more recent investigations show an extremely small risk of GBS with the current vaccines, which is slightly more than one extra case per 1 million vaccinees (100).
Immediate allergic reactions. Hives, angioedema, or systemic anaphylaxis rarely occur after vaccination

(115). These hypersensitivity reactions are most likely due to residual egg-protein exposure to sensitive patients.

Special Considerations

Egg allergies. The majority of egg-allergic subjects can safely receive immunization, but those with a history of anaphylactic reaction to eggs or previous influenza vaccines should discuss their history of such allergies with their physician before a decision is made regarding vaccination (100).

New Developments in Influenza Vaccines

A new intranasal vaccine was recently approved as an alternative form of influenza vaccination. The cold-adapted, live attenuated, trivalent influenza virus vaccine (FluMist) is able to replicate in the cooler nasal passages and stimulate mucosal as well as systemic immunity, similar to natural infection. However, the altered virus is unable to grow in the warmer temperatures of the lower respiratory tract. Clinical studies in children have shown the vaccine to be 93% effective in preventing culture-positive influenza A and B infections (116). Also, the vaccinated group had 21% fewer febrile illnesses and 30% fewer cases of febrile otitis media when compared with placebo. Adverse reactions were mild and included rhinorrhea, fever, and lethargy. A similar study in adults demonstrated 23% fewer days of severe febrile illness and 25% fewer days of febrile upper respiratory tract illness (117). This resulted in 28% fewer missed work days and 41% fewer physician visits. The intranasal vaccine first became available for the 2003–2004 influenza season.

HEPATITIS A VIRUS VACCINE

Both inactivated and attenuated forms of hepatitis A vaccines have been developed and studied. However, the inactivated vaccine is the only type licensed and available in the United States (Havrix and Vaqta). These vaccines are propagated in human diploid fibroblast culture and inactivated by formalin. Immunization generally involves 2 doses given 6–12 months apart in adults and children 2 years old and older. Studies of both available inactivated vaccines show excellent, as well as comparable, immunogenicity and efficacy rates. Overall, 97–99% of recipients have developed protective levels of antibodies 1 month after the first dose, and 99–100% of recipients were protected 1 month after the second dose (118–123). When studied in placebo-controlled clinical trials in Thailand (which has high rates of hepatitis A), two doses of the inactivated vaccine were 94% effective in protecting against hepatitis A infection (124). A similar study in New York children showed 100% efficacy after a single dose of vaccine (125). Because of limited long-term data on this vaccine, the duration of immunity is yet to be determined. In one study of a three-dose series in adults, detectable antibodies were documented in all subjects 4 years after immunization (126). Kinetic models of antibody concentration decline have estimated that protective levels of hepatitis A antibodies can be expected to persist for 20 years (127), and perhaps up to 30 years (128). A separate mathematical evaluation of long-term immunity after a primary dose and booster dose for hepatitis A has calculated that protective antibody levels should persist for 24–47 years (129). It is not known whether vaccine-induced immunity will persist beyond the loss of detectable antibody levels, as occurs with hepatitis B immunization, but this has been suggested to occur (129).

The hepatitis A vaccine is recommended for persons at least 2 years of age living in or traveling to areas of high endemicity for hepatitis A. It is also recommended for persons with chronic liver disease due to causes other than hepatitis A, persons engaging in high-risk sexual activity, residents of a community experiencing an outbreak of hepatitis A, and users of illicit injectable drugs. In addition, the hepatitis A vaccine is currently recommended for routine pediatric use in some states and regions. The need for hepatitis A vaccination for the general public was highlighted by the fact that the largest single outbreak of hepatitis A in U.S. history was reported in November 2003. In this outbreak, 555 persons became ill with hepatitis A (and 3 persons died) after eating green onions at a restaurant in Pennsylvania (130).

Adverse Effects

Adverse effects with hepatitis A vaccination are generally mild, and no serious side effects have been attributed to the vaccine in clinical trials (126).

> **Injection site.** Soreness.
> **Headache.** Headache occurs in 14% of vaccines.
> **Malaise.** Malaise occurs in 7% in adults.
> **Children.** Feeding problems (8%) and headaches (4%) occur in children.

Special Consideration

Travelers or those at risk for exposure for both hepatitis A and B might want to consider taking the combined hepatitis A and B vaccines. The combination reduces the number of injections from 5 to 3, taken over a 6-month period.

HEPATITIS B VIRUS VACCINE

Hepatitis B is described in Chapter 3. Immunization for hepatitis B became a reality in 1981 when the plasma-derived vaccine was licensed in the United States. This vaccine was highly effective in inducing immunity, but was associated with several drawbacks. The supply of suitable carrier plasma needed to make the vaccine was not sufficient for large-scale production. Also, despite the chemical treatment of plasma products for safety, there was some concern about the risk, albeit small, of HIV transmission (131). Both of these issues were addressed in 1986, when the yeast recombinant hepatitis B vaccine was licensed. This particular vaccine has been a major breakthrough for the field of medicine. It was the first licensed recombinant viral vaccine prototype, as well as the first effective viral vaccine for a sexually transmitted disease. This vaccine is produced by recombinant DNA technology, which inserts the gene for HBsAg (hepatitis B surface antigen) into the yeast *Saccharomyces cerevisiae* (baker's yeast). Clinical studies in high-risk homosexual men demonstrated three-dose vaccine efficacy of 82–93% in preventing acute hepatitis B (132,133). Overall, approximately 5% of immunocompetent adults fail to develop significant antibody titers after hepatitis B vaccination. Nearly 99% of children respond to vaccination (134), while only 50–70% of those over age 60 acquire immunity (135,136). Variables associated with a lower likelihood of seroconversion include immunosuppression, renal failure, prematurity with low birth weight, age older than 40 years, obesity, and smoking (137–139). Because of the decreased rates of seroconversion in specific populations, additional research is focusing on methods of increasing immunogenicity to hepatitis B vaccines. Alternative delivery systems, such as adenoviruses and vaccinia vectors, are under evaluation. Clinical trials are currently investigating the addition of adjuvants to the current recombinant vaccine in order to increase the host immune response (140,141). Several different types of vaccines are also in development, such as DNA vaccines (142) and Pre-S vaccines (143–145).

The duration of immunity afforded by vaccination merits further long-term studies, but according to present data, long-term efficacy is expected (139). Antibody levels decline rapidly in the first year after vaccination, and then level off to a slow pace of decline (146). The loss of detectable antibodies to hepatitis B years after vaccination does not necessarily indicate a lack of immunity. The majority of individuals are protected by immunological memory in B lymphocytes, which mount an anamnestic response to natural infection (147). Rare cases of hepatitis B infection in previously vaccinated patients have been described (148,149). These patients generally have subclinical disease, and none have developed chronic infection or serious complications (139).

The regimen for immunization includes three doses, given at months 0, 1, and 6. Hepatitis B vaccination is recommended for adults at risk (i.e., persons living in or traveling to areas of high endemicity of hepatitis B, health-care personnel, morticians, persons engaging in high risk sexual activity, persons with chronic liver disease due to causes other than hepatitis B, prisoners, users of illicit injectable drugs, and police and fire department personnel who render first aid) and all children aged 0–18 years. Because of the current widespread use in children, a thimerosal-free vaccine was recently approved by the FDA. Thimerosal is a mercury-containing preservative, which has prompted the limitation of its use in children (150). In persons in whom vaccine-induced protection is less complete, such as in hemodialysis patients, the need for a booster dose should be assessed by annual antibody testing.

Adverse Effects

Adverse effects after hepatitis B vaccination are generally mild and well-tolerated.

Fatigue. Fatigue is most commonly reported (15%).
Headache. Headache occurs in 9% of subjects.
Fever. Fever occurs in 1–9% of vaccinees (151,152).

A post-marketing clinical surveillance of 4.5 million doses of hepatitis B vaccine over 5 years revealed no serious or severe reactions attributable to the vaccine (153).

Rarely occurring adverse effects include:

Thrombocytopenic purpura (154–156).
Vasculitis (157,158).
Rheumatoid arthritis (159).
Lichen planus (160).
Lichenoid reaction (161).

However, it appears that these conditions do not occur at a higher rate than in the unvaccinated population. Large-scale hepatitis B vaccination programs have been unable to establish any association between the vaccine and severe adverse effects other than rare episodes of anaphylaxis (152,162).

On May 14, 2000, the FDA announced approval of a new combination vaccine that protects people at least 18 years of age against hepatitis A virus and hepatitis B virus. This vaccine, Twinrix®, combines two already approved vaccines, Havrix® and Engerix-B®, so that persons at high risk for exposure to both viruses can be immunized against both at the same time. The combination reduces the number of injections from 5 to 3.

RABIES VIRUS VACCINE

Rabies is a zoonotic virus transmitted to humans by bite, scratch, or vaporization to mucous membranes. Other terrestrial mammals are vectors. Once infection occurs, a series of progressive neoneuronal symptoms occur, such as nausea and vomiting, abdominal pain, headaches, photophobia, etc. These tend to progress to more serious symptoms involving muscle weaknesses, slurred speech, muchal rigidity, copious oral secretions, and agitation. Fever may vary by case from low grade to high (e.g., 104°F). Progressive encephalopathy ensues with coma preceding death.

Rabies continued to be a feared disease for centuries, even after Louis Pasteur developed the first vaccine (1885) for post-exposure treatment of rabies (163). This and several other rabies vaccines that followed contained brain or nerve tissue, which posed a serious risk of neurological complications. In addition, some of these vaccines led to pathogenic infections because of imperfect inactivation of the vaccine virus. Safer duck embryo vaccines were later introduced, but proved to be less immunogenic. After years of development and studies, the cell culture-derived vaccines have become the "gold standard" for rabies immunization. The human diploid cell vaccine (HDCV) was licensed in the United States in 1980, and contains concentrated and purified inactivated rabies virus from the Pitman-Moore strain.

When compared with brain tissue vaccine and duck embryo vaccine, human diploid cell cultures are superior, as they express: 1) high antigenicity; 2) rapid development of antibodies; and 3) absence of adverse reactions, even in later-administered booster inoculation (164).

Worldwide, greater than 95% of the 50,000 cases of human rabies occur annually as a result of accidental exposure to rabid bats. In the United States, domestic animals that were exposed to stray or wild animals were once the main cause of rabies infection. Rabies control through pet vaccination and removal of stray or unwanted animals reduced confirmed cases of rabies in dogs from nearly 7,000 in 1947 to 89 in 2001. Rabies vaccines are currently approved for dogs, cats, sheep, cattle, horses, and ferrets (165). In additional, reduced handling of wildlife, non-removal of wildlife to a domestic setting, pet vaccination, use of oral rabies vaccine for coyotes and grey foxes distributed aerially, and prompt treatment of wounds have significantly reduced human rabies. Of concern are those species that appear to act as a latent reservoir for the host; skunks, raccoons, and bats are prime examples (166). Of the U.S. rabies cases reported for 2002, several commonalities exist. Primarily, the patient did not report contact with a non-domestic animal and the possibility or actual exposure to a rabid animal. Only after the neurological events were irreversible did acquaintances relate some contact with an animal that could have had rabies. These are highlighted in Table 4.4.

In several clinical studies of the rabies vaccine regimens for pre- and postexposure prophylaxis, all subjects developed antibody responses within 2–4 weeks (167–169). The antibody response typically develops in 7–10 days and lasts for at least 2 years (170). Preexposure prophylaxis is intended for those at high risk of contracting rabies (bites by carnivorous wild animals or bats; bites by dogs or cats that develop symptoms during 10 days of observation, or are rabid, suspected rabid, or unknown (i.e., escaped); or any bite from an unprovoked attack), and is given in three doses on days 0, 7, and 21 or 28. Postexposure prophylaxis is given to those who are exposed to suspected or confirmed rabid animals, according to recommendations by the CDC (170). This regimen is given in conjunction with rabies immune globulin and consists of 5 vaccinations given on days 0, 3, 7, 14, and 28. Previously immunized individuals who have been exposed to rabid animals require only vaccination given in 2 doses 3 days apart.

Adverse Effects

For each of the currently utilized vaccines approved for use worldwide, adverse events differ. Vaccines are listed in order of efficacy and safety with the most safe vaccine listed first. HDCV and RVA are interchangeable when used as recommended.

Table 4.4 Summary of Contact and Rapidity of Disease Progression of Human Rabies (2002)

Age/Sex	State	Exposure	Date of Exposure	Date Seeking Medical Help	Date Died
28/Male	California	Killed bat in his house. Bat colony in attic. Bite denied.	March 10	March 18	March 31
13/Male	Tennessee	Found bat on ground and brought it home. Animal bite? Family not aware bats carry rabies.	July 1	August 21	August 31
49/Male	California	Bat found in home and patient removed it.	?	September 15	September 20
54/Male	New York	Arrived in United States from Ghana a few days earlier; patient bitten by dog in Ghana.	?	September 22	October 3
26/Male	Georgia	Bats had been in house and landing on him as he slept.	?	October 3	October 10
47/Male	Minnesota	Woke to find bat on hand and was bitten while killing it.	October 8	October 14	October 25
69/Male	Wisconsin	Removed bats from house with bare hands.	Before October 7	October 14	October 16

HDCV (Human Diploid Cell Vaccine)

Nausea, abdominal pain, headache, dizziness, and muscle aches. Reported by 20% of recipients (171).

Allergic reaction. Urticaria or anaphylactic shock are rarely reported (172).

Neurological complication. Rarely reported, although there have been three cases of Guillain-Barré syndrome reported (170).

Booster shots of HDCV. May cause an immune complex-like reaction within 2–21 days after vaccination. Reactions may include generalized urticaria, angioedema, nausea, vomiting, fever, malaise, arthralgia, or arthritis (173,174).

RVA (Rabies Vaccine Absorbed)

Anaphylactic reaction. Has not been reported among users.

Local reaction. Occurs in 65–70% of patients, with 10% reporting mild symptoms.

Immune complex-like illness. Rare ($\leq$1%).

Serious neurological condition. Rare.

PCECV (Purified Chick-Embryo Cell-Culture Vaccine)

Anaphylactic shock. Two cases of anaphylaxis have occurred among 11.8 million doses worldwide.

Egg allergy. Reaction is a concern for those with egg allergies.

Local and mild systemic reaction. Occurs the least in PCECV. No immune complex-like illnesses have been reported.

Brain or Nerve Tissue

Neurological complication. Serious risk of neurological complications.

Pathogenic infection. Caused by imperfect inactivation of vaccine virus.

Special Considerations

Immunosuppressive agents. Corticosteroids and other immunosuppressive agents may suppress antibody development following vaccinations. Unless they are absolutely necessary, these should not be administered during postexposure therapy.

Antimalarials. Chloroquine phosphate, mefloquine, and other antimalarials can diminish response to rabies treatment. Intramuscular injection of the vaccine enhances response in those taking antimalarials.

Immunosuppressed patients. In patients preparing to undergo transplants or chemotherapy, or who have immunosuppressive diseases, some physicians have recommended doubling the dose of rabies vaccine to achieve an acceptable immune response (175–177).

Recent and Continuing Developments in Rabies Vaccines

Because of the higher cost associated with the HDC vaccine, the development of other cell-culture vaccines has been pursued intensely. The purified chick-embryo cell-culture vaccine (PCECV) has been licensed in the United States for both prophylactic and postexposure immunization. This vaccine is produced by the growth of fixed rabies virus strain Flury LEP in chicken-embryo fibroblast culture. Clinical studies have shown it to be as effective and well-tolerated as HDCV, with antibody responses in over 99% of recipients (178,179). Compared with HDCV, no type III hypersensitivity reactions have been observed with PCECV (180), but serious anaphylactic reactions or neuroparalytic events have been reported rarely. Rabies vaccine absorbed (RVA) is another available rabies vaccine, which is produced by growth of the Kissling strain of Challenge Virus Standard rabies virus in fetal rhesus lung diploid cell culture. All three types of the inactivated rabies vaccine currently available are considered comparable in safety and efficacy (170).

Indian scientists have produced a new rabies vaccine that is ready for human trials. The new vaccine is the world's first combination DNA vaccine against rabies. The procedure is new, as it combines inoculating a DNA vaccine and a low dose of an inactivated virus vaccine. Scientists expect the vaccine to be less costly. If the vaccine is administered to a rabies-infected dog, its bite to a human will not transmit the disease. However, testing of the vaccine and continued refinement have been delayed due to animal-rights activists who have protected the use of stray animals for vaccine testing. This appears to be enigmatic when one considers that the vaccine, once approved, can be given to strays to enhance reservoir/vector control of rabies. DNA vaccines may be stored at room temperature, an added benefit in areas where availability of constant refrigeration may be questionable. Currently, India uses nerve tissue vaccine, which is now banned in most countries (181).

POLIOVIRUS VACCINES

Polioviruses occur as three serotypes. They are highly contagious and paralysis can occur. Infection of one person may lead to infection of other household members or others in close contact in 73–96% of the cases, depending on the contactee's age. The virus is spread by the fecal-oral route with some transmissions being oral-oral. The virus first replicates in the mucosal membranes of the pharynx and gastrointestinal tract, then, 3–35 days later, in the blood stream and, to a lesser degree, in the central nervous system. Polio was the dreaded summer disease up until the 1960s. While up to 95% of cases are subclinical, paralytic poliomyelitis accounted for 2% of the cases. From 2–5% of young children and from 15–30% of adults who acquired paralytic polio died. Before the development of preventive vaccines, treatment of paralytic polio consisted of medications, iron lungs, limb and back braces, and rehabilitation therapy.

The inactivated poliovirus vaccine (IPV) was developed by Jonas Salk in the early 1950s and was introduced for use in the United States in 1955. Although this vaccine was shown to be safe and efficacious, its use quickly declined after introduction of the oral poliovirus vaccine (OPV) in the early 1960s.

An enhanced version of the inactivated vaccine was developed in 1978 (182) and later licensed in the United States in 1987. This more potent formulation results in improved immunity in children and adults (183). In children given the three dose regimen, 99–100% developed antibody responses to all three types of poliovirus two months after the second dose (184). Significant increases in antibody concentrations were observed after administration of the third dose. In separate clinical studies, 99–100% of subjects developed protective antibodies after three doses (185,186). The use of IPV results in less gastrointestinal immunity than OPV (163), although the newer enhanced formulation induces a significant degree of mucosal immunity that has been demonstrated to produce effective protection (185,188). The duration of immunity induced by IPV is unknown, but is thought to be long-term (Table 4.5). A study in Sweden using 4 doses of less potent IPV indicated that over 90% of vaccine recipients had persistent antibodies after 25 years (189).

The oral polio vaccine was first licensed in the United States in 1963 and consists of live attenuated strains of the three serotypes of poliovirus, all grown in monkey kidney cell culture. In the 1960s, OPV quickly became the favored vaccine because of its ease of oral administration, consistent production of gastrointestinal immunity, expected long-lasting immunity, and spread of the vaccine virus to unvaccinated contacts (190). After three doses of OPV, over 95% of recipients produce immunity to all three serotypes of poliovirus (184). This immunity is considered to be long-lasting, and likely lifelong. Because of fecal shedding of the vaccine virus after OPV administration, this vaccine can immunize unvaccinated contacts (191). However, viral shedding of mutated virus may also lead to vaccine-associated paralytic poliomyelitis (VAPP) in unvaccinated contacts, particularly the immunosuppressed.

Since the introduction and widespread use of the two polio vaccines, the number of poliovirus infections and complications has dramatically decreased. In 1994, the Western Hemisphere was certified to be free of indigenous wild poliovirus (192). The last case of indigenously acquired wild poliovirus infection in the United States occurred in 1979 (193).

Table 4.5 Variability in Poliovirus Vaccine Administered and Response

Factor	Oral Poliovirus Vaccine (OPV)	Inactivated Poliovirus Vaccine (IPV)	OPV/IPV
Type	Live, attenuated virus	Inactivated virus	Combination of OPV/IPV
Administration	Oral	Injection	Oral and Injection
Doses	3	3	IPV 2 mo; 4 mo OPV 12–18 mo; 4–6 yrs
Immunogenicity[a]	95%	90%	—
Occurrence of vaccine associated paralytic polio (VAPP)	8–9 cases per year	None	2–5 cases per year[b]
Immunity of gastrointestinal mucosa	High	Low	High
Secondary transmission of vaccine virus	Yes	No	Some
Extra injections or office visits needed	No	Yes	Yes

[a] Immunogenicity appears to be variable for OPV, particularly in underdeveloped areas. Factors associated with 1) maternal antibody level; 2) season; 3) diarrhea at time of vaccination; 4) exposure to other recipients; and 5) breastfeeding.
[b] Estimated.

Since that time, an average of 8–9 cases of paralytic polio have been reported each year in the United States due to the use of the oral, live attenuated polio vaccine (OPV) (194). VAPP occurs in one case per 2.4 million doses, but is more common after the first vaccine dose (one case per 750,000 first OPV doses) (194).

The World Health Organization developed a strategy for global eradication of poliomyelitis by the end of the year 2000, which unfortunately was not met. Significant progress has been achieved toward that goal, with a 90% reduction of poliomyelitis cases between 1988 and 1996 (195). In 1988, poliovirus was found on every continent except Australia. However, in 1998, only three major foci of disease remained including the regions of South Asia, West Africa, and Central Africa (196). Worldwide, there were 2979 new cases in 2000 and 537 in 2001 (197). Global eradication continues to be elusive as local customs and fear affect vaccination rates. As an example, parents in Nigeria recently were refusing to allow children to be vaccinated for fear that the vaccine might contain HIV or make their children infertile. The vaccine is viewed as a Western ploy to curb population growth. Nigeria is one country where polio eradication is in danger of failure (198).

In 2002, India had over 85% of the new cases of polio worldwide despite national immunization days and house-to-house visits to administer OPV (199).

Adverse Effects

Vaccine-associated paralytic poliomyelitis (VAPP). Between 1980 and 1994, 125 cases of VAPP were reported in the United States: 49 cases occurred in healthy vaccine recipients; 40 cases developed in healthy contacts of the vaccine recipient; 23 cases occurred in immunodeficient vaccines; 7 cases developed in immunodeficient contacts of vaccine recipients; and the remaining 6 cases developed in community contacts (194). VAPP more frequently occurs in adults, immunodeficient persons, and those receiving the first dose of OPV (187). Because of the diminished risk for wild poliovirus disease in the United States, the risk for VAPP is now considered to be less acceptable (194). It is now recommended that, to eliminate the risk for VAPP, an all-IPV schedule be used for routine childhood vaccination in the United States. All children should receive four doses of IPV: at age 2 months, age 4 months, between ages 6 and 18 months, and between ages 4 and 6 years.

Inactivated polio vaccine (IPV). No serious adverse effects have been reported with IPV. This vaccine contains

trace amounts of polymyxin B, neomycin, and strepto-
mycin and may cause hypersensitivity reactions in persons allergic to these substances.

Oral poliovirus vaccine (OPV). OPV has no serious
adverse effects other than VAPP.

Guillain-Barré syndrome. Evidence indicates that neither OPV nor IPV increases the risk for Guillain-Barré
syndrome (194).

Special Considerations

Oral poliovirus vaccine (OPV). If available, OPV may
be used only for the following special circumstances:

Mass vaccination campaigns to control outbreaks of
paralytic polio.

Unvaccinated children who will be traveling within 4
weeks to areas where polio is endemic or epidemic.

Children of parents who do not accept the recommended number of vaccine injections; these children
may receive OPV only for the third or fourth dose or
both. In this situation, health-care providers should
administer OPV only after discussing the risk for
VAPP with parents or caregivers.

As a result, OPV supplies are expected to be very limited in the United States after inventories are depleted
(200).

**Monkeyvirus SV40 and rare cancer (pleural me-
sothelioma).** High levels of SV40 cause tumors when
injected in rodents. There is no association between
prior childhood vaccination of strains of SV40 in polio
vaccine and pleural mesothelioma. Persons least likely
to have been immunized (age >75 yrs) were those with
increased rates of plural mesothelioma (201).

Pleconaril. Pleconaril was used to treat three acute flaccid
paralysis cases: two vaccine-mediated and one wild-
type with a good clinical and virological response (202).

Immunocompromised. Live vaccines are contraindicated in people who are infected with HIV because of

the risk of infection from attenuated microorganisms. Benefits of OPV outweigh the risks and should continue to be used in countries where HIV infections are endemic.

YELLOW FEVER VIRUS VACCINE

Yellow fever is considered to be the original viral hemorrhagic fever. Although most individuals experience only mild illness, approximately 15% of infected persons develop serious disease, with hepatorenal dysfunction, myocardial injury, and hemorrhage (203). 20–80% of serious infections end in death. There is no antiviral therapy specifically targeted to yellow fever (204).

The incidence of yellow fever has been increasing dramatically in the past two decades (205). Between 1985–1996, 23,543 cases and 6421 deaths were reported to the World Health Organization, although many more cases are believed to go unreported (203). An outbreak in Guinea in 2000 involved 688 cases with 225 deaths. A massive vaccination program was hampered by insufficient stocks, leading UNICEF to stockpile 2 million doses of 17D vaccine to be used in response to outbreaks (206). Yellow fever is found in tropical South America and sub-Saharan Africa. Two clinically identical forms of yellow fever exist (urban and jungle) and both are spread by *Aedes aegypti*. The urban form is transmitted from human to human by the *A. aegypti* mosquitoes. In areas that control *A. aegypti*, yellow fever has disappeared (204). The jungle form is transmitted among nonhuman primates by various mosquitoes, and humans are incidentally infected. However, the rarity of infections may be an artifact of poor reporting of cases in the past.

The live attenuated yellow fever vaccine was first developed 1936, and is produced by growth of the 17D virus strain in chick embryos. It is the only vaccine strain for yellow fever and serious events occur at less than 1 in 1 million. It is so low that it is not feasible, at this time, to develop a new vaccine (207).

Seroconversion rates with the vaccine are 95–98% in both adults and children. Vaccinations consist of a single subcutaneous injection of 0.5 ml of vaccine. Immunity has been documented for at least 30–35 years and is thought to be lifelong (205). Regardless, a certificate of yellow fever immunization for international travel to certain countries is only valid for 10 years, requiring revaccination thereafter. Immunization for yellow fever is indicated for anyone ≥9 months of age living or traveling in endemic areas (tropical South America or sub-Saharan Africa) (208). Vaccination may also be required for entry into particular countries, and current information is available from health departments.

Adverse Effects

Despite recent reports of incidents resembling classic yellow fever after vaccination, the yellow fever vaccine is considered to be extremely safe with few side effects (207). Those persons who develop some side effects (2–5%) usually recover in 5–10 days, and immediate hypersensitivity reactions occur at a rate of approximately 1 in 1 million doses (209).

As with all vaccinations, some adverse events are reported. Improved surveillance since the 1990s has brought some previously unreported problems to light. The most recent is the description of 20 incidents that resemble classic yellow fever. It is not known if some of the vaccine recipients had recent prior exposure to wild yellow fever virus before receiving the vaccine. However, the cases occurred in production lots of virus from three different manufacturers. Reversion virulence among several different manufacturers seems unlikely. There may be an idiosyncratic host susceptibility that permits virulence-associated mutations during a prolonged viremic phase (207). Advanced age may also be a risk factor, but those persons having a repeat vaccination are less likely to have a severe reaction (207,210).

General side effects lasting 5–10 days:

Low-grade fevers.
Mild headaches.
Myalgia.

Hypersensitivity (immediate reactions) is often associated with egg allergy or the gelatin stabilizer used in the vaccine:

Rash.

Urticaria.

Asthma symptoms.

Vaccine-associated neurotrophic disease. Worldwide vaccinations (200 million) have resulted in 22 cases of encephalitis with laboratory analysis of the presence of the vaccine virus (211).

Vaccine-associated viscerotropic disease (VAVD). May be associated with 10 cases and ranges from moderate illness with focal organ dysfunction to severe disease with overt multiple organ system failure and death (204).

Special Considerations

Children. The majority of encephalitis cases were reported in children <4 months of age. Recommendations are that children not be vaccinated until they are >9 months of age.

Pregnant women. Vaccination for yellow fever should not occur in pregnant women (207).

Immunocompromised. Immunization should be withheld from immunosuppressed individuals.

Asymptomatic HIV infection. In the United States, asymptomatic infection with HIV is not considered a contraindication (209). In the United Kingdom, HIV is a contradiction (207).

Better surveillance and documentation of yellow fever symptoms resulting from yellow fever vaccine is needed. Additional tests to monitor organ function for viscerotropic complications should be considered. Reactions to the vaccine need to be characterized to determine which ones are vaccine-mediated or which ones resulted from individual risk factors (allergies, immunosuppression, etc.). Behavioral research into why travelers to areas of concentrated yellow fever cases are not properly vaccinated prior to traveling may help decrease the number of travelers' cases of yellow fever.

JAPANESE ENCEPHALITIS VIRUS VACCINE

Japanese encephalitis (JE) is a mosquito-born infection endemic to parts of Asia. The flaviviral neurologic infection is closely related to St. Louis encephalitis and West Nile virus. This infection causes an average of 35,000 reported cases and 10,000 deaths each year (209), although the majority of infections are subclinical. Viremia develops after a bite from an infected mosquito and 1 out of 250 infections leads to symptomatic disease (211). Most infections clear before the virus enters the central nervous system. However, once neurologic invasion occurs, large areas of the brain may be involved. The resulting encephalitis is typically severe, with a 25–40% fatality rate (212,213). Residual neurologic sequelae are evident in 10–30% of cases (212). Japanese encephalitis is seasonal with most cases occurring after infection during the rainy season; in temperate areas, this is from June through September. In the more tropical areas, the season begins in March and extends until October.

Several findings related to JE infection are:

1. Poorer performance on standardized tests (compared with uninfected subjects).
2. Those who had dengue fever infection earlier may have decreased morbidity and mortality rates, possibly due to the presence of other antiflavivirus antibodies.
3. Risk factors for death include documented virus in CSF, low levels of IgG or IgM, and decreased sensorium.

Control of vectors and reservoirs of infection aid in decreasing cases of JE. These measures are: 1) control of mosquitoes and avoidance of areas where mosquitoes are likely to occur; 2) draining or spraying of swamps and other areas with standing water; 3) humans and other mammals may be dead-end hosts requiring no containment; and 4) agricultural animals (pigs) and endemic birds (egrets and herons) may be amplifying hosts with high-grade viremia.

Three vaccines are available worldwide. The one used commercially for travelers is derived from mouse brain and is a formaldehyde inactivated vaccine. The vaccine contains a Beijing-1

Table 4.6   Japanese Encephalitis: Comparison of Vaccine Types

	InV	LAV
Efficacy	90–97%	90–97%
Immunogenicity	High after 2 doses in endemic areas and 3 doses in nonendemic area	High after 1–2 doses in endemic area
Safety	Severe allergic reactions and neurologic complications	No adverse effects
Cost for Asia (US $/dose)	$5.00/dose	$0.75/dose

strain, thimersol, gelatin, and other components. The vaccine
is administered as 3 doses on days 0, 7, and 30. More frequent
inoculations may be given (5–7 days apart) when there is a
need for a quick immunization schedule, although antibody
response is lower and may not last as long. The vaccine is
licensed for persons ≥1 year of age in the United States
(214,215). The vaccine is recommended for travelers to Asia
who will be spending a month or longer in endemic areas during the transmission season of the virus (which varies according to geographic region) (213). Two other JE vaccines are
licensed in China: an inactivated JE vaccine derived from
hamster kidney and a live attenuated vaccine from the same
source combined with the SA14-14-2 viral strain. The latter
is less costly and is replacing the inactivated virus vaccine.
The efficacy record of this vaccine is reported to be greater
(Table 4.6).

Adverse Effects

> **Systemic side effects.** Fever, headache, malaise, chills,
> dizziness, rash, myalgia, abdominal pain, and nausea
> and vomiting are reported.
> **Adverse neurologic events.** Encephalitis, peripheral
> neuropathy, or other adverse neurologic events occur in
> 1.0 to 2.3 cases per 1 million vaccinations (216).

Allergic mucocutaneous reactions. The mouse brain vaccine has been associated with 73 allergic mucocutaneous reactions (217).

Adverse allergic reaction. May occur within minutes or as late as 17 days after vaccination; most occur within 48 hours. Those with a history of allergic rhinitis or urticaria development (insect stings or bites) have a great risk (218,219).

General. 1 of 260 vaccinees complains of a general rash, itching, or swelling, especially in the areas of the face, lips, and throat, and/or the extremities.

Special Considerations

Travelers. A 10-day period following vaccination is recommended before traveling due to possibility of adverse events.

Live virus vaccines. Should live virus vaccines (such as MMR) be necessary, it is better to administer two doses of JE vaccines before the live virus vaccines for maximum efficacy.

Malaria. The efficacy of JE vaccine is lessened if chloroquine is being taken for prophylaxis against malaria.

ADENOVIRUS VACCINES

Adenoviruses were first isolated from adenoid tissue from tonsillectomies of children and from military patients with febrile illness (1953). There are more than 49 human serotypes, several of which have oncogenic potential. The virus can become latent in lymphoid tissue and reactivated at a later date. Reactivation occurs during immunosuppression but it is unclear how long the virus persists (220,221).

Adenoviruses can cause acute respiratory illness, including pneumonia in military recruits or groups of infants. Most people have been infected with one serotype of adenovirus by age 15. Infants are susceptible to pharyngitis, gastroenteritis, and, more rarely, acute hemorrhagic cystitis and hepatitis. More recently, an outbreak in a boarding vocational school indicates that adenoviruses may prevail anywhere there are concentrated crowded conditions and new groups of potentially susceptible persons are frequently introduced (222). Adenovirus is also a less common cause of pneumonia in hospitalized children as well as gastroenteritis in infants and children, although immunization is not recommended for this population. Adenoviruses have received considerable attention as a defective vector to carry and express foreign genes for therapeutic purposes (223). The genome is easy to manipulate in vitro. Vaccines have been available since 1971 as live, oral, enteric-coated tablets, available in two different strains: type 4 and type 7 adenovirus vaccines. At one time, all military recruits received adenovirus vaccine. Several studies of vaccine recipients demonstrated a significant decrease, generally a 94–100% reduction, in acute respiratory disease due to adenovirus (224). Unfortunately, production of these vaccines was discontinued in 1996. Between 10–12% of unvaccinated military recruits become ill with adenovirus infection during basic training. The Department of Defense is currently searching for an alternate source of the product (225).

INVESTIGATIONAL VACCINES

Many of the virus vaccines currently under investigation will more than likely expand the focus of immunization. All of the vaccines available up to the end of the 20th century have been used solely to prevent disease. However, several new candidate vaccines are being developed and evaluated for the treatment of already acquired viral infections.

Rotavirus

Approximately 3 million children, worldwide, die of diarrhea annually, with 680,000 of these deaths caused by rotavirus. Most of these deaths occur in developing countries (226), where a child's risk of death from the rotavirus approaches 0.5%. In 1998, the rhesus-human reassortant tetravalent (RRV-TV) rotavirus vaccine (Rotashield) was licensed for use in the United States. It is an oral vaccine which consists of live attenuated Rhesus rotavirus serotype 3 and human-rhesus reassortants that express serotypes 1, 2, and 4. In clinical trials, three doses of rotavirus vaccine resulted in 49–57% efficacy against disease. The vaccine also prevented dehydration in 100% of recipients and reduced physician visits by 73%. It is expected that widespread implementation of rotavirus immunization in the United States would reduce physician office visits and reduce by two-thirds the number of rotavirus-related hospitalizations and deaths.

The rotavirus vaccine was FDA approved for administration of 3 doses at 2, 4, and 6 months of age. Soon after public availability of the vaccine, several cases of intussusception in recent vaccinees were reported. Because of strong concerns over the possible association between the rhesus-based rotavirus vaccine and intussusception, the CDC recommended postponement of rotavirus vaccination until further studies are complete. Thus, this vaccine is no longer available.

Discontinuance has created a moral dilemma for those who work in developing countries. Ethicists argue that, even with a 25% fatality rate from intussusception that would cause 2000–3000 deaths/year, this is far less that the 600,000–800,00 annual deaths from rotavirus infection.

Adverse Effects

Fever. 20% of infants develop fever after rotavirus vaccination, generally 3–5 days after the first dose. Older infants have a higher incidence of febrile reactions, which restricted the use of this vaccine to the first 6 months of life.

Irritability. Irritability and decreased appetite and activity have been reported as adverse effects in some trials.

Intussusception. The rate of intussusception in recent vaccinees was approximately 220–300 cases per 100,000 infant-years, compared with 45–50 cases per 100,000 infant-years in unvaccinated infants (227).

According to the Vaccine Adverse Event Reporting System, the majority of infants developed this complication after the first vaccine dose and developed symptoms within 1 week of immunization.

Discontinuance of the rotavirus vaccine is an example of making the standards of care for the United States a worldwide standard of care. What is an unsuitable adverse event risk for children receiving the rotavirus vaccine in the United States is a death wish for children who live in countries where there is no adequate treatment for the diarrhea.

Another human-animal reassortant vaccine is undergoing clinical trials (228). It is based on a bovine rotavirus parent strain (WC-3), and has thus far proved to be safe and effective, although there is concern that some children may be genetically predisposed to intussusception when they are given oral vaccine (226). An altogether different live rotavirus vaccine has shown promising efficacy rates in phase II clinical trials. The human rotavirus vaccine 89–12 was 89% effective in preventing disease in infants after only 2 doses (229). Serologic evidence of immunity was demonstrated in 94% of recipients. It has been suggested that the use of an attenuated human rotavirus strain may induce greater immunity than animal strains or reassortants. Mild fever has been the only adverse reaction experienced to date. Any rotavirus vaccine should be designed for use in children. Some of the early failures of vaccines to control infantile diarrhea may be due to a lack of understanding of children's mucosal immune response, reassortment of viral strains in nature, and seasonal emergence of different types of strains in the field (230). Oral immunization may induce mucosal immunity in gut mucosa (231). Parenteral administration of virus-like particles (VLPs) provides active immunogenic protection (232). Development of a new vaccine may take decades with many more children dying from rotavirus than intussusception.

Concerns expressed by pediatricians were fear of adverse reactions, high cost of vaccine, and time for educating parents on efficacy and safety of a new vaccine (227). The future of rotavirus vaccine development depends on the reasons for the association of intussusception (233).

Varicella-Zoster Virus Vaccine

The two pronged consequences of VZV have been previously discussed in Chapter 3. In brief, childhood chickenpox is one manifestation of VZV. Children develop immunity to the latent virus. The major risk after this event is that one's immunity will wane over time and the VZV reactivates, causing painful shingles. As one ages, the probability that the VZV will reactivate approaches 50% for those 85 and older. There are numerous major benefits from the VZV or "chickenpox" vaccine:

1. Prevention of chickenpox in young children.
2. As widespread immunization occurs, there will be a reduced reservoir for the wild virus.
3. Reduction in infant hydrocephaly associated with maternal VZV infection early in pregnancy (234).
4. Vaccination in the elderly to attenuate the course of herpes zoster (235,236).
5. Vaccination of others whose immune systems are impaired (236).

It is evident that waning cellular immunity is strongly correlated with the development of herpes zoster (237–239). The live attenuated varicella vaccine was approved for anyone aged 1 year or older by the FDA in 1995. The vaccine was developed in Japan over 30 years ago, yet the United States is the only country using it as a universal vaccine against chickenpox. Cases of chickenpox and complications from chickenpox (hospitalizations) have been reduced. Children usually receive 1 dose of vaccine, while those 13 years of age or older receive 2 doses 1–2 months apart.

One issue has been the degree of efficacy of the vaccine. Breakthrough varicella is reported in 10–15% of vaccinees. Vaccine effectiveness, based on case studies and clinical trials, may range from <45–90% (240). Another issue has been the lasting degree of high immunity. Vaccine efficacy seems to be reduced by improper handling and storage of the vaccine and individual response characteristics, such as a history of asthma or age of <14 months at time of immunization, and short interval (<30 days) between MMR inoculation and VZV immunization. Efficacy may be improved by administering a higher dosage of vaccine and/or more than one dose in children. When older children (>13 years of age) and adults are given two doses of VZV vaccine, higher antibody titers are evident 6 weeks after immunization. In small children, higher antibody titers occur when a booster dose is given (241).

Vaccination with the Oka or vaccine strain of VZV rarely causes rash. Breakthrough cases due to wild virus tend to be less severe than cases in the non-vaccinated. Breakthrough cases are less likely to cause secondary infection (241).

Investigators are currently evaluating the potential for the live-attenuated vaccine to act as a booster for the compromised cellular immune response in older individuals. A phase III clinical trial is underway to investigate this effect and to determine any clinical significance with regard to the reduction of severity or prevention of herpes zoster. The vaccine under investigation is a more potent version of the one currently licensed for immunization in children.

In later life, VZV plagues the elderly as painful shingles. Especially painful are those that occur on the face and involve the trigeminal nerve. Levin et al. (242) have previously studied the immune response of elderly persons who received the live attenuated vaccine and found that approximately 10–15% of the vaccinees failed to develop increased immunity. Overall, the calculated half-life of the enhanced immunity in this study was 54 months. The long-term duration of the booster effect had a positive correlation with the dose of the administered vaccine. In a follow-up study 6 years after vaccination, Levin et al. (243) found that the varicella-zoster virus-responding T cell frequency was still significantly improved over initial baseline measurements, as well as expected measurements for this age cohort. In this vaccinated population, the frequency of herpes zoster was within the range of expected incident for this age cohort. However, in all cases of herpes zoster in the study, the number of lesions was small, the associated pain was minimal, and postherpetic neuralgia did not occur. This preliminary study suggests that vaccination in the elderly may be able to attenuate the course of herpes zoster (235).

Adverse Effects

Fever. Fever is common (37.7°C or 100°F), but a fever over 39°C (102°F) may be of more concern. Patients should check with their physician.

Injection site. The injection site may be tender or erythematous but this should diminish over 2–3 days.

Varicella-like rash. Patients should check with their doctor if a rash appears in areas other than the injection site.

These signs and symptoms are less common, but patients should check with their doctor if they continue for an extended period of time or are more bothersome than usual:

Abdominal pain.
Common cold or sore throat.
Congestion or cough.
Nausea or diarrhea.
Rare events.

- Black, tarry stools
- Blood in urine or stools
- Reddening of skin, especially around the ears
- Airway or swallowing difficulty
- Hives
- Irritability
- Peripheral itching (feet or hands)
- Unusual bleeding or bruising
- Sudden or severe tiredness or weakness
- Muscle or joint pain
- Pinpoint red macules on skin
- Stiff neck
- Confusion
- Severe or continuing headache
- Facial swelling (eyelids, face, or nasal passage ways, swollen glands)
- Vomiting
- Patients should check with their doctor as soon as possible if any of these rare events occurs.

Special Considerations

Leukemia. Immunized children with leukemia are less likely to develop chickenpox or shingles.

Allergies to neomycin or gelatin. May be contraindicated for vaccine administration.

Pregnancy or intent to become pregnant. Varicella vaccine is not known to harm the fetus, but tests have not been done. However, wild viral infection can sometimes cause birth defects.

Breastfeeding. Mothers who receive the vaccine and wish to breastfeed should consult first with their doctor.

Tuberculosis. Although wild virus infection may exacerbate tuberculosis, there are no reports that the vaccine causes tuberculosis to worsen.

Immune deficiency. Decreased immunity may increase the chance and degree of side effects of the vaccine and/or decrease the efficacy of the vaccine.

Febrile illness. Febrile illness symptoms may be confused with possible side effects of the vaccine.

Human Immunodeficiency Virus Vaccine

A review of HIV infection and transmission can be found in Chapter 2. As the AIDS epidemic persists and spreads unabated in much of the world, the search for an effective HIV vaccine is becoming critical. In 1997, President Clinton challenged scientists to develop an effective HIV vaccine by the year 2007. Since clinical trials first began in 1987, at least 34 different HIV candidate vaccines have begun phase I trials, and a handful of these have progressed to phase II or III trials (212). 74 additional HIV vaccine candidates are reported to be in research and development or preclinical testing in animals, and this number has likely increased (212).

Recombinant subunit HIV vaccines are genetically engineered from HIV surface envelope proteins, such as gp120 or gp160. Because they do not contain live virus or DNA, there is no risk of causing infection. A therapeutic trial was carried out with gp160 subunit immunization every 3 months for 3 years in HIV-positive persons in addition to antiretroviral therapy

(244). Results demonstrated a modest effect on CD4 counts, but no clinical benefit. These results were consistent with similar earlier studies (245,246). A recombinant gp120 candidate vaccine (AIDSVAX) was evaluated in phase III trials for the prevention of HIV. This three-year placebo-controlled trial enlisted 5000 high-risk seronegative persons. A similar vaccine was studied in Thailand in 2500 HIV-negative drug users. Earlier research suggested that this subunit vaccine stimulates antibody production, but may not induce cellular immunity. HIV research has shown that the induction of cytotoxic T lymphocytes may be an important correlate for protective efficacy of HIV vaccines (247). Unfortunately, this candidate vaccine was not able to prevent infection in seronegative individuals.

Recombinant live-virus vector vaccines use virus carriers which are genetically engineered to express particular HIV genes. The first candidate to be tested was a vaccinia vector with the insertion of HIV gp160 gene. The vaccine alone induced little antibody (212). However, when used as a primer followed by boosting with the recombinant gp160 vaccine, results showed strong induction of cellular immunity and antibody responses (248). Phase I trials are underway for a recombinant vaccinia HIV primer followed by boosting with a recombinant gp120 vaccine (212).

Because of concerns over shedding of the vaccinia virus and possible disseminated disease in immunosuppressed persons, more attention has been focused on canarypox and adenovirus vectors which can infect humans but cannot replicate. Replication in humans continues long enough to produce the necessary HIV proteins before abortion of the cycle (249). Early results have shown that recombinant canarypox vector vaccines can induce humoral and cellular immune responses, including cytotoxic lymphocytes (250). The greatest interest for these vaccine candidates lies in the prime and boost approach. The canarypox vaccine primer induces a strong cellular immunity, followed by a recombinant subunit vaccine which boosts the antibody response (249). The combination of both vaccines induces a stronger immune response than either one alone (247,251). Recent results from a phase II trial

(252) showed that 93% of subjects who received the combination of vaccines developed neutralizing antibodies. Also, almost one-third of the recipients developed a cytotoxic lymphocyte response. Additional studies have investigated canarypox vectors expressing gp160 or gp120/gag/pol HIV-1 antigens given along with recombinant gp160 or gp120 subunit vaccines (253). When comparing data from different trials of several candidate canarypox vector HIV vaccines, more than half of the recipients developed durable, HIV-specific cytotoxic T-lymphocyte responses (254). Researchers suggest that a broader recombinant vector vaccine would likely increase the percentage of responders (254).

A trial in Uganda studying the effect of a canarypox vector vaccine alone commenced in February 1999 (255). The vaccine, called ALVAC vCP205, contains three HIV genes in a weakened version of canarypox virus. The particular genes come from clade B viruses, which are the predominant subtype of HIV found in the United States and Europe. However, the majority of HIV infections that occur in Uganda are due to clades A and D. This study will first evaluate the cross-reactivity among these viral subunits and compare the immune responses in recipients. DNA (or nucleic acid) vaccines are another promising prospect for HIV immunization. With this approach, purified DNA that encodes for particular immunogenic antigens is injected. This antigen is presented to the host immune system in its native form and is processed similar to that for a natural viral infection (250). Therapeutic immunization with a plasmid/gp160 and gag+ pol DNA vaccine in HIV-positive chimpanzees revealed a significant decrease in viral load and a boost in the immune response (256). Studies in seronegative primates demonstrated the induction of neutralizing antibodies and cytotoxic T-lymphocyte responses, but the vaccine did not protect against infection (212). A phase I clinical trial of two DNA vaccine candidates is currently in progress (212).

Several other approaches to HIV vaccine development are under investigation. Live-attenuated virus vaccines are known to generate a broad and durable immune response, but these have not been tested in humans due to potential safety concerns with live HIV virus (212). Whole-inactivated vaccines are generally thought to be safer than live-attenuated ones. However, inactivation of the virus often leads to a vaccine that is less potent or immunogenic. Studies of whole-killed virus vaccines in chimpanzees thus far have not been able to demonstrate protection from HIV infection (212). In addition, there is concern that inadvertently incomplete inactivation could lead to HIV infection of vaccine recipients. Virus-like particles (VLP) are a safer option, since they consist of a noninfectious HIV look-alike that does not contain the HIV genome. One such candidate, known as p17/p24:TY, has reached the stage of clinical trials. Early results have shown that this vaccine leads to low levels of HIV binding antibodies and T-cell memory responses, but induces very little cytotoxic T-lymphocyte activity (212). Other VLP candidates are under development. Many important controversies exist in HIV vaccine development, such as the issue of whether neutralizing antibodies as typically measured are relevant to clinical protection.

HERPES SIMPLEX VIRUS VACCINE

Herpes simplex (HSV-1 and-2) viruses are discussed in Chapter 3. The search for a vaccine for herpes simplex virus (HSV-1 and-2) spans eight decades. In the 1920s, untreated vesicular fluid from herpes lesions was injected into patients in an attempt to induce immunity (212). This method, to say the least, did not withstand the test of time. Inactivated whole virus vaccines were developed in the 1930s and were made from HSV-infected animal tissue, such as rabbit brain (257). Despite the many advances made with inactivated virus vaccines through the years, none of the candidates proved to be sufficiently immunogenic. With increasing technology, several different approaches for HSV vaccines are currently in development and evaluation.

A number of vaccine strategies could be implemented to prevent and protect against HSV disease. For example, a vaccine that prevents infection at the route of entry would be effective in combating establishment of latent reservoirs that could reactivate.

Also, a vaccine that challenged mucocutaneous tissues would be a good paradigm for human HSV infection. Vaccines for prevention are the primary goal, but the question of whether vaccines can be used to reduce the severity of the disease if it cannot completely eliminate HSV infection is also improtant (258).

Two separate recombinant subunit vaccines have been investigated in phase III trials. One such candidate developed by Chiron contained HSV-2 surface glycoproteins gB and gD and the adjuvant MF59. The development of this vaccine was halted prematurely because results demonstrated overall lack of efficacy for both preventive and therapeutic use (259,260). A second recombinant vaccine contains the glycoprotein gD and the adjuvant monophosphoryl lipid A immunostimulant (MPL). Results of clinical trials with this candidate indicate that it has clinical efficacy in protecting women who are serologically negative for both HSV-1 and HSV-2 from acquiring HSV-2 disease (261).

A report of mixed HSV-1 glycoproteins (ISCOMS) protected mice from latent HSV-1 infection, with a reduction of latent infection in the brain of 93% of vaccinated mice. Only 59% of the controls were free of HSV in the brain (262). This may be a promising area of future study in humans.

Another approach combines the safety profile of a killed vaccine with the immunogenic potential of a live virus vaccine (263). The disabled infectious single cycle (DISC) vaccine lacks the glycoprotein H (gH) gene necessary for virus entry into cells. After a single replication cycle, the virus is unable to spread to surrounding cells and thus remains noninfectious. Studies in guinea pigs demonstrated encouraging results for both preventive and therapeutic treatment (263,264). After phase I studies demonstrated DISC to be safe and well tolerated, phase II trials are currently underway to evaluate the vaccine as a therapeutic agent in infected persons. Trials are also planned to evaluate the efficacy in preventing infection in seronegative partners of discordant couples (212).

DNA vaccines are also in development for HSV immunization. Animal studies involving inoculations of plasmid DNA carrying the desired viral genes have shown promising results for the prevention of infection (265,266). These vaccines are only able to express one or two viral antigens, but can induce cell-mediated immunity without the need for potent adjuvants. One such candidate which encodes glycoprotein D2 (gD2) is currently in phase I clinical trials, and several others are in preclinical development.

Live attenuated HSV vaccines have been rather difficult to develop, as viruses that are the safest and most attenuated tend to lack immunogenicity. Research in the past has shown that stable attenuation of HSV was not achieved after passage in cell culture. After immunization, the vaccine strain would then have the potential to revert to its virulent state and cause disease. A genetically engineered HSV mutant vaccine was found to be safe and effective in animal studies (267), but in humans was overly attenuated and lacked sufficient immunogenicity (268). New genetically engineered strains are currently under development.

Human Papillomavirus Vaccine

Because certain subtypes of human papillomavirus (HPV) are associated with the development of cervical cancer, the search for a prophylactic or therapeutic HPV vaccine has been an important endeavor. Although more than 30 types of HPV are known to be sexually transmittable, the major types associated with malignancy (HPV-16, -18, -31, -33, -45, -52, and -58) and condylomata (HPV-6 and -11) are relatively few in number, allowing for more focused strategies for immunization against these specific subtypes. Vaccine development has been hampered in the past because of the inability to culture HPV. However, an in vitro culture system for HPV has more recently been developed, furthering the prospect for advancements in this field (269). Virus-like particle (VLP) vaccines are produced by recombinant DNA technology and are designed to self-assemble into conformations that resemble natural HPV. These vaccines contain no viral DNA and carry no risk of infection or oncogenic exposure. VLP vaccines have been designed for all of the major HPV subtypes and clinical trials are currently underway for HPV-11 L1 VLP (270), HPV-6 L1 VLP (271), and HPV-16 L1 VLP (272).

Fusion protein vaccines are currently under evaluation for the immunotherapy of cervical cancer and genital warts. TA-HPV is a live recombinant vaccinia virus which has been engineered to express the E6 and E7 protein genes for HPV-16 and -18 as a treatment for cervical cancer (212). This method also utilizes the viral vector approach, using vaccinia as a vehicle. Viral vector vaccines can be polyvalent and have the potential to produce immunity similar to that induced by live attenuated vaccines. A phase I/II clinical trial of TA-HPV (273) has shown encouraging results, and further studies are underway. TA-GW is a recombinant fusion protein vaccine consisting of HPV-6 L2 and E7 proteins, which is under investigation for the treatment of genital warts. A phase IIa clinical trial showed the vaccine to be immunogenic, with encouraging clinical responses (274). A third protein vaccine, TA-CIN, is in preclinical development for the treatment of cervical dysplasia (212).

Peptide-based vaccines have been shown to be protective against HPV-induced tumors in mice, although the T-cell repertoires in mice and humans differ. Two early-stage human clinical trials are underway, one involving HLA A*0201 binding HPV-16 E7 peptides, to assess the possible therapeutic implications these vaccines may offer (275). Other investigational approaches to HPV immunization include DNA vaccines (275), bacterial vectors (276–278), and dendritic cells pulsed with HPV epitopes (279). Koutsky reported in a study of 2392 young women that a HPV-16 VLP vaccine was 100% effective in preventing HPV-16 infection. In addition, the vaccine was safe, with no serious side effects reported. Therefore, immunization of HPV-16–negative women may eventually reduce the incidence of cervical cancer (280).

Cytomegalovirus Vaccine

Although cytomegalovirus (CMV) produces an uncommon mononucleosis-like syndrome in immunocompetent patients, its potential effects in the newborn and immunocompromised patient can be devastating. Congenital CMV is the most common intrauterine infection in the United States, and an estimated 8000 American infants develop neurologic or fatal complications each year because of this disease (281). This infection represents a common problem for HIV-infected persons, typically leading to neurologic syndromes or retinitis. CMV is also the most significant infectious agent in organ transplant recipients, and is often a factor in graft rejection. Hematopoietic stem cell transplant recipients are immunocompromised for a period of time and may develop progressive CMV infection (282). Over two-thirds of transplant recipients develop CMV infection or reactivation within 4 months of transplantation (212). CMV is further described in Chapter 3.

Several types of CMV vaccines are currently under evaluation. The first of these is the live attenuated Towne strain vaccine, which was first developed in the mid-1970s. Clinical studies in seronegative renal allograft recipients showed that the vaccine did not prevent infection, but significantly reduced the incidence of severe disease by approximately 85% (283,284). Another study evaluated the effect of CMV vaccine in preventing child-to-mother transmission of CMV acquired in daycare centers (285). The infection rate for vaccinated mothers was no different than placebo, while naturally seropositive mothers were protected. These disappointing results showed that the Towne strain vaccine did not induce immunity as effectively as natural infection. Concerns continue to focus on the use of a live virus that constitutes a major risk in a transplant patient. Current work is underway to develop improved versions of the Towne strain vaccine (286,287).

Subunit glycoprotein B (gB) vaccines that circumvent the use of viral vectors have also been evaluated for CMV immunization. This approach may use full-length proteins that are incorporated into a cell as endogenous proteins. CMV gB can be combined with an adjuvant called MF59 and, in one trial, stimulated the neutralizing antibody for at least 12 months (288). Clinical studies of the vaccine in healthy toddlers and adults have shown good immune response, but neutralizing antibodies rapidly declined in the 6 months following the third dose (289,290). A fourth dose in adults led to higher antibody levels, though titers declined again in 6 months (290). Further long-term data on this study is not yet available. A clinical vaccine efficacy study in mothers is currently underway to evaluate the effects on the antibody response (291). The canarypox-gB recombinant vaccine has been developed and evaluated as a candidate CMV vaccine. Initial trials have demonstrated a weak antibody response after multiple doses, but additional studies are currently evaluating its potential as a primer for boosting of subsequent Towne strain injections (292). Normal CD8+ cytotoxic T lymphocyte response to CMV involves a few proteins that could be candidates for vaccines (282). Polysaccharide nanoparticles may be useful in stimulating CMV-specific T_H cells and CMV-specific CD8+ cytotoxic T lymphocytes. This system is promising in that it is nonviral. It remains to be tested in humans to determine efficacy (282). Other potentially hopeful avenues for CMV vaccines include DNA plasmids (293), an HLA-restricted peptide-based vaccine (294), and lipopeptides.

Respiratory Syncytial Virus Vaccine

Respiratory syncytial virus (RSV) is the most common cause of severe lower respiratory tract infection in infants and young children which results in nearly 100,000 hospitalizations and 4500 dead in the United States each year (295).

Premature infants and those with chronic lung disease or congential heart disease are most susceptible, as are bone-marrow transplant recipients and the elderly (296–302). RSV epidemics are thought to be fueled by reinfection with RSV and incomplete immunity from RSV (303). More information on RSV may be obtained in Chapter 3. To meet the challenge of providing some type of immunization to the very weak (premature newborns), the immunologically challenged (transplant recipients), and the elderly, unique mechanisms of innoculation must be encouraged. For example, many newborns retain some maternal immunity. Therefore, a safe carrier of RSV vaccine to the mother prior to or during pregnancy might provide more resistance to RSV in the newborn. Vaccinating a newborn with traditional administration routes could be difficult; and it must be determined when to administer the vaccine to an already-at-risk premature infant. Also, a proposed nasal spray vaccine has the potential to induce better mucosal immunity with less trauma than from the innoculation (295).

Formalin-inactivated vaccines. Development of a formalin-inactivated (FI) vaccine suffered several set-backs in the 1960s when clinical trials led to severe, unexpected illnesses associated with exposure to wild-type RSV (304,305). There was one observation, however, that older children vaccinated with FI-RSV did not develop wild-type RSV later. This suggested that the older children had had a previous wild-type infection. A live RSV vaccine may be more effective by reducing the risk of subsequent disease as seen in the FI-RSV vaccine. Difficulties with the FI-RSV suggest that a successful vaccine should induce sufficient levels of neutralizing antibody, CD8+ RSV T-cells, and CD4 responses that are similar to the profile of those stimulated by wild-type RSV. One thought has been to combine a non-replicating vaccine with unique adjuvants or cytokines to achieve a better immunologic status. (306,307).

Live-attenuated RSV vaccines. A variety of strategies for a live-attenuated vaccine led to investigations of multiple host range mutants, cold-passaged mutants, and temperature-sensitive mutants. Problems associated with the temperature sensitive mutants and the cold-passaged mutants were reversions to the wild-type virus, overattenuation, and underattentuation. If live-attenuated vaccines are delivered intranasally, there is the potential for both local mucosal and systemic immunity that should protect against upper and lower respiratory tract disease. However, progress in the understanding of immunity to wild-type virus vaccine versus live-attenuated virus vaccine has led to the current cold-passaged, temperature-sensitive vaccine. One particular candidate, cpts-248/404, has been shown to be safe and immunogenic in children older than 6 months, but led to nasal congestion in infants 1–2 months of age (308). Additional live-attenuated vaccine candidates are currently under evaluation in animal models with some promising results (212). Advanced technologies may be able to provide live-attenuated vaccines which are genetically engineered (309).

cDNA clones of RSV. The discovery that cDNA could produce infectious virus meant that the viral genome has the capability to be manipulated (310). By introducing single mutations into cDNA and evaluating the results in vitro, recombinant gene technology could delete a nonessential gene (such as the SH glycoprotein) or insert an additional gene.

Sub-unit vaccines. The genome for RSV has 10 genes that encode 22 proteins. The two major surface glycoproteins are a fusion protein (F) and an attachment glycoprotein (G). In animal models subunit vaccines consisting of purified RSV glycoproteins are another promising avenue for RSV immunizations. Two separate purified F subunit protein vaccines have demonstrated efficacy and safety in clinical trials involving healthy adults, elderly subjects, RSV-seropositive children over 12 months of age, and children with pulmonary disease (311–317). Further clinical studies are planned. A subunit vaccine with the G protein fragment of RSV-A is also under investigation (212). A purified F protein subunit was recently evaluated and found to reduce the overall incidence of RSV infections, but further testing is needed (318). Subunit vaccines would be very useful if they could be used to immunize pregnant women to enhance the protection of their newborns and in other high risk groups.

Parainfluenza Virus Vaccine

The human parainfluenza virus (HPIV) contains two viral glycoproteins in the viral envelope. Human parainfluenza viruses are closely related to the measles, mumps, and respiratory syncytial viruses. Human parainfluenza virus type 3 is the second leading cause of infant and childhood respiratory disease (after RSV). Currently, no vaccine or antiviral is available. The human parainfluenza virus was first discovered in the 1950s (Japan: Sendai virus). Since then, 4 types with numerous subtypes and subgroups/genotypes have been identified.

HPIV-3. Several approaches to vaccine development have been evaluated in recent years. Two separate live-attenuated vaccines have been under evaluation. The cold-passaged (cp) HPIV-3 vaccines are cold-adapted, temperature-sensitive prospects. In early studies, the cp-18 strain was not sufficiently attenuated for children, but the cp-45 strain showed more promising results. When given intranasally to children, the vaccine candidate was immunogenic and safe (319). The antigenically-related bovine parainfluenza-3 (BPIV-3) vaccine has also been evaluated in early clinical trials (320,321). Results revealed that this vaccine is safe, immunogenic, and poorly transmittable. In addition, serum hemagglutination-inhibition antibody responses were increased with BPIV-3 when compared with those induced by cold-passaged HPIV-3. Trivalent subunit vaccines (322) as well as recombinant vaccines (323,324) are also under evaluation as potential parainfluenza vaccine candidates.

HPIV strains are seasonal. HPIV-1 and -2 usually cause respiratory outbreaks in the autumn. HPIV-3 may cause croup, but it may produce symptoms that mimic respiratory syncytial virus infection with bronchiolitis and pneumonia being common symptoms. HPIV-3 is associated with spring outbreaks. HPIV-4 causes mild respiratory infections and is rarely observed. HPIV is very common and almost all children have had HPIV in at least one form by age 6 years. Children are most at risk, although bouts of HPIV are reported in foreign travelers. Hence, the elderly and other immunosuppressed individuals are at risk.

Parainfluenza virus infections after hematopoietic stem cell transplantation occur in 7–8% of cases with 78% of these infections being community acquired. Three-fourths of these patients died from pneumonia within 180 days after pneumonia was diagnosed. Ribavirin and intravenous immunoglobulin were not effective treatments (325).

OTHER VACCINES

Vaccines for several other viral diseases are currently in the early stages of development. At least four different types of hepatitis C vaccines are in preclinical development. However, research for these candidate vaccines is hampered by the lack of reproducible tissue culture or a convenient small animal model for testing (212). Early studies in chimpanzees with several hepatitis C vaccines are currently underway.

Three different Epstein-Barr virus vaccine types are reported to be in phase I studies, including a glycoprotein subunit (gp350) vaccine, a vaccinia recombinant vaccine expressing gp350, and peptide induction of cutaneous T lymphocytes (212). It is yet unknown if the specific antigenic components of these vaccines are sufficient to prevent infection.

At least 14 different vaccines are under development for dengue virus. While most are in preclinical stages, a combined quadrivalent vaccine is in phase I trials. The live-attenuated vaccines have shown encouraging promise in the prevention of infection (212).

Viral vaccine development continues to move away from classical live-attenuated vaccines towards whole inactivated virus vaccines, peptide-based vaccines, DNA-based vaccines, use of viral vectors to insert recombinant information in vaccines, human immune globulins, monoclonal antibodies, and recombinant humanized vaccines, such as product production standardization, sustained immunological response, technical feasibility, less reactogenic, and nontransmissable or nonpathogenic to humans. However, there are challenges to the use of these new technologies, such as reliable efficacy and potency, need for an adjuvant or delivery system, or establishement of proof of principal.

Perhaps the greatest challenge is the expectation that a vaccine will be 100% effective and safe for every vaccinee. One death among 1 million vaccinees is considered excessive. However, without the vaccine, many more may die from the disease. Such is the case with the withdrawn approval of the rotavirus vaccine, when up to 600,000 children from developing countries die each year from dehydration and diarrhea. Adjuvants enhance the effect of the vaccine and may permit lower dosage levels and lower number of dosages. They may provide better mucosal immunity, more protection for the immunocompromised, and better antibody response (326).

IMMUNOGLOBULINS

Antibodies that occur in mucosal secretions play two major roles in antiviral immunity. One mechanism is to prevent the virus from reaching host target cells, thus providing immunity by exclusion. Usually the presence of a mucosal barrier prevents the virus from establishing an infection. A second mechanism is to neutralize viral infectivity by binding an antibody to a virus particle (Figure 4.2). Neutralization can occur via mucosal antibodies and within the cell. Antibodies may bind to virus particles rendering them unable to infect the cell. Neutralizing antibodies not only prevent infection but may aid in clearing already established infection. Other factors also may protect the host, such as innate immunity, specific antibody in mucosal fluids, antibody-dependent cellular cytotoxicity, and cytolytic T cells (321). IgA and IgG are present in high concentrations and contribute to intracellular neutralization and cell lysis. The antibodies can move through interstitial fluid and may enter through breaks in the epithelium.

One mechanism for administering immunoglobulins has been the nasal spray/respiratory inhaler as antibody in the respiratory tract prevents or lessens the viral infection and may even cure some viral infections. A number of human studies have been conducted to test the efficacy of intranasal antibody treatment to prevent viral respiratory tract infection. Treatments were by nose drops, aerosol application, or nasal spray.

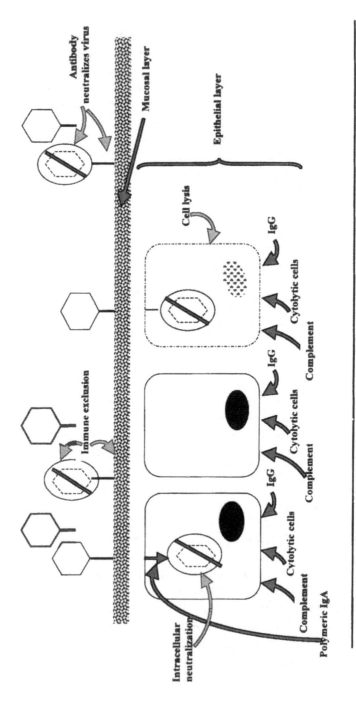

Fig. 4.2 Mechanisms for protection against viral diseases by immunoglobulins.

Generally, various treatments of coxsackie virus, influenza, and rhinovirus infections were effective in decreasing viral shedding. Human IgA treatments tended to decrease rhinitis and upper respiratory tract infection. The treatment of RSV with IgG (aerosol) and monoclonal antibody IgA (nose drops) was deemed safe with a trend for decreased illness (321).

Intravenous applications of immunoglobulin therapy as a treatment adjuvant or as immunoprophylaxis protect against RSV. Prophylactic use of immunoglobulins has significantly reduced morbidity and mortality of infectious diseases (Table 4.7).

Table 4.7 Immunoglobulin Systems Currently Utilized

Disease	Source of Immunoglobulins	Administration	Uses
Cytomega-lovirus	Specific human antibodies	Intravenous	Used as a prophylaxis for bone marrow and liver transplantation
Hepatitis A	Pooled human antibodies	Intramuscular	Pre- and postexposure prophylaxis
Hepatitis B	Specific human antibodies	Intramuscular	Hepatitis B postexposure prophylaxis
Human rabies	Specific human antibodies	Intramuscular injection and injection around wound	Rabies postexposure if patient was not immunized previously for rabies
Measles	Pooled human antibodies	Intramuscular	Postexposure prophylaxis
Vaccinia	Specific human antibodies	Intramuscular	Treatment of eczema vaccinatum, vaccinia necrosum and ocular vaccinia
Varicella-zoster	Specific human antibodies	Intramuscular	Susceptible pregnant women and perinatally exposed newborns; postexposure prophylaxis for the immunocompromised

Immunoglobulins are proteins made by B lymphocytes and plasma cells as part of the humoral portion of the immune system. Commercial sterile preparations are made from pooled human plasma of several thousand donors, and consist of purified IgG with small amounts of other globulins. These preparations were first used to treat immune deficiency diseases in 1952, following the discovery of Bruton's agammaglobulinemia (328). Early preparations were associated with frequent side effects when given intravenously, and thus required frequent and painful intramuscular administration. In 1981, an improved preparation of immunoglobulin was licensed for intravenous use (IVIG). FDA-approved indications include the following six conditions: 1) primary immunodeficiencies; 2) immune-mediated thrombocytopenia; 3) Kawasaki syndrome; 4) recent bone marrow transplantation (in persons at least 20 years of age); 5) chronic B-cell lymphocytic leukemia; and 6) pediatric HIV-1 infection (329). IVIG is also used in clinical practice for numerous other conditions, such as multiple sclerosis. Intravenous preparations are manufactured by several different companies and, due to differences in the production process and donor populations, the products available may vary considerably (330).

The intramuscular form of immunoglobulin is still available and is approved for the prophylaxis of hepatitis A and measles. Several immunoglobulin preparations with high titers to individual viruses are also available for the prophylaxis of specific viral infections. These hyperimmune globulins are available for rabies, varicella, CMV, respiratory syncytial virus, and hepatitis B. For the immunotherapy of viral infections, IVIG is predominantly used for cytomegalovirus prophylaxis in transplant recipients. Prophylactic treatment in bone marrow transplant recipients does not prevent CMV infection, but does lessen the risk of symptomatic disease, interstitial pneumonia, and death due to CMV (331,332). On comparing the use of IVIG and CMV hyperimmune globulin, there were no differences in clinical outcome to suggest the preferential use of CMV-IG (332,333). For bone marrow recipients with established CMV pneumonia, a combination treatment of IVIG and ganciclovir has been shown to improve survival (334,335). However, studies of IVIG alone for this situation have shown minimal efficacy (336,337). Studies of CMV prophylaxis with IVIG in renal transplant recipients have also shown favorable results, with either a decrease in the risk of infection and/or attenuation of clinical disease (338,339).

IVIG has also been shown to be of potential benefit for HIV-infected children. This population frequently suffers from bacterial infections with common encapsulated bacteria, whereas infected adults more frequently develop opportunistic infections (340). Several small studies have demonstrated decreased bacterial infections and sepsis as well as improved survival in HIV-positive children (341–343). Another study of HIV-infected children on zidovudine showed a benefit with the use of IVIG, but only in those subjects not receiving trimethoprim-sulfamethoxazole as antibiotic prophylaxis (344). The exact role of IVIG in this situation remains unclear.

Intramuscular immunoglobulin can be given for the prevention of measles in susceptible individuals (those with no previous infection or immunization). It is indicated for exposed persons with an increased risk of complications from disease, such as immunocompromised patients or children less than 1 year old. This treatment should be given within 6 days of exposure. The second indication for intramuscular immunoglobulin is the prophylaxis of hepatitis A. The protective effect is of most value if given prior to or immediately after exposure, and within 2 weeks of exposure. If given within several days of exposure, the immunoglobulin prevents infection in 80–95% of patients (345,346). This treatment was also indicated for travelers who planned to stay in areas with poor sanitation, but the HAV vaccine is now the preferred method for HAV prevention in travelers (347).

Rabies immune globulin is given once locally as well as systemically at the initiation of postexposure prophylaxis. It provides immediate antibodies to previously unvaccinated persons. Seven days after vaccination, recipients begin actively producing antibodies.

Hepatitis B immune globulin is given with hepatitis B vaccine in certain situations as part of the recommended post-exposure prophylaxis regimen. The following susceptible persons who were exposed to hepatitis B virus should receive hepatitis B hyperimmune globulin in addition to immunization: persons with acute exposure to HBsAg-positive blood; infants with perinatal exposure to HBsAg-positive mothers; persons with sexual exposure to HBsAg-positive partners; and infants with an HBsAg-positive primary care-giver. Hepatitis hyperimmune globulin has been evaluated for the prophylactic treatment of HBsAg-positive liver transplant recipients. High-dose, long-term treatment has led to increased survival and decreased serological recurrence in a number of studies (348,349). However, maintenance treatment is required for the prevention of recurrence and long-term treatment is expensive (350).

Varicella-zoster immune globulin should be administered to susceptible persons exposed to varicella virus who have an increased risk for complications (i.e., immunocompromised individuals). The postexposure prophylaxis should be administered as soon as possible and no later than 96 hours after exposure (351). The duration of protection lasts at least 3 weeks after the injection.

RSV immune globulin is indicated for prophylaxis in high-risk infants. A clinical trial by Groothuis et al. (352) evaluated monthly RSV-IG prophylaxis in at-risk infants with bronchopulmonary dysplasia, congenital heart disease, or prematurity. Results showed that the RSV-IG prophylaxis led to a reduction in the number of hospitalizations, hospital days, and intensive care unit days. These results were confirmed by a second clinical trial (353). Adverse reactions with any of the immunoglobulin preparations are rare. The incidence of systemic side effects is generally less than 5%, and these reactions are typically mild and self-limited. Fever, chills, headache, backache, nausea, vomiting, chest tightness, myalgias, and dyspnea have all been reported. With intravenous preparations, slowing of the infusion rate can be of benefit in alleviating the side effects. Hydrocortisone and antihistamines are also useful. Anaphylactic reactions may also occur in IgA-deficient patients receiving IVIG, but this is a rare complication (354). From 1985–1998, acute renal failure has been described in 120 IVIG recipients worldwide (330). Acute renal failure appears most closely associated with IVIG preparations with high sucrose content. The majority of affected patients developed renal failure within 7 days of IVIG administration, and 40% required dialysis due to the degree of failure. Although this complication remains infrequent, it is associated with significant morbidity and mortality.

Because these biological products are derived from human plasma, viral contamination poses a potential, though small, risk. In 1994, two different IVIG preparations were associated with hepatitis C contamination, leading to numerous cases of acute hepatitis C infection (more than 100 cases in the United States). The manufacturers added a solvent-detergent treatment for viral inactivation, and the products no longer are considered to be at risk for hepatitis C (355). All current IVIG preparations come from donors who are screened for hepatitis B and C, HIV, and elevated liver enzymes. Also, the majority of manufacturers include a viral inactivation step in the production process. No cases of HIV transmission have been reported with IVIG.

MONOCLONAL ANTIBODIES

Monoclonal antibodies are a more recent approach to antiviral immunotherapy. These antibodies have been developed for viruses such as HIV, although extensive evaluation has yet to be undertaken. A specific monoclonal antibody against cellular IL-2 receptors (daclizumab) has been developed and evaluated for the prevention of graft rejection in renal transplant recipients (356). In these graft recipients, daclizumab led to a decreased incidence of CMV infection when added to conventional dual immunosuppressive therapy, but had no effect when added to triple therapy. Additional development and studies will be needed.

The only licensed form of monoclonal antibodies available is palivizumab (Synagis) for RSV infection. This is a humanized preparation of monoclonal antibodies directed at the F glycoprotein, a specific surface protein of RSV (357). Because palivizumab is not produced from human blood products, it carries no risk of infectious contamination. Administration of the preparation is more convenient than RSV-IG, requiring 1 intramuscular injection rather than a 4-hour intravenous infusion of the hyperimmune globulin. In addition, product shortages are not expected since the preparation can easily be produced in large batches.

In a large, placebo-controlled clinical trial of high-risk infants, palivizumab led to a 55% reduction in RSV hospitalization, a 42% reduction in the number of hospitalization days, and a 57% reduction in intensive-care unit days due to RSV infection (358). Adverse effects are rare and minimal. When comparing palivizumab and placebo, there were no significant differences in the rates of side effects or the development of antibodies to monoclonal antibody (359), but an increase in aminotransferase levels was noted in the palivizumab group compared with placebo (290). Viral resistance has not yet been detected with the use of palivizumab (360).

CONCLUSION

The implementation of routine immunizations not only has a significant impact on the overall incidence of disease, but also markedly decreases the direct and indirect costs associated with health care. For instance, a 1994 study on the cost-effectiveness of a varicella vaccination program in the United States estimated a savings of $384 million per year (361). The cost savings with varicella are mostly due to a decrease in time lost from work by caregivers, although this is significant. Vaccines for more serious diseases that often require hospitalization, such as RSV in infants, will likely result in a more beneficial cost-effective profile. The cost savings of the eradication of smallpox, a disease which killed millions of people, approaches the level of infinity when considering the millions more that would have been affected. A similar situation exists for poliomyelitis, which is expected to be eradicated worldwide in the near future. The cost savings for an HIV vaccine would also be phenomenal, when considering the long-term treatment and numerous complications that are involved with this chronic infection.

Immunization has successfully led to the reduction in incidence of numerous diseases. Careful development and clinical evaluation have provided safe and effective vaccines with few adverse effects. Many reported adverse reactions following vaccination may be coincidental and have no proven direct relationship with the vaccine in question. Although serious side effects may rarely occur from vaccines, a much greater risk for morbidity and mortality results from the failure to become immunized. One vaccine, however, was recently removed from the market due to safety issues. Rotashield® was a live, oral tetravalent, rotavirus vaccine that was associated with several cases of intussusception and is considered to be causal (362).

Most associations between vaccines and adverse events are not, however, demonstrated to be causal. For example, the measles mumps rubella (MMR) vaccine was reported recently not to have a causal relationship to autism (363,364). Likewise, a causal relationship between the hepatitis B vaccine and a variety of autoimmune diseases has been disproven. This vaccine does not increase the risk of multiple sclerosis (365) nor does it cause a relapse of preexisting multiple sclerosis (366). Nevertheless, suspected relationships between vaccines and adverse events need to be reported to the "Vaccine Adverse Event Reporting System" (1-800-822-7967) so that the excellent safety record of vaccines can be maintained.

The technology of vaccine development has progressed dramatically in the last decade. While more conventional methods have consisted of whole-killed or live-attenuated viruses, more recent advancements include genetically engineered vectors and virus-like particles, among many others. Anticipated vaccine developments in the future show exciting promise in several areas, such as immunization with plants.

Potatoes, tomatoes, and bananas are currently undergoing genetic engineering to express immunizing antigens against infections such as hepatitis B virus and Norwalk virus (367, 368). This form of vaccination would offer a convenient, painless, and inexpensive approach to widespread control of disease and would thus be accessible to developing countries.

It is anticipated that the future will bring safe and effective vaccines for a variety of viral diseases, e.g., HIV, hepatitis C, HSV, and HPV. Although no vaccine is available for the therapy of a viral disease, the concept of vaccines is now being expanded by ongoing clinical trials of therapeutic vaccines, e.g., for HIV, HSV, and HPV.

REFERENCES

1. Wright, P. F., R. J. Kim-Farley, C. A. de Quadros, S. E. Robertson, R. M. Scott, N. A. Ward, and R. H. Henderson. 1991. Strategies for the global eradication of poliomyelitis by the year 2000. *N. Engl. J. Med.* 325:1774–1779.

2. Plotkin, S. A. 2001. Immunologic correlates of protection induced by vaccination. *Pediatr. Infect. Dis. J.* 20:63–75.

3. Henderson, D. A., and B. Moss. 1999. Smallpox and vaccinia. In: S. A. Plotkin and W. A. Orenstein (eds.). Vaccines, 3rd edition. Philadelphia: WB Saunders Company, 1999, pp. 74–97.

4. Is smallpox history? [editorial]. 1999. *Lancet* 353:1539.

5. LeDuc, J. W., and J. Becher. 1999. Current status of smallpox vaccine [letter]. *Emerg. Infect. Dis.* 5:593.

6. Frey, S. E., R. B. Couch, C. O. Tacket, J. J. Treanor, M. Wolff, F. K. Newman, R. L. Atmar, R. Edelman, C. M. Nolan, and R. B. Belshe, for the National Institute of Allergy and Infectious Diseases Smallpox Vaccine Study Group. 2002. Clinical responses to undiluted and diluted smallpox vaccine. *N. Engl. J. Med.* 346:1265–1274.

7. Frelinger, J. A., and M. L. Garba. 2002. Responses to smallpox vaccine [comment]. *N. Engl. J. Med.* 347:689–690.

8. Sauri, M. A. 2002. Responses to smallpox vaccine [comment]. *N. Engl. J. Med.* 347:689–690.

9. Bicknell, W. J. 2002. The case for voluntary smallpox vaccination. *N. Engl. J. Med.* 346:1323–1325.

10. Roizman, B., W. Joklik, B. Fields, and B. Moss. 1994. The destruction of smallpox virus stocks in national repositories: a grave mistake and a bad precedent. *Infect. Agents Dis.* 3:215–217.

11. Joklik, W. 1996. The remaining smallpox virus stocks are too valuable to be destroyed. *Scientist* 10:11.

12. Breman, J. G., and D. A. Henderson. 1998. Poxvirus dilemmas—monkeypox, smallpox, and biologic terrorism. *N. Engl. J. Med.* 339:556–559.

13. Weir, E. 2001. Does smallpox still pose a threat? *JAMC* 165:1380.

14. Lofquist, J. M., N. A. Weimert, and M. S. Hayney. 2003. Smallpox: a review of clinical disease and vaccination. *Am. J. Health-Syst. Pharm.* 60:749–758.

15. Meltzer, M. I., I. Damon, J. W. LeDuc, and J. D. Millar. 2001. Modeling potential responses to smallpox as a bioterrorist weapon. *Emerging Infect. Dis.* 7:959–969.

16. Kaplan, E. H., K. D. L. Craft, and L. M. Wein. 2002. Emergency response to a smallpox attack: the case for mass vaccination. *PNAS* 99:10935–10940.

17. Charatan, F. 2002. U. S. draws up plans for smallpox outbreak after terrorist attack. *Br. Med. J.* 324:1540.

18. Hanrahan, J. A., M. Jakubowycz, and B. R. Davis. 2003. A smallpox false alarm. *N. Engl. J. Med.* 348:467–468.

19. Smallpox, vaccine. 2003. *The Medical Letter* 45:1–2.

20. Frey, S. E., F. K. Newman, J. Cruz, W. B. Shelton, J. M. Tennant, T. Polach, A. L. Rothman, J. S. Kennedy, M. Wolff, R. B. Belshe, and F. A. Ennis. 2002. Dose-related effects of smallpox vaccine. *N. Engl. J. Med.* 346:1275–1280.

21. Sepkowitz, K. A. 2003. How contagious is vaccinia? *N. Engl. J. Med.* 348:439–446.

22. Kempner, A. R., M. M. Davis, and G. L. Freed. 2002. Expected adverse events in a mass smallpox vaccination campaign. *Eff. Clin. Pract.* 5:84–90.

23. Booss, J., and L. E. Davis. 2003. Smallpox and smallpox vaccination. *Neurology* 60:1241–1245.

24. Hoey, J. 2002. Smallpox vaccination advice. *JAMC* 167:1148.

25. Le, C. T., 2001. Combination vaccines: choices or chaos? a prac-
tioner's perspective. *Clin. Infect. Dis.* 35:S367–371.

26. Wharton, M., S. L. Cochi, and W. W. Williams. 1990. Measles,
mumps, and rubella vaccines. *Infect. Dis. Clin. North Am.*
4:47–73.

27. Centers for Disease Control and Prevention. 1998. Measles,
mumps, and rubella—vaccine use and strategies for elimination of measles, rubella, and congenital rubella syndrome and
control of mumps: recommendations of the Advisory Committee
on Immunization Practices (ACIP). *Morbid. Mortal Weekly Rep.*
47(No. RR-8):1–57.

28. Khakoo, G. A., and G. Lack. 2000. Recommendations for using
MMR vaccines in children allergic to eggs. *Br. Med. J.* 320:
929–932.

29. James, J. M., A. W. Burks, P. K. Roberson, and H. A. Sampson.
1995. Safe administration of the measles vaccine to children
allergic to eggs. *N. Engl. J. Med.* 332:1262–1266.

30. Gellin, B. G., and S. L. Katz. 1974. Putting a stop to a serial
killer: measles. *J. Infect. Dis.* 170:S1–S2.

31. Hope-Simpson, R. E. 1952. Infectiousness of communicable
diseases in the household (measles, chicken pox, and mumps).
Lancet 2:549–554.

32. Centers for Disease Control and Prevention. 1997. Measles
eradication: recommendations from a meeting cosponsored by
the World Health Organization, the Pan American Health Organization, and CDC. *Morbid. Mortal Weekly Rep.* 46(No. RR-
11):1–20.

33. Centers for Disease Control and Prevention. 2003. Measles—
United States, 2003. *Morbid. Mortal Weekly Rep.* 52:1211.

34. Murray, C. J., and A. D. Lopez. 1997. Mortality by cause for
eight regions of the world: global burden of disease study.
Lancet 349:1269–1276.

35. Krause, P. J., J. D. Cherry, J. M. Carney, M. J. Nalditch, and
K. O'Connor. 1980. Measles-specific lymphocyte reactivity and
serum antibody in subjects with different measles histories.
Am. J. Dis. Child. 134:567–571.

36. Watson, J. C., J. A. Pearson, L. E. Markowitz, A. L. Baughman, D. D. Erdman, W. J. Bellini, et al. 1996. An evaluation of measles revaccination among school-entry-aged children. *Pediatrics* 97:613–618.

37. Davis, R. M., E. D. Whitman, W. A. Orenstein, S. R. Preblud, L. E. Markowitz, and A. R. Hinman. 1987. A persistent outbreak of measles despite appropriate control measures. *Am. J. Epidemiol.* 126:438–449.

38. Krugman, S. 1983. Further-attenuated measles vaccine: characteristics and use. *Rev. Infect. Dis.* 5:477–481.

39. Mathias, R. G., W. G. Meekison, T. A. Arcand, and M. T. Schechter. 1989. The role of secondary vaccine failures in measles outbreaks. *Am. J. Public Health* 79:475–478.

40. Reyes, M. A., M. F. de Borrero, J. Roa, G. Bergonzoli, and N. G. Saravia. 1987. Measles vaccine failure after documented seroconversion. *Pediatr. Infect. Dis. J.* 6:848–851.

41. Centers for Disease Control and Prevention. 2003. Measles epidemic attributed to inadequate vaccination coverage—Campania, Italy, 2002. *Morbid. Mortal Weekly Rep.* 52:1044–1047.

42. Pelota., H., and O. P. Heinonen. 1986. Frequency of true adverse reactions to measles-mumps-rubella vaccine: a double-blind placebo-controlled trial in twins. *Lancet* 1:939–942.

43. Centers for Disease Control and Prevention. 1989. Measles—United States, 1988. *Morbid. Mortal Weekly Rep.* 38:601–605.

44. Modlin, J. F., J. T. Jabbour, J. J. Witte, and N. A. Halsey. 1977. Epidemiologic studies of measles, measles vaccine, and subacute sclerosing panencephalitis. *Pediatrics* 59:505–512.

45. Centers for Disease Control and Prevention. 1982. Subacute sclerosing panencephalitis surveillance—United States. *Morbid. Mortal Weekly Rep.* 31:585–588.

46. Dyken, P. R. 1985. Subacute sclerosing panencephalitis, current status. *Neurol. Clin.* 3:179–196.

47. Bennett, J. V., J. F. de Castro, J. L. Valdespino-Gomez, M. de Lourdes Garcia-Garcia, R. Islas-Romero, G. Echaniz-Aviles, and A. Jimenez-Corona. 2002. Aerosolized measles and measles-rubella vaccines induce better measles antibody booster

responses than injected vaccines: randomized trials in Mexican schoolchildren. *Bull. World Health Org.* 80:806–812.

48. Hilleman, M. R., E. B. Buynak, R. E. Weibel, and J. Stokes, Jr. 1968. Live, attenuated mumps vaccine. *N. Engl. J. Med.* 278:227–232.

49. Weibel, R. E., J. Stokes, Jr., E. B. Buynak, J. E. Whitman, Jr., and M. R. Hilleman. 1967. Live attenuated mumps-virus vaccine: 3. Clinical and serologic aspects in a field evaluation. *N. Engl. J. Med.* 276:245–251.

50. Sugg, W. C., J. A. Finger, R. H. Levine, and J. S. Pagano. 1968. Field evaluation of live virus mumps vaccine. *J. Pediatr.* 72:461–466.

51. Chaiken, B. P., N. M. Williams, S. R. Preblud, W. Parkin, and R. Altman. 1987. The effect of a school entry law on mumps activity in a school district. *J. Am. Med. Assoc.* 257:2455–2458.

52. Kim-Farley, R., S. Bart, H. Stetler, W. A. Orenstein, K. Bart, K. M. Sullivan, T. Halpin, and B. Sirotkin. 1985. Clinical mumps vaccine efficacy. *Am. J. Epidemiol.* 121:593–597.

53. Sullivan, K. M., T. J. Halpin, J. S. Marks, and R. Kim-Farley. 1985. Effectiveness of mumps vaccine in a school outbreak. *Am. J. Dis. Child.* 139:909–912.

54. Wharton, M., S. L. Cochi, R. H. Hutcheson, J. M. Bitowish, and W. Schaffner. 1988. A large outbreak of mumps in the postvaccine era. *J. Infect. Dis.* 158:1253–1260.

55. Hersh, B. S., P. E. Fine, W. K. Kent, S. L. Cochi, L. H. Kahn, E. R. Zell, P. L. Hays, and C. L. Wood. 1991. Mumps outbreak in a highly vaccinated population. *J. Pediatr.* 119:187–193.

56. Centers for Disease Control and Prevention. 1995. Mumps surveillance—United States, 1988–1993. *Morbid. Mortal Weekly Rep.* 44(SS-3):1–14.

57. Weibel, R. E., E. B. Buynak, A. A. McLean, and M. R. Hilleman. 1978. Persistence of antibody after administration of monovalent and combined live attenuated measles, mumps, and rubella virus vaccines. *Pediatrics* 61:5–11.

58. Chang, T. W., S. DesRosiers, and L. Weinstein. 1970. Clinical and serologic studies of an outbreak of rubella in a vaccinated population. *N. Engl. J. Med.* 283:246–248.

59. Bakshi, S. S., and L. Z. Cooper. 1990. Rubella and mumps vaccines. *Pediatr. Clin. North Am.* 37:651–668.

60. Plotkin, S. A., J. D. Farquhar, and P. L. Ogra. 1973. Immunologic properties of RA 27-3 rubella virus vaccine: a comparison with strains presently licensed in the United States. *J. Am. Med. Assoc.* 225:585–590.

61. Gershon, A. A., H. M. Frey, W. Borkowsky, and S. Steinberg. 1980. Live attenuated rubella virus vaccine: comparison of responses to HPV-77-DE5 and RA 27/3 strains. *Am. J. Med. Sci.* 279:95–97.

62. Hilleman, M. R., R. E. Weibel, E. B. Buynak, J. Stokes, Jr., and J. E. Whitman, Jr. 1967. Live attenuated mumps-virus vaccine: 4. Protective efficacy as measured in a field evaluation. *N. Engl. J. Med.* 276:252–258.

63. Chu, S. Y., R. H. Bernier, J. A. Stewart, K. L. Herrmann, J. R. Greenspan, A. K. Henderson, and A. P. Liang. 1988. Rubella antibody persistence after immunization: sixteen-year follow-up in the Hawaiian islands. *J. Am. Med. Assoc.* 259:3133–3136.

64. O'Shea, S., J. M. Best, J. E. Banatvala, W. C. Marshall, and J. A. Dudgeon. 1982. Rubella vaccination: persistence of antibodies for up to 16 years. *Br. Med. J. (Clin. Res. Ed.)* 285:253–255.

65. Kimberlin, D. W. 1997. Rubella immunization. *Pediatr. Ann.* 26:366–370.

66. Freestone, D. S., J. Prydie, S. G. Smith, and G. Laurence. 1971. Vaccination of adults with Wistar RA 27/3 rubella vaccine. *J. Hyg. (Lond.)* 69:471–477.

67. Polk, B. F., J. F. Modlin, J. A. White, and P. C. De Girolami. 1982. A controlled comparison of joint reactions among women receiving one of two rubella vaccines. *Am. J. Epidemiol.* 115:19–25.

68. Preblud, S. R., M. K. Serdula, J. A. Frank, Jr., A. D. Brandling-Bennet, and A. R. Hinman. 1980. Rubella vaccination in the United States: a ten-year review. *Epidemiol. Rev.* 2:171–194.

69. Panagiotopoulos, T., I. Antoniadore, and E. Valessi-Adam. 1999. Increase in congential rubella. *B. Med. J.* 319:1462–1467.

70. Centers for Disease Control and Prevention. 1999. Prevention of varicella: updated recommendations of the Advisory Committee

on Immunization Practices (ACIP). *Morbid. Mortal Weekly Rep.* 48(No. RR-6):1–5.

71. Arvin, A. M. 2001. Varicella vaccine—the first six years. *N. Engl. J. Med.* 344:1007–1009.

72. Vazquez, M., P. S. LaRussa, A. A. Gershon, S. O. Steinberg, K. Freudigman, and E. D. Shapiro. 2001. The effectiveness of the varicella vaccine in clinical practice. *N. Engl. J. Med.* 344: 955–960.

73. Wise, R. P., M. E. Salive, M. M. Braun, G. T. Mootrey, J. F. Seward, L. G. Rider, and P. R. Krause. 2000. Postlicensure safety surveillance for varicella vaccine. *J. Am. Med. Assoc.* 284:1271–1279.

74. White, C. J. 1997. Varicella-zoster virus vaccine. *Clin. Infect. Dis.* 24:753–763.

75. Takahashi., M. 1986. Clinical overview of varicella vaccine: development and early studies. *Pediatrics* 78:736–741.

76. Asano, Y., S. Suga, T. Yoshikawa, I. Kobayashi, T. Yazaki, M. Shibata, Shibata M., K. Tsuzuki, and S. Ito. 1994. Experience and reason: twenty-year follow-up of protective immunity of the Oka strain live varicella vaccine. *Pediatrics* 94:524–526.

77. Weibel, R. E., B. J. Neff, B. J. Kuter, H. A. Guess, C. A. Rothenberger, A. J. Fitzgerald, K. A. Connor, A. A. McLean, M. R. Hilleman, E. B. Buynak, et al. 1984. Live attenuated varicella virus vaccine: efficacy trial in healthy children. *N. Engl. J. Med.* 310:1409–1415.

78. Kuter, B. J., R. E. Weibel, H. A. Guess, H. Matthews, D. H. Morton, B. J. Neff, P. J. Provost, B. A. Watson, S. E. Starr, and S. A. Plotkin. 1991. Oka/Merck varicella vaccine in healthy children: final report of a 2-year efficacy study and 7-year follow-up studies. *Vaccine* 9:643–647.

79. Watson, B. M., P. M. Keller, R. W. Ellis, and S. E. Starr. 1990. Cell-mediated immune responses after immunization of healthy seronegative children with varicella vaccine: kinetics and specificity. *J. Infect. Dis.* 162:794–799.

80. White, C. J., B. J. Kuter, C. S. Hildebrand, K. L. Isganitis, H. Matthews, W. J. Miller, P. J. Provost, R. W. Ellis, R. J. Gerety, and G. B. Calandra. 1991. Varicella vaccine (VARIVAX) in

healthy children and adolescents: results from clinical trials, 1987 to 1989. *Pediatrics* 87:604–610.

81. Watson, B., C. Boardman, D. Laufer, S. Piercy, N. Tustin, D. Olaleye, A. Cnaan, and S. E. Starr. 1995. Humoral and cell-mediated immune responses in healthy children after one or two doses of varicella vaccine. *Clin. Infect. Dis.* 20:316–319.

82. Watson, B., R. Gupta, T. Randall, and S. Starr. 1994. Persistence of cell-mediated and humoral immune responses in healthy children immunized with live attenuated varicella vaccine. *J. Infect. Dis.* 169:197–199.

83. Asano, Y., T. Nagai, T. Miyata, T. Yazaki, S. Ito, K. Yamanishi, and M. Takahashi. 1985. Long-term protective immunity of recipients of the OKA strain of live varicella vaccine. *Pediatrics* 75:667–671.

84. Kuter, B. J., A. Ngai, C. M. Patterson, B. O. Staehle, I. Cho, H. Matthews, P. J. Provost, and C. J. White, for the Oka/Merck Varicella Vaccine Study Group. 1995. Safety, tolerability, and immunogenicity of two regimens of Oka/Merck varicella vaccine (Varivax) in healthy adolescents and adults. *Vaccine* 13:967–972.

85. Hardy, I., A. A. Gershon, S. P. Steinberg, and P. LaRussa for the Varicella Vaccine Collaborative Study Group. 1991. The incidence of zoster after immunization with live attenuated varicella vaccine. A study in children with leukemia. *N. Engl. J. Med.* 325:1545–1550.

86. Heller, L., G. Berglund, L. Ahström, K. Hellstrand, and B. Wahren. 1985. Early results of a trial of the Oka-strain varicella vaccine in children with leukaemia or other malignancies in Sweden. *Postgrad. Med. J.* 61(Suppl 4):79–83.

87. Gershon, A. A., S. P. Steinberg, L. Gelb, G. Galasso, W. Borkowsky, P. LaRussa, and A. Farrara. 1984. Live attenuated varicella vaccine-efficacy for children with leukemia in remission. *J. Am. Med. Assoc.* 252:355–362.

88. Tsolia, M., A. A. Gershon, S. P. Steinberg, and L. Gelb, for the National Institute of Allergy and Infectious Diseases Varicella Vaccine Collaborative Study Group. 1990. Live attenuated varicella vaccine: evidence that the virus is attenuated and the importance of skin lesions in transmission of varicella-zoster virus. *J. Pediatr.* 116:184–189.

89. White, C. J., B. J. Kuter, A. Ngai, C. S. Hildebrand, K. L. Isganitis, C. M. Patterson, A. Capra, W. J. Miller, D. L. Krah, P. J. Provost, et al. 1992. Modified cases of chickenpox after varicella vaccination: correlation of protection with antibody response. *Pediatr. Infect. Dis. J.* 11:19–23.

90. Clements, D. A., C. B. Armstrong, A. M. Ursano, M. M. Moggio, E. B. Walter, and C. M. Wilfert. 1995. Over five-year follow-up of Oka/Merck varicella vaccine recipients in 465 infants and adolescents. *Pediatr. Infect. Dis. J.* 14:874–879.

91. Bernstein, H. H., E. P. Rothstein, B. M. Watson, K. S. Reisinger, M. M. Blatter, C. O. Wellman, S. A. Chartrand, I. Cho, A. Ngai, and C. J. White. 1993. Clinical survey of natural varicella compared with breakthrough varicella after immunization with live attenuated Oka/Merck varicella vaccine. *Pediatrics* 92:833–837.

92. Hammerschlag, M. R., A. Gershon, S. Steinberg, L. Clarke, and L. Gelb. 1989. Herpes zoster in an adult recipient of live attenuated varicella vaccine. *J. Infect. Dis.* 160:535–537. [Erratum, *J. Infect. Dis.* 160:1095, 1989.]

93. Gelb, L. D., D. E. Dohner, A. A. Gershon, S. P. Steinberg, J. L. Waner, M. Takahashi, P. H. Dennehy, and A. E. Brown. 1987. Molecular epidemiology of live, attenuated varicella virus vaccine in children and in normal adults. *J. Infect. Dis.* 155:633–640.

94. White, C. J. 1996. Clinical trials of varicella vaccine in healthy children. *Infect. Dis. Clin. North Am.* 10:595–608.

95. Watson, B., J. Seward, A. Yang, P. Witte, J. Lutz, C. Chan, S. Orlin, and R. Levenson. 2000. Postexposure effectiveness of varicella vaccine. *Pediatrics* 105:84–88.

96. Wood, J. M. 2001. Developing vaccines against pandemic influenza. *Phil. Trans. R. Soc. Lond. B Biol. Sci.* 356:1953–1960.

97. Fiers, W., S. Neirynchk, T. Derov, X. Saelens, and W. M. Jon. 2001. Soluble recombinant influenza vaccine. *Phil. Trans. R. Soc. Lond. B Biol. Sci.* 356:1961–1963.

98. Rimmelzuvan, G. F., and A. D. Osterhaust. 2001. Influenza vaccines: new development. *Current Opin. Pharmacol.* 1:491–496.

99. La Montagne, J. R., G. R. Noble, G. V. Quinnan, G. T. Curlin, W. C. Blackwelder, J. I. Smith, F. A. Ennis, and F. M. Bozeman. 1983.

Summary of clinical trials of inactivated influenza vaccine—1978. *Rev. Infect. Dis.* 5:723–776.

100. Centers for Disease Control and Prevention. 1999. Prevention and control of influenza: recommendations of the Advisory Committee on Immunization Practices (ACIP). *Morbid. Mortal Weekly Rep.* 48(No. RR-4):1–28.

101. Neuzil, K. M., W. D. Dupont, P. F. Wright, and K. M. Edwards. 2001. Efficacy of inactivated and cold-adapted vaccines against influenza A infection, 1985 to 1990: the pediatric experience. *Pediatr. Infect. Dis. J.* 20:732–740.

102. Gross, P. A., A. W. Hermogenes, H. S. Sacks, J. Lau, and R. A. Levandowski. 1995. The efficacy of influenza vaccine in elderly persons: a meta-analysis and review of the literature. *Ann. Intern. Med.* 123:518–527.

103. Mullooly, J. P., M. D. Bennett, M. C. Hornbrook, W. H. Barker, W. W. Williams, P. A. Patriarca, and P. H. Rhodes. 1994. Influenza vaccination programs for elderly persons: cost-effectiveness in a health maintenance organization. *Ann. Intern. Med.* 121:947–952.

104. Meiklejohn, G. 1983. Viral respiratory disease at Lowry Air Force Base in Denver, 1952–1982. *J. Infect. Dis.* 148:775–784.

105. Davenport, F. M. 1961. Inactivated influenza virus vaccines: past, present, and future. *Am. Rev. Respir. Dis.* 83(Suppl):146–150.

106. Palache, A. M. 1997. Influenza vaccine: a reappraisal of their use. *Drugs* 54:841–856.

107. Goronzy, J. J., J. W. Fulbright, C. S. Crowson, G. A. Poland, W. M. O'Fallon, and C. M. Weyand. 2001. Value of immuno-logical markers in predicting responsiveness to influenza vaccination in elderly individuals. *J. Virol.* 75:12182–12187.

108. Govaert, T. M., C. T. Thijs, N. Masurel, M. J. Sprenger, G. J. Dinant, and J. A. Knottnerus. 1994. The efficacy of influenza vaccination in elderly individuals: a randomized double-blind placebo-controlled trial. *J. Am. Med. Assoc.* 272:1661–1665.

109. Patriarca, P. A., J. A. Weber, R. A. Parker, W. N. Hall A. P. Kendal, D. J. Bregman, and L. B. Schonberger. 1985. Efficacy of influenza vaccine in nursing homes: reduction in illness and complications during an influenza A (H3N2) epidemic. *J. Am. Med. Assoc.* 253:1136–1139.

110. Arden, N. H., P. A. Patriarca, and A. P. Kendal. 1986. Experiences in the use and efficacy of inactivated influenza vaccine in nursing homes. In: A. P. Kendal and P. A. Patriarca (eds.). Options for the Control of Influenza. New York: Alan R. Liss, Inc; 1986, pp. 155–168.

111. Kilbourne, E. D., and N. H. Arden. 1999. Inactivated influenza vaccines. In: S. A. Plotkin and W. A. Orenstein (eds.). Vaccines, 3rd edition. Philadelphia: WB Saunders Company; 1999, pp. 531–551.

112. Influenza vaccine, 1999–2000. 1999. *Med. Lett. Drugs. Ther.* 41:82–83.

113. Nichol, K. L., A. Lind, K. L. Margolis, M. Murdoch, R. McFadden, M. Hauge, S. Magnan, and M. Drake. 1995. The effectiveness of vaccination against influenza in healthy, working adults. *N. Engl. J. Med.* 333:889–893.

114. Schonberger, L. B., D. J. Bregman, J. Z. Sullivan-Bolyai, R. A. Keenlyside, D. W. Ziegler, H. F. Retailliau, D. L. Eddins, and J. A. Bryan. 1979. Guillain-Barré syndrome following vaccination in the National Influenza Immunization Program, United States, 1976–1977. *Am. J. Epidemiol.* 110:105–123.

115. Bierman, C. W., G. G. Shapiro, W. E. Pierson, J. W. Taylor, H. M. Foy, and J. P. Fox. 1977. Safety of influenza vaccination in allergic children. *J. Infect. Dis.* 136 (Suppl):S652–S655.

116. Belshe, R. B., P. M. Mendelman, J. Treanor, J. King, W. C. Gruber, P. Piedra, D. I. Bernstein, F. G. Hayden, K. Kotloff, K. Zangwill, D. Iacuzio, and M. Wolff. 1998. The efficacy of live attenuated, cold-adapted, trivalent, intranasal influenza virus vaccine in children. *N. Engl. J. Med.* 338:1405–1412.

117. Nichol, K. L., P. M. Mendelman, K. P. Mallon, L. A. Jackson, G. J. Gorse, R. B. Belshe, W. P. Glezen, and J. Wittes. 1999. Effectiveness of live, attenuated intranasal influenza virus vaccine in healthy, working adults. *J. Am. Med. Assoc.* 282: 137–144.

118. Balcarek, K. B., M. R. Bagley, R. F. Pass, E. R. Schiff, and D. S. Krause. 1995. Safety and immunogenicity of an inactivated hepatitis A vaccine in preschool children. *J. Infect. Dis.* 171 (Suppl 1):S70–S72.

119. Clemens, R., A. Safary, A. Hepburn, C. Roche, W. J. Stanbury, and F. E. André. 1995. Clinical experience with an inactivated hepatitis A vaccine. *J. Infect. Dis.* 171(Suppl 1):S44–S49.

120. Horng, Y. C., M. H. Chang, C. Y. Lee, A. Safary, F. E. André, and D. S. Chen. 1993. Safety and immunogenicity of hepatitis A vaccine in healthy children. *Pediatr. Infect. Dis. J.* 12: 359–362.

121. Westblom, T. U., S. Gudipati, C. DeRousse, B. R. Midkiff, and R. B. Belshe. 1994. Safety and immunogenicity of an inactivated hepatitis A vaccine: effect of dose and vaccination schedule. *J. Infect. Dis.* 169:996–1001.

122. Block, S. L., J. A. Hedrick, R. D. Tyler, R. A. Smith, G. Calandra, C. Patterson, J. Lewis, R. Sitrin, W. Miller, S. Schwartz, et al. 1993. Safety, tolerability and immunogenicity of a formalin-inactivated hepatitis A vaccine (VAQTA) in rural Kentucky children. *Pediatr. Infect. Dis. J.* 12:976–980.

123. Werzberger, A., B. Mensch, B. Kuter, L. Brown, J. Lewis, R. Sitrin, W. Miller, D. Shouval, B. Wiens, G. Calandra, et al. 1992. A controlled trial of a formalin-inactivated hepatitis A vaccine in healthy children. *N. Engl. J. Med.* 327:453–457.

124. Innis, B. L., R. Snitbhan, P. Kunasol, T. Laorakpongse, W. Poopatanakool, C. A. Kozik, S. Suntayakorn, T. Suknuntapong, A. Safary, D. B. Tang, et al. 1994. Protection against hepatitis A by an inactivated vaccine. *J. Am. Med. Assoc.* 271:1328–1334.

125. Centers for Disease Control and Prevention. 1996. Prevention of hepatitis A through active or passive immunization: recommendations of the Advisory Committee on Immunization Practices (ACIP). *Morbid. Mortal Weekly Rep.* 45(No. RR-15): 1–30.

126. Wiens, B. L., N. R. Bohidar, J. G. Pigeon, J. Egan, W. Hurni, L. Brown, B. J. Kuter, and D. R. Nalin. 1996. Duration of protection from clinical hepatitis A disease after vaccination with VAQTA. *J. Med. Virol.* 49:235–241.

127. Van Damme, P., S. Thoelen, M. Cramm, K. De Groote, and A. Safary, and A. Meheus. 1994. Inactivated hepatitis A vaccine: reactogenicity, immunogenicity, and long-term antibody persistence. *J. Med. Virol.* 44:446–451.

128. Wiedermann, G., M. Kundi, F. Ambrosch, A. Safary, E. D'Hondt, and A. Delem. 1997. Inactivated hepatitis A vaccine: long term antibody persistence. *Vaccine* 15:612–615.

129. Nalin, D. R., B. J. Kuter, L. Brown, C. Patterson, G. B. Calandra, A. Werzberger, D. Shouval, E. Ellerbeck, S. L. Block, R. Bishop, et al. 1993. Worldwide experience with the CR326F-derived inactivated hepatitis A virus vaccine in pediatric and adult populations: an overview. *J. Hepatol.* 18(Suppl 2): S51–S55.

130. Centers for Disease Control and Prevention. 2003. Hepatitis A outbreak associated with green onions at a restaurant—Monaca, Pennsylvania, 2003. *Morbid. Mortal Weekly Rep.* 52:1155–1157.

131. Douglas, R. G. 1996. The heritage of hepatitis B vaccine. *J. Am. Med. Assoc.* 276:1796–1798.

132. Francis, D. P., S. C. Hadler, S. E. Thompson, J. E. Maynard, D. G. Ostrow, N. Altman, E. H. Braff, P. O'Malley, D. Hawkins, F. N. Judson, K. Penley, T. Nylund, G. Christie, F. Meyers, J. N. Moore, Jr., A. Gardner, I. L. Doto, J. H. Miller, G. H. Reynolds, B. L. Murphy, C. A. Schable, B. T. Clark, J. W. Curran, and A. G. Redeker. 1982. The prevention of hepatitis B with vaccine: report of the Centers for Disease Control multicenter efficacy trial among homosexual men. *Ann. Intern. Med.* 97:362–366.

133. Szmuness, W., C. E. Stevens, E. J. Harley, E. A. Zang, W. R. Oleszko, D. C. William, R. Sadovsky, J. M. Morrison, and A. Kellner. 1980. Hepatitis B vaccine: demonstration of efficacy in a controlled trial in a high-risk population in the United States. *N. Engl. J. Med.* 303:833–841.

134. Katkov, W. N., and J. L. Dienstag. 1995. Hepatitis vaccines. *Gastroenterol. Clin. North Am.* 24:147–159.

135. Denis, F., M. Mounier, L. Hessel, J. P. Michel, N. Gualde, F. Dubois, F. Barin, and A. Goudeau. 1984. Hepatitis-B vaccination in the elderly. *J. Infect. Dis.* 149:1019.

136. Heyward, W. L., T. R. Bender, B. J. McMahon, D. B. Hall, D. P. Francis, A. P. Lanier, W. L. Alward, J. L. Ahtone, B. L. Murphy, and J. E. Maynard. 1985. The control of hepatitis B virus infection with vaccine in Yupik Eskimos: demonstration of safety, immunogenicity, and efficacy under field conditions. *Am. J. Epidemiol.* 121:914–923.

137. Roome, A. J., S. J. Walsh, M. L. Cartter, and J. L. Hadler. 1993. Hepatitis B vaccine responsiveness in Connecticut public safety personnel. *J. Am. Med. Assoc.* 270:2931–2934.

138. Wood, R. C., K. L. MacDonald, K. E. White, C. W. Hedberg, M. Hanson, and M. T. Osterholm. 1993. Risk factors for lack of detectable antibody following hepatitis B vaccination of Minnesota health care workers. *J. Am. Med. Assoc.* 270: 2935–2949.

139. Zimmerman, R. K., F. L. Ruben, and E. R. Ahwesh. 1997. Hepatitis B virus infection, hepatitis B vaccine, and hepatitis B immune globulin. *J. Fam. Pract.* 45:295–315.

140. Thoelen, S., P. Van Damme, C. Mathei, G. Leroux-Roels, I. Desombere, A. Safary, P. Vandepapeliere, M. Slaoui, and A. Meheus. 1998. Safety and immunogenicity of a hepatitis B vaccine formulated with a novel adjuvant system. *Vaccine* 16:708–714.

141. Heineman, T. C., N. L. Clements-Mann, G. A. Poland, R. M. Jacobson, A. E. Izu, D. Sakamoto, J. Eiden, G. A. Van Nest, and H. H. Hsu. 1999. A randomized, controlled study in adults of the immunogenicity of a novel hepatitis B vaccine containing MF59 adjuvant. *Vaccine* 17:2769–2778.

142. Jilg, W. 1998. Novel hepatitis B vaccines. *Vaccine* 16(Suppl): S65–S68.

143. Hourvitz, A., R. Mosseri, A. Solomon, Y. Yehezkelli, J. Atsmon, Y. L. Danon, R. Koren, and D. Shouval. 1996. Reactogenicity and immunogenicity of a new recombinant hepatitis B vaccine containing Pre S antigens: a preliminary report. *J. Viral. Hepat.* 3:37–42.

144. Yap, I., R. Guan, and S. H. Chan. 1992. Recombinant DNA hepatitis B vaccine containing Pre-S components of the HBV coat protein—a preliminary study on immunogenicity. *Vaccine* 10:439–442.

145. Bertino, J. S. Jr., P. Tirrell, R. N. Greenberg, H. L. Keyserling, G. A. Poland, D. Gump, M. L. Kumar, and K. Ramsey. 1997. A comparative trial of standard or high-dose S subunit recombinant hepatitis B vaccine versus a vaccine containing S subunit, Pre-S1, and Pre-S2 particles for revaccination of healthy adult nonresponders. *J. Infect. Dis.* 175:678–681.

146. Jilg, W., M. Schmidt, and F. Deinhardt. 1988. Persistence of specific antibodies after hepatitis B vaccination. *J. Hepatol.* 6:201–207.

147. Stevens, C. E., P. E. Taylor, M. J. Tong, and P. T. Toy. 1984. Hepatitis B vaccine; an overview. In: G. N. Vyas, J. L. Dienstag, and J. H. Hoofnagle (eds.). Viral Hepatitis and Liver Disease. Orlando: Grune & Stratton, 1984, pp. 275–291.

148. Hadler, S. C., D. P. Francis, J. E. Maynard, S. E. Thompson, F. N. Judson, D. F. Echenberg, D. G. Ostrow, P. M. O'Malley, K. A. Penley, N. L. Altman, et al. 1986. Long-term immunogenicity and efficacy of hepatitis B vaccine in homosexual men. *N. Engl. J. Med.* 315:209–214.

149. Stevens, C. E., P. T. Toy, P. E. Taylor, T. Lee, and H. Y. Yip. 1992. Prospects for control of hepatitis B virus infection: implications of childhood vaccination and long-term protection. *Pediatrics* 90:170–173.

150. Centers for Disease Control and Prevention. 1999. Notice to readers: availability of hepatitis B vaccine that does not contain thimerosal as a preservative. *Morbid. Mortal Weekly Rep.* 48:780–782.

151. Andre, F. E., and A. Safary. 1987. Summary of clinical findings on Engerix-B, a genetically engineered yeast derived hepatitis B vaccine. *Postgrad. Med. J.* 63(Suppl 2):169–178.

152. Centers for Disease Control and Prevention. 1996. Update: vaccine side effects, adverse reactions, contraindications and precautions: recommendations of the Advisory Committee on Immunization Practices (ACIP). *Morbid. Mortal Weekly Rep.* 45(No. RR-12):1–35.

153. Andre, F. E. 1990. Overview of 5 year clinical experience with a yeast-derived hepatitis B vaccine. *Vaccine* 8(Suppl):74–78.

154. Neau, D., F. Bonnet, M. Michaud, Y. Perel, M. Longy-Boursier, J. M. Ragnaud, and J. M. Guillard. 1998. Immune thrombocytopenic purpura after recombinant hepatitis B vaccine: retrospective study of seven cases. *Scand. J. Infect. Dis.* 30:115–118.

155. Ronchi, F., P. Cecchi, F. Falcioni, A. Marsciani, G. Minak, G. Muratori, P. L. Tazzari, and S. Beverini. 1998. Thrombocytopenic purpura as adverse reaction to recombinant hepatitis B vaccine. *Arch. Dis. Child.* 78:273–284.

156. Poullin, P., and B. Gabriel. 1994. Thrombocytopenic purpura after recombinant hepatitis B vaccine [letter]. *Lancet* 334:1293.

157. Le Hello, C., P. Cohen, M. G. Bousser, P. Letellier, and L. Guillevin. 1999. Suspected hepatitis B vaccination related vasculitis. *J. Rheumatol.* 26:191–194.

158. Allen, M. B., P. Cockwell, and R. L. Page. 1993. Pulmonary and cutaneous vasculitis following hepatitis B vaccination. *Thorax* 48:580–581.

159. Pope, J. E., A. Stevens, W. Howson, and D. A. Bell. 1998. The development of rheumatoid arthritis after recombinant hepatitis B vaccination. *J. Rheumatol.* 25:1687–1693.

160. Rebora, A., F. Rongioletti, F. Drago, and A. Parodi. 1999. Lichen planus as a side effect of HBV vaccination. *Dermatology* 198:1–2.

161. Saywell, C. A., R. A. Wittal, and S. Kossard. 1997. Lichenoid reaction to hepatitis B vaccination. *Australas. J. Dermatol.* 38:152–154.

162. Chen, DS. 1991. Control of hepatitis B in Asia: mass immunization program in Taiwan. In: F. B. Hollinger, S. M. Lemon, and H. S. Margolis (eds.). Viral Hepatitis and Liver Disease. Baltimore: Williams & Wilkins, 1991, pp. 616–619.

163. Hoenig, L. J. 1986. Triumph and controversy—Pasteur's preventive treatment of rabies as reported in the JAMA. *Arch. Neurol.* 34:397–399.

164. Wiktor, T. J. 1976. Production and control of rabies vaccines made on diploid cells. *Dev. Biol. Stand.* 37:265–266.

165. National Association of State Public Health Veterinarians, Inc. 2003. Comprendium of animal rabies prevention and control, 2003. *Morbid. Mortal Weekly Rep.* 52:1–6.

166. Oral Rabies Vaccination Programs (ORVP). Texas Department of Health 11/19/02.

167. Anderson, L. J., R. K. Sikes, C. W. Langkop, J. M. Mann, J. S. Smith, W. G. Winkler, and M. W. Deitch. 1980. Postexposure trial of a human diploid cell strain rabies vaccine. *J. Infect. Dis.* 142:133–138.

168. Kuwert, E. K., I. Marcus, J. Werner, P. G. Hoher, O. Thraenhart, E. Hierholzer, A. Iwand, E. B. Helm, T. J. Wiktor, and H.

Koprowski. 1977. [Postexposure use of human diploid cell culture rabies vaccine.] *Zentralbl. Bakteriol.* [Orig A] 239(4): 437–458.

169. Strady, A., J. Lang, M. Lienard, C. Blondeau, R. Jaussaud, and S. Plotkin. 1998. Antibody persistence following preexposure regimens of cell-culture rabies vaccines: 10-year follow-up and proposal for a new booster policy. *J. Infect. Dis.* 177:1290–1295.

170. Centers for Disease Control and Prevention. 1999. Human rabies prevention—United States, 1999: recommendations of the Advisory Committee on Immunization Practices (ACIP). *Morbid. Mortal Weekly Rep.* 48(No. RR-1):1–21.

171. Centers for Disease Control and Prevention. 1984. Rabies prevention—United States, 1984: recommendations of the Advisory Committee on Immunization Practices (ACIP). *Morbid. Mortal Weekly Rep.* 33:393–408.

172. Centers for Disease Control and Prevention. 1980. Adverse reactions to human diploid cell rabies vaccine. *Morbid. Mortal Weekly Rep.* 29:609–610.

173. Centers for Disease Control and Prevention. 1984. Systemic allergic reactions following immunization with human diploid cell rabies vaccine. *Morbid. Mortal Weekly Rep.* 33:185–187.

174. Dreesen, D. W., K. W. Bernard, R. A. Parker, Deutsch, and J. Brown. 1986. Immune complex-like disease in 23 persons following a booster dose of rabies human diploid cell vaccine. *Vaccine* 4:45–49.

175. Tantawichien, T., W. Jaijaroensup, P. Khawplod, and V. Sitprija. 2001. Failure of multiple-site intradermal postexposure rabies vaccination in patients with human immunodeficiency virus with low lymphocyte counts. *Clin. Inf. Dis.* 33:E122–E124.

176. Gibbons, R. V., and C. E. Rupprecht. 2001. Postexposure rabies prophylaxis in immunosuppressed patients [letters]. *J. Am. Med. Assoc.* 285:1574–1575.

177. Hay, E., H. Derazon, N. Bukish, S. Scharf, and S. Rishpon. 2001. Postexposure rabies prophylaxis in a patient with lymphoma. *J. Am. Med. Assoc.* 285:166–167.

178. Dreesen, D. W., D. B. Fishbein, D. T. Kemp, and J. Brown. 1989. Two-year comparative trial on the immunogenicity and adverse

effects of purified chick embryo cell rabies vaccine for pre-exposure immunization. *Vaccine* 7:379–400.

179. Vodipiyi, I., P. Sureau, and M. Lafon. 1986. An evaluation of second generation tissue culture rabies vaccine for use in man: a four-vaccine comparative immunogenicity study using a pre-exposure vaccination schedule and an abbreviated 2-1-1 post-exposure schedule. *Vaccine* 4:245–248.

180. Marwick, C. 1985. Changes recommended in use of human diploid cell rabies vaccine [news]. *J. Am. Med. Assoc.* 245:14–15.

181. Riti, M. D. 2002. DNA and a new rabies vaccine Rediff.com, 25 November 2002. (http://indiabroad.rediff.com/news/2002/nov/25spec.html).

182. van Wezel A. L., C. A. van der Velden-de Groot, and J. A. van Herwarden. 1980. The production of inactivated poliovaccine on serially cultivated kidney cells from captive-bred monkeys. Proceedings of the 3rd General Meeting of ESACT, Oxford, 1979. *Dev. Biol. Stand.* 46:151–158.

183. International Association of Biological Standardization. 1980. Proceedings of the International Symposium on Reassessment of Inactivated Poliomyelitis Vaccine, Bilthoven, The Netherlands. *Dev. Biol. Stand.* 1981:47.

184. McBean, A. M., M. L. Thoms, P. Albrecht, J. C. Cuthie, and R. Bernier. 1988. Serologic response to oral polio vaccine and enhanced-potency inactivated polio vaccines. *Am. J. Epidemiol.* 128:615–628.

185. Faden, H., J. F. Modlin, M. L. Thoms, A. McBean, M. B. Ferdon, and P. L. Ogra. 1990. Comparative evaluation of immunization with live attenuated and enhanced-potency inactivated trivalent poliovirus vaccines in childhood: systemic and local immune responses. *J. Infect. Dis.* 162:1291–1297.

186. Modlin, J. F., N. A. Halsey, M. L. Thoms, C. K. Meschievitz, and P. A. Patriarca, for the Baltimore Area Polio Vaccine Study Group. 1997. Humoral and mucosal immunity in infants induced by three sequential inactivated poliovirus vaccine-live attenuated poliovirus vaccine immunization schedules. *J. Infect. Dis.* 175(Suppl 1):S228–S234.

187. Zimmerman, R. K., and S. J. Spann. 1999. Poliovirus vaccine options. *Am. Fam. Physic.* 59:113–118.

188. Salk, D. 1980. Eradication of poliomyelitis in the United States: II Experience with killed poliovirus vaccine. *Rev. Infect. Dis.* 2:243–257.

189. Bottiger, M. 1987. A study of the sero-immunity that has protected the Swedish population against poliomyelitis for 25 years. *Scand. J. Infect. Dis.* 19:595–601.

190. Nathanson, N. 1982. Eradication of poliomyelitis in the United States. *Rev. Infect. Dis.* 4:940–950.

191. Soto, N. E., and L. I. Lutwick. 1999. Poliovirus immunizations: what goes around, comes around. *Infect. Dis. Clin. North Am.* 13:265–278.

192. Centers for Disease Control and Prevention. 1994. Certification of poliomyelitis elimination—the Americas, 1994. *Morbid. Mortal Weekly Rep.* 43:720–722.

193. Strebel, P. M., R. W. Sutter, S. L. Cochi, R. J. Biellik, E. W. Brink, O. M. Kew, M. A. Pallansch, W. A. Orenstein, and A. R. Hinman. 1992. Epidemiology of poliomyelitis in the United States one decade after the last reported case of indigenous wild virus-associated disease. *Clin. Infect. Dis.* 14:568–579.

194. Centers for Disease Control and Prevention. 1997. Poliomyelitis prevention in the United States: introduction of a sequential vaccination schedule of inactivated poliovirus vaccine followed by oral poliovirus vaccine: recommendations of the Advisory Committee of Immunization Practices (ACIP). *Morbid. Mortal Weekly Rep.* 46(No. RR-3):1–25.

195. World Health Organization. 1997. Global eradication of poliomyelitis: report of the second meeting of the Global Technical Consultative Group (TCG), 28 April 1997. www.who.int/gpv-documents/DocsPDF/www9814.pdf (accessed 21 September, 1999).

196. World Health Organization. 1999. Polio eradication: the beginning of the end. www.who.int/gpv-polio (accessed 21 September 1999).

197. Vass, A. 2002. Eradication of polio threatened by $275m [million] funding shortfall. *Br. Med. J.* 324:936.

198. Raufa, A. 2002. Polio cases rise in Nigeria as vaccine is shunned for fear of AIDS. *Br. Med. J.* 324:1414.

199. Kohler, K. A., K. Banerjee, W. G. Hlady, J. K. Andrus, and R. W. Sutter. 2002. Vaccine-associated paralytic poliomyelitis in India during 1999: decreased risk despite massive use of oral polio vaccine. *Bulletin-of-the World Health Org.* 80:210–216.

200. Poliomyelitis prevention in the United States: updated recommendations of the Advisory Committee on Immunization Practices (ACIP). 2002. *Morbid. Mortal Weekly Rep.* 49:1–22.

201. Strickler, H. D., J. J. Goedert, S. S. Devesa, J. Lahey, J. F. Fraumeni, Jr., and P. S. Rosenberg. 2003. Trends in U.S. pleural mesothelioma incidence rates following simian virus 40 contamination of early poliovirus vaccines. *J. Natl. Cancer Inst.* 95:38–45.

202. Arya S. C. 2003. Response to polio elimination through massive immunization programs. *Br. Med. J.* 326:354.

203. Monath, T. P., J. A. Giesberg, and E. G. Fierros. 1998. Does restricted distribution limit access and coverage of yellow fever vaccine in the United States? *Emerg. Infect. Dis.* 4:698–702.

204. Cetron, M. S., A. A. Marfin, K. G. Julian, D. J. Gubler, D. J. Sharp, R. S. Barwick, L. H. Weld, R. Dhen, R. D. Clover, J. Deseda-Tous, V. Marchessault, P. A. Offit, and T. P. Monath. 2002. Yellow fever vaccine: recommendations of the Advisory Committee on Immunization Practices (ACIP), 2002. *Morbid. Mortal Weekly Rep.* 51:1–10.

205. Poland, J. D., C. H. Calisher, T. P. Monath, W. G. Downs, and K. Murphy. 1981. Persistence of neutralizing antibody 30–35 years after immunization with 17D yellow fever vaccine. *Bull. World Health Org.* 56:895–900.

206. Nathan, N., M. Barry, M. Van Herp, and H. Zeller. 2001. Shortage of vaccines during a yellow fever outbreak in Guinea. *Lancet* 358:2129–2130.

207. Mortimer, P. P. 2002. Yellow fever vaccine *Br. Med. J.* 324:439.

208. Centers for Disease Control and Prevention. 1990. Yellow fever vaccine: recommendations of the Immunization Practices Advisory Committee (ACIP). *Morbid. Mortal Weekly Rep.* 39(No. RR-6):1–6.

209. Igarashi, A. 1992. Epidemiology and control of Japanese encephalitis. *World Health Stat Q* 45:299–305.

210. Martin, M., L. H. Weld, T. F. Tsai, G. T. Mootrey, R. T. Chen, M. Niu, and M. S. Centron, for the Geosentinel Yellow Fever Working Group. 2001. Advanced age a risk factor for illness termporarily associated with yellow fever vaccination. *Emerg. Infect. Dis.* 7:945–951.

211. Gajanana, A., V. Thenmozhi, P. Samuel, and R. Reuben. 1995. A community-based study of subclinical flavivirus infections in children in an area of Tamil Nadu, India, where Japanese encephalitis is endemic. *Bull. World Health Org.* 73: 237–244.

212. The Jordan report: accelerated development of vaccines, 1998. Bethesda, Maryland. National Institute of Allergy and Infectious Diseases.

213. Centers for Disease Control and Prevention. 1993. Inactivated Japanese encephalitis virus vaccine: recommendations of the Advisory Committee on Immunization Practices (ACIP). *Morbid. Mortal Weekly Rep.* 42(No. RR-1):1–15.

214. Hsu, T. C., L. P. Chow, H. Y. Wei, et al. 1972. A completed field trial for an evaluation of the effectiveness of mouse-brain Japanese vaccine. In: W. McDHammon, M. Kitaoka, and W. G. Downs (eds.). Immunization for Japanese Encephalitis. Amsterdam: Excerpta Medica, 1972, pp. 285–291.

215. Hoke, C. H., A. Nisalak, N. Sangawhipa, S. Jatanasen, T. Laorakapongse, B. L. Innis, S. Kotchasenee, J. B. Gingrich, J. Latendresse, K. Fukai, et al. 1988. Protection against Japanese encephalitis by inactivated vaccines. *N. Engl. J. Med.* 319: 608–614.

216. Kitaoka, M. 1972. Follow-up on use of vaccine in children in Japan. In: W. McDHammon, M. Kitaoka and W. G. Downs (eds.). Immunization for Japanese Encephalitis. Amsterdam: Excerpta Medica, 1972, pp. 275–277.

217. Plesner, A. M., and T. Ronne. 1977. Allergic mucocutaneous reactions to Japanese encephalitis. *Vaccine* 15:1239–1243.

218. Berg, S. W., B. S. Mitchell, R. K. Hanson, R. P. Olafson, R. P. Williams, J. E. Tueller, R. J. Burton, D. M. Novak, T. F. Tsai, and Wignall F. S. 1997. Systemic reactions in U. S. Marine Corps personnel who received Japanese encephalitis vaccine. *Clin. Infect. Dis.* 24:265–266.

219. Nothdurft, H. D., T. Jelinek, A. Marschang, H. Maiwald, A. Kapaun, and T. Losche. 1996. Adverse reactions to Japanese encephalitis vaccine in travelers. *J. Infect.* 32:119–122.

220. Shirali, G. S., J. Ni, R. E. Chinnock, J. K. Johnston, G. L. Rosenthal, N. E. Bowles, and J. A. Towbin. 2001. Association of viral genome with graft loss in children after cardiac transplantation. *N. Engl. J. Med.* 344:1498–1503.

221. Avery, R. K. 2001. Viral triggers of cardiac-allograft dysfunction. *Br. Med. J.* 344:1545–1547.

222. Centers for Disease Contorl and Prevention. 1998. Civilian outbreak of adenovirus acute respiratory disease—South Dakota, 1997. *Morbid. Mortal Weekly Rep.* 47:567–570.

223. Russell, W. C. 2000. Update on adenovirus and its vector. *J. Gen. Virol* 81:2573–2604.

224. Lee, S. G., and P. P. Hung. 1993. Vaccines for control of respiratory disease caused by adenoviruses. *Med. Virol.* 209:209–216.

225. Gaydos, C. A., and J. C. Gaydos. 1999. Adenovirus vaccines. In: S. A. Plotkin and W. A. Orenstein (eds.). Vaccines, 3rd edition. Philadelphia: WB Saunders Company, 1999 pp. 609–628.

226. Weijer, C. 2000. The future of research into a rotavirus vaccine (editorial). *Br. Med. J.* 321:525–526.

227. Iwamoto, M., T. N. Saari, S. R. McMahon, H. R. Yusuf, M. S. Massoudi, J. M. Stevenson, S. Y. Chu, and L. K. Pickering. 2003. A survey of pediatricians on the reintroduction of rotavirus vaccine. *Pediatrics* 112:e6–e10.

228. Clark, H. F., P. A. Offit, R. W. Ellis, J. J. Eiden, D. Krah, A. R. Shaw, M. Pichichero, J. J. Treanor, F. E. Borian, L. M. Bell, and S. A. Plotkin. 1996. The development of multivalent bovine rotavirus (strain WC3) reassortant vaccine for infants. *J. Infect. Dis.* 174(Suppl 1):S73–S80.

229. Bernstein, D. I., D. A. Sack, E. Rothstein, K. Reisinger, V. E. Smith, D. O'Sullivan, D. R. Spriggs, and D. L. Ward. 1999. Efficacy of live, attenuated, human rotavirus vaccine 89–12 in infants: a randomised, placebo-controlled trial. *Lancet* 354: 287–290.

230. Naik, T. N., and T. Krishnan. 1996. Rotavirus vaccine: current status and future prospect. *Indian J. Med. Res.* 104:76–85.

231. Chen, S. C., D. H. Jones, E. F. Fynan, G. H. Farrar, JCS Clegg, H. B. Greenberb, and J. E. Herrmann. 1998. Protective immunity induced by oral immunization with a rotavirus DNA vaccine encapsulated in microparticles. *J. Virol.* 72:5757–5761.

232. Ciarlet, M., S. E. Crawford, C. Barone, A. Bertolotti-Ciarlet, R. F. Ramig, M. K. Estes, and M. E. Conner. 1998. Subunit rotavirus vaccine administered parenterally to rabbits induces active protective immunity. *J. Virol.* 72:9244–9246.

233. Dennehy, P. H., and J. S. Bresee. 2001. Rotavirus vaccine and intussusceptions: where do we go from here? *Infect. Dis. Clin. North Am.* 15:189–207.

234. Mazzella, M., C. Arioni, C. Bellini, A. E. M. Allegri, and C. Savioli. 2003. Severe hydrocephalus associated with congenital varicella syndrome. *CMAJ* 168:561–563.

235. Levin, J. M. 2001. Use of varicella vaccines to prevent herpes zoster in older individuals. *Arch. Virol. Suppl.* 39:151–160.

236. Hata, A., H. Asanuma, M. Rinki, M. Sharp, R. M. Wong, Blume K., and A. M. Arvin. 2002. Use of an inactivated varicella vaccine in recipients of hematopoietic-cell transplants. *N. Engl. J. Med.* 347:26–34.

237. Miller, A. E. 1980. Selective decline in cellular immune response to varicella-zoster in the elderly. *Neurology* 30:582–587.

238. Burke, B. L., R. W. Steele, and O. W. Beard. 1982. Immune responses to varicella-zoster in the aged. *Arch. Intern. Med.* 142:291–293.

239. Hayward, A., M. Levin, W. Wolf, and G. Angelova. 1991. Varicella-zoster virus-specific immunity after herpes zoster. *J. Infect. Dis.* 163:873–875.

240. Hoey, J. 2003. Varicella vaccine update: need for a booster? *CMAJ* 165:589.

241. Gershon, A. A. 2002. Varicella vaccine: are two doses better than one? [editorial]. *N. Engl. J. Med.* 347:1962–1963.

242. Levin, M. J., M. Murray, G. O. Zerbe, C. J. White, and A. R. Hayward. 1994. Immune responses of elderly persons 4 years after receiving a live attenuated varicella vaccine. *J. Infect. Dis.* 170:522–526.

243. Levin, M. J., D. Barber, E. Goldblatt, M. Jones, B. LaFleur, C. Chan, D. Stinson, G. O. Zerbe, and A. R. Hayward. 1998. Use of a live attenuated varicella vaccine to boost varicella-specific immune responses in seropositive people 55 years of age and older: duration of booster effect. *J. Infect. Dis.* 178(Suppl 1): S109–S112.

244. Sandstöm, E., and B. Wahren, for the Nordic VAC-04 Study Group. 1999. Therapeutic immunisation with recombinant gp160 in HIV-1 infection: a randomised double-blind placebo-controlled trial. *Lancet* 353:1735–1742.

245. Birx, D. L., C. Davis, N. Ruiz, et al. 1996. Results of a phase II double-blind multicenter, placebo controlled HIV therapeutic vaccine trial. XI International Conference on AIDS, Vancouver, July 1996, Abstract TuA 175.

246. Tsoukas, C. M., J. Raboud, N. F. Bernard, J. S. Montaner, M. J. Gill, A. Rachlis, I. W. Fong, W. Schlech, O. Djurdjev, J. Freedman, R. Thomas, R. Lafreniere, M. A. Wainberg, S. Cassol, M. O'Shaughnessy, J. Todd, F. Volvovitz, and G. E. Smith. 1998. Immunization of patients with HIV infection: a study of the effect of VaxSyn, a recombinant HIV envelope subunit vaccine, on progression of immune deficiency. *AIDS Res. Hum. Retroviruses* 14:483–490.

247. Evans, T. G., M. C. Keefer, K. J. Weinhold, M. Wolff, D. Montefiori, G. J. Gorse, B. S. Graham, M. J. McElrath, M. J. Clements-Mann M. L., M. J. Mulligan, P. Fast, M. C. Walker, J. L. Excler, A. M. Duliege, and J. Tartaglia. 1999. A canarypox vaccine expressing multiple human immunodeficiency virus type 1 genes given alone or with Rgp120 elicits broad and durable CD8+ cytotoxic T lymphocyte responses in seronegative volunteers. *J. Infect. Dis.* 180:290–298.

248. Graham, B. S., T. J. Matthews, R. B. Belshe, M. L. Clements, R. Dolin, P. F. Wright, G. J. Gorse, D. H. Schwartz, M. C. Keefer, and D. P. Bolognesi, for the NIAID AIDS Vaccine Clinical Trials Network. 1993. Augmentation of human immunodeficiency virus type 1 neutralizing antibody by priming with gp160 recombinant vaccinia and boosting with rgp160 in vaccinia-naïve adults. *J. Infect. Dis.* 167:533–537.

249. Frey, S. E. 1999. HIV vaccines. *Infect. Dis. Clin. North Am.* 13:95–112.

250. Oxford, J. S., M. Addawe, and R. Lambkin. 1998. AIDS vaccine development: let a thousand flowers bloom. *J. Clin. Pathol.* 51:725–730.

251. Clements-Mann, M. L., K. Weinhold, T. J. Matthews, B. S. Graham, G. J. Gorse, M. C. Keefer, M. J. McElrath, R. H. Hsieh, J. Mestecky, S. Zolla-Pazner, J. Mascola, D. Schwartz, R. Siliciano, L. Corey, P. F. Wright, R. Belshe, R. Dolin, S. Jackson, S. Xu, P. Fast, M. C. Walker, D. Stablein, J. L. Excler, J. Tartaglia, and E. Paoletti, for the NIAID AIDS Vaccine Evaluation Group. 1998. Immune responses to human immunodeficiency virus (HIV) type 1 induced by canarypox expressing HIV-1MN gp120, HIV-1SF2 recombinant gp120, or both vaccines in seronegative adults. *J. Infect. Dis.* 177:1230–1246.

252. Belshe, R. B., C. Stevens, G. Gorse, et al. 1999. Phase II evaluation of a live recombinant canarypox (ALVAC) vector HIV-1 vaccine with or without gp120 subunit HIV-1 vaccine. 13th Meeting of the International Society for Sexually Transmitted Diseases Research, Denver, Colorado, 11–14 July 1999, Abstract 227.

253. Ferrari, G., W. Humphrey, M. J. McElrath, A. M. Duliege, M. L. Clements, L. C. Corey, D. P. Bolognesi, and K. J. Weinhold. 1997. Clad B-based HIV-1 vaccines elicit cross-clade cytotoxic T lymphocyte reactivities in uninfected volunteers. *Proc. Natl. Acad. Sci. USA* 94:1396–1401.

254. Evans, T., L. Corey, M. L. Clements-Mann, et al. 1998. CD8+CTL induced in AIDS Vaccine Evaluation Group Phase I trials using canarypox vectors (ALVAC) encoding multiple HIV gene products (vCP125, vCP205, vCP300) given with or without subunit boost. [slide presentation]. 12th World AIDS Conference, Geneva, Switzerland, June 28–July 3, 1998.

255. Doepel, L. K. 1999. NIAID opens first AIDS vaccine trial in Africa. National Institute of Allergy and Infectious Diseases. NIAID News, 8 February 1999. www.niaid.nih.gov/newsroom/uganda.html (accessed 18 September 1999).

256. Boyer, J. D., K. E. Ugen, B. Wang, M. Agadjanyan, L. Gilbert, M. L. Bagarazzi, et al. 1997. Protection of chimpanzees from high-dose heterologous HIV-1 challenge by DNA vaccination. *Nature Med.* 3:526–532.

257. Frank, S. B. 1938. Formulized herpes virus therapy and neutralizing substance in herpes simplex. *J. Invest. Dermatol.* 1:267–282.

258. Deatly, A. M. 2001. Vaccines to protect against HSV diseases [commentary]. *Neurobiol. Aging* 22:715–716.

259. Straus, S. E., A. Wald, R. G. Kost, R. McKenzie, A. G. Langenberg, P. Hohman, J. Lekstrom, E. Cox, M. Nakamura, R. Sekulovich, A. Izu, C. Dekker, and L. Corey. 1997. Immunotherapy of recurrent genital herpes with recombinant herpes simplex virus type 2 glycoproteins D and B: results of a placebo-controlled vaccine trial. *J. Infect. Dis.* 176:1129–1134.

260. Corey, L., A. G. Langenberg, R. Ashley, R. E. Sekulovich, A. E. Izu, J. M. Douglas Jr., H. H. Handsfield, T. Warren, L. Marr, S. Tyring, R. DiCarlo, A. A. Adimora, P. Leone, C. L. Dekker, R. L. Burke, W. P. Leong, and S. E. Straus, for the Chiron HSV Vaccine Study Group. 1999. Recombinant glycoprotein vaccine for the prevention of genital HSV-2 infection: two randomized controlled trials. *J. Am. Med. Assoc.* 282:331–340.

261. Stanberry, L. R., S. L. Spruance, L. Cunningham, D. I. Bernstein, A. Mindel, S. Sacks, S. K. Tyring, F. Y. Aoki, M. Slaoui, M. Denis, P. Vandepapeliere, and G. Dubin. 2002. Glycoprotein D adjuvant vaccine to prevent genital herpes. *N. Engl. J. Med.* 347: 1652–1661.

262. Lin, W-R., R. Jennings, T. L. Smith, M. A. Wozniak, and R. F. Itzhaki. 2001. Vaccination prevents latent HSV1 infection of mouse brain [commentary]. *Neurobiol.* 22:699–703.

263. Boursnell, M. E., C. Entwisle, D. Blakely, C. Roberts, I. A. Duncan, S. E. Chisholm, G. M. Martin, R. Jennings, D. Ni Challanain, I. Sobek, S. C. Inglis, and C. S. McLean. 1997. A genetically inactivated herpes simplex virus type 2 (HSV-2) vaccine provides effective protection against primary and recurrent HSV-2 disease. *J. Infect. Dis.* 175:16–25.

264. McLean, C. S., D. Ni Challanin, I. Duncan, M. E. Boursnell, R. Jennings, and S. C. Inglis. 1996. Induction of a protective immune response by mucosal vaccination with a DISC HSV-1 vaccine. *Vaccine* 14:987–992.

265. McClements, W. L., M. E. Armstrong, R. D. Keys, and M. A. Liu. 1996. Immunization with DNA vaccines encoding glycoprotein

D or glycoprotein B, alone or in combination, induces protective immunity in animal models of herpes simplex virus-2 disease. *Proc. Natl. Acad. Sci. USA* 93:11414–11420.

266. Rouse, B. T., S. Nair, R. J. Rouse, Z. Yu, N. Kuklin, K. Karem, and E. Manickan. 1998. DNA vaccines and immunity to herpes simplex virus. *Curr. Top. Microbiol. Immunol.* 226:69–78.

267. Meignier, B., R. Longnecker, and R. Roizman. 1988. In vivo behavior of genetically engineered herpes simplex viruses R7017 and R 7020: construction and evaluation in rodents. *J. Infect. Dis.* 58:602–614.

268. Cadoz, M., M. Micoud, and J. M. Seigneurin. 1992. Phase I trial of R7020: a live-attenuated recombinant herpes simplex virus (HSV) candidate vaccine. 32nd Interscience Conference on Antimicrobial Agents and Chemotherapy, Anaheim, CA, 1992.

269. The Jordan report: accelerated development of vaccines, 1994. Bethesda, Maryland. National Institute of Allergy and Infectious Diseases.

270. Reichman, R., J. Balsley, D. Carlin, et al. 1999. Evaluation of the safety and immunogenicity of a recombinant HPV-11 L1 virus like particle vaccine in healthy adult volunteers. Proceedings of the 17th International Papillomavirus Conference, Charleston, SC, 9–15 January 1999.

271. Zhang, L. F., J. Zhou, C. Shao, et al. 1999. A phase 1 trial of HPV 6 B virus like particles as immunotherapy for genital warts. Proceedings of the 17th International Papillomavirus Conference, Charleston, SC, 9–15 January 1999.

272. Da Silva, D. M., J. D. Nieland, H. L. Greenstone, J. T. Schiller, and W. M. Kast. 1999. Chimeric papillomavirus virus-like particles induce antigen-specific therapeutic immunity against tumours expressing the HPV-16 E7 protein. Proceedings of the 17th International Papillomavirus Conference, Charleston, SC, 9–15 January 1999.

273. Borysiewicz, L. K., A. Fiander, M. Nimako, S. Man, G. W. Wilkinson, D. Westmoreland, A. S. Evans, M. Adams, S. N. Stacey, M. E. Boursnell, E. Rutherford, J. K. Hickling, and S. C. Inglis. 1996. A recombinant vaccinia virus encoding human papillomavirus types 16 and 18, E6 and E7 proteins as immunotherapy for cervical cancer. *Lancet* 347:1523–1527.

274. Lacey, C. J., E. F. Monteiro, H. S. Thompson, et al. 1997. A phase IIa study of a therapeutic vaccine for genital warts. Medical Society for the Study of Venereal Disease Spring Meeting, Oxford, UK, July 1997.

275. Duggan-Keen, M. F., M. D. Brown, S. N. Stacey, and P. L. Stern. 1998. Papillomavirus vaccines. *Front. Biosci.* 3:1192–208.

276. Nardelli-Haefliger, D., R. B. Roden, J. Benyacoub, R. Sahli, J. P. Kraehenbuhl, J. T. Schiller, P. Lachat, A. Potts, and P. De Grandi. 1997. Human papillomavirus type 16 virus-like particles expressed in attenuated Salmonella typhimurium elicit mucosal and systemic neutralizing antibodies in mice. *Infect. Immun.* 65:3328–3336.

277. Jensen, E. R., R. Selvakumar, H. Shen, R. Ahmed, F. O. Wettstein, and J. F. Miller. 1997. Recombinant Listeria monocytogenes vaccination eliminates papillomavirus-induced tumors and prevents papilloma formation from viral DNA. *J. Virol.* 71:8467–8474.

278. Krul, M., E. Tijhaar, J. Kleijne, A. Van Loon, M. Nievers, and H. Schipper. 1996. Induction of an antibody response in mice against human papillomavirus (HPV) type 16 after immunization with HPV recombinant Salmonella strains. *Cancer Immunol. Immunother.* 43:44–48.

279. Ossevoort, M. A., M. C. Feltkemp, K. J. VanVeen, C. J. Melief, and W. M. Kast. 1995. Dendritic cells as carriers for a cytotoxic T-lymphocyte epitope-based peptide vaccine in protection against a human papillomavirus type 16-induced tumor. *J. Immunother.* 18:86–94.

280. Koutsky, L. A., K. A. Ault, C. M. Wheeler, D. R. Brown, E. Barr, F. B. Alvarez, L. M. Chiacchierini, and K. U. Jansen, for Proof of Principle Study Investigators. 2002. A controlled trial of a human papillomavirus type 16 vaccine. *N. Engl. J. Med.* 347:1645–1651.

281. Fowler, K. B., S. Stagno, R. F. Pass, W. J. Britt, T. J. Boll, and C. A. Alford. 1992. The outcome of congenital cytomegalovirus infection in relation to maternal antibody status. *N. Engl. J. Med.* 326:663–673.

282. Zaia, J. A., J. G. Sissons, S. Riddell, D. J. Diamond, M. R. Wills, A. J. Carmichael, M. P. Weekes, M. Gandhi, C. La Rosa,

M. Villacres, S. Lacey, S. Markel, and J. Sun. 2000. Status of cytomegalovirus prevention and treatment in 2000. *Hematology (Am. Soc. Hematol. Educ. Program)* 2000:339–355.

283. Plotkin, S. A., S. E. Starr, H. M. Friedman, K. Brayman, S. Harris, S. Jackson, N. B. Tustin, R. Grossman, D. Dafoe, and C. Barker. 1991. Effect of Towne live virus vaccine on cytomegalovirus disease after renal transplant: a controlled trial. *Ann. Intern. Med.* 114:525–531.

284. Plotkin, S. A., R. Higgins, and J. B. Kurtz. 1994. Multicenter trial of Towne strain attenuated virus vaccine in seronegative renal transplant recipients. *Transplantation* 58:1176–1178.

285. Adler, S. P., S. E. Starr, S. A. Plotkin, S. H. Hempfling, J. Buis, M. L. Manning, and A. M. Best. 1995. Immunity induced by a primary cytomegalovirus infection protects against secondary infection among women of childbearing age. *J. Infect. Dis.* 171:26–32.

286. Adler, S. P., S. H. Hempfling, S. E. Starr, S. Plotkin, and S. Riddell. 1998. Evaluation of the safety and immunogenicity of the Towne strain of cytomegalovirus among women of childbearing age and children. *Pediatr. Infect. Dis.* 17:200–206.

287. Cha, T. A., E. Tom, G. W. Kemble, G. M. Duke, E. S. Mocarski, and R. R. Spaete. 1996. Human cytomegalovirus clinical isolates carry at least 19 genes not found in laboratory strains. *J. Virol.* 70:78–83.

288. Diamond, D. J., J. York, J. Y. Sun, C. L. Wright, and S. J. Forman. 1997. Development of a candidate HLA A 0201 restricted peptide-based vaccine against human cytomegalovirus infection. *Blood* 90:1751–1767.

289. Mitchell, D., S. J. Holmes, R. L. Burke, et al. 1997. Immunogenicity of a recombinant human cytomegalovirus (CMV) gB vaccine in toddlers [abstract]. Sixth International Cytomegalovirus Workshop, Perdido Beach, AL, 5–9 March 1997.

290. Pass, R., A. M. Duliége, R. Sekulovich, et al. 1997. Antibody response to a fourth dose of CMV gB vaccine in healthy adults [abstract]. Sixth International Cytomegalovirus Workshop, Perdido Beach, AL, 5–9 March 1997, Abstract 159.

291. Plotkin, S. A. 1999. Vaccination against cytomegalovirus, the changeling demon. *Pediatr. Infect. Dis. J.* 18:313–326.

292. Adler, S. P., S. A. Plotkin, E. Gonczol, M. Cadoz, C. Meric, J. B. Wang, P. Dellamonica, A. M. Best, J. Zahradnik, S. Pincus, K. Berencsi, W. I. Cox, and Z. Gyulai. 1999. A canarypox vector expressing cytomegalovirus (CMV) glycoprotein B primes for antibody responses to a live attenuated CMV vaccine (Towne). *J. Infect. Dis.* 180:843–846.

293. Endresz, V., L. Kari, K. Berencsi, C. Kari, Z. Gyulai, C. Jeney, et al. 1999. Induction of human cytomegalovirus (HCMV)-glycoprotein B (gB)-specific neutralizing antibody and phosphorprotein 65 (pp65)-specific cytotoxic T lymphocyte responses by naked DNA immunization. *Vaccine* 17:50–58.

294. Boldogh, I., J. A. Patel, and T. Chonmaitree. 2002. Cytomegalovirus. In: S Tyring (ed.). Mucocutaneous Manifestations of Viral Diseases. New York: Marcel Dekker; 2002, pp. 173–195.

295. Dudas, R. A., and R. A. Karron. 1998. Respiratory syncytial virus vaccines. *Clin. Microb. Rev.* 11:430–439.

296. Fouillard, L., L. Mouthon, J. P. Laporte, F. Isnard, J. Stachowiak, M. Aoudjhane, J. D. Lucet, M. Wolf, F. Bricourt, L. Douay, M. Lopez, C. Marche, A. Najman, and N. C. Gorin. 1992. Severe respiratory syncytial virus pneumonia after autologous bone marrow transplantation: a report of three cases and review. *Bone Marrow Transplant.* 9:97–100.

297. Dowell, S. F., L. J. Anderson, H. E. Gary, D. D. Erdman, J. F. Plouffe, T. M. File, B. J. Marston, and R. F. Breiman. 1996. Respiratory syncytial virus is an important cause of community-acquired lower respiratory infection amoung hospitalized adults. *J. Infect. Dis.* 174:456–462.

298. Falsey, A. R., C. K. Cunningham, W. H. Barker, R. W. Kouides, J. B. Yuen, M. Menegus, L. B. Weiner, C. A. Bonville, and R. F. Betts. 1995. Respiratory syncytial virus and influenza A infections in the hospitalized elderly. *J. Infect. Dis.* 172:389–394.

299. Falsey, A. R., J. J. Treanor, R. F. Betts, and E. E. Walsh. 1998. Relationship of serum antibody to risk of respiratory syncytial virus infection in elderly adults. *J. Infect. Dis.* 177:463–466.

300. Falsey, A. R., and E. E. Walsh. 1998. Reslationship of serum antibody to risk of respiratory syncytial virus infection in elderly adults. *J. Infect. Dis.* 177:463–466.

301. Mlinaric-Galinovic, G., A. R. Falsey, and E. E. Walsh. 1996. Respiratory syncytial virus infection in the elderly. *Eur. J. Clin. Microbial Infect. Dis.* 15:777–781.

302. Cunningham, C. K., J. A. McMillan, and S. J. Gross. 1991. Rehospitalizaiton for respiratory illness in infants of less than 32 weeks' gestation. *Pediatrics* 88:527–532.

303. Baker, K. A., and M. E. Ryan. 1999. RSV infection in infants and young children. *Postgrad. Med.* 106:97–111.

304. Kapikian, A. Z., R. H. Mitchell, R. M. Chanock, R. A. Shvedoff, and C. E. Stewart. 1969. An epidemiologic study of altered clinical reactivity to respiratory syncytial (RS) virus infection in children previously vaccinated with an inactivated R. S. virus vaccine. *Am. J. Epidemiol.* 89:405–421.

305. Kim, H. W., J. G. Canchola, C. D. Brandt, G. Pyles, R. M. Chanock, K. Jensen, and R. H. Parrott. 1969. Respiratory syncytial virus disease in infants despite prior administration of antigenic inactivated vaccine. *Am. J. Epidemiol.* 89:422–434.

306. Neuzil, K. M., J. E. Johnson, Y. Tang, J. Prieel, M. Slaoui, N. Gar, and B. S. Graham. 1997. Adjuvants influence the quantitative and qualitative immune response in BALB/c mice immunized with respiratory syncytial virus F. G. subunity vaccine. *Vaccine* 15:525–532.

307. Tang, Y. W., and G. S. Graham. 1995. Interleukin-12 treatment during immunization elicits a T helper cell type 1-like immune response in mice challenged with respiratory syncytial virus and improves vaccine immunogenicity. *J. Infect. Dis.* 172:734–738.

308. Karron, R. A., P. F. Wright, J. E. Crowe, Jr., M. L. Clements-Mann, J. Thompson, M. Makhene, R. Casey, and B. R. Murphy. 1997. Evaluation of two live, cold-passaged, temperature-sensitive respiratory syncytial virus vaccines in chimpanzees and in human adults, infants, and children. *J. Infect. Dis.* 176:1428–1436.

309. Polack, F. P., and R. A. Karron. 2004. The future of respiratory syncytial virus vaccine development. *Pediatr. Infect. Dis. J.* 23(Suppl 1):S65–S73.

310. Collins, P. L., M. G. Hill, E. Camargo, H. Grosfeld, R. M. Chanock, and B. R. Murphy. 1995. Production of infectious human respiratory syncytial virus from cloned cDNA confirms an essential

role for the transcription elongation factor form the 5' proximal open reading frame of the M2 mRNA in gene expression and provides a capability for vaccine development. *Proc. Natl. Am. Soc. USA* 92:11563–11567.

311. Paradiso, P. R., S. W. Hildreth, D. A. Hogerman, D. J. Speelman, E. B. Lewin, J. Oren, and D. H. Smith. 1994. Safety and immunogenicity of a subunit respiratory syncytial virus vaccine in children 24 to 48 months old. *Pediatr. Infect. Dis. J.* 13: 792–798.

312. Falsey, A. R., and E. E. Walsh. 1997. Safety and immunogenicity of a respiratory syncytial virus subunit vaccine (PFP-2) in the institutionalized elderly. *Vaccine* 15:1130–1132.

313. Tristram, D. A., R. C. Welliver, C. K. Mohar, D. A. Hogerman, S. W. Hildreth, and P. Paradiso. 1993. Immunogenicity and safety of respiratory syncytial virus subunit vaccine in seropositive children 18–36 months old. *J. Infect. Dis.* 167: 191–195.

314. Belshe, R. B., E. L. Anderson, and E. E. Walsh. 1993. Immunogenicity of purified F glycoprotein of respiratory syncytial virus: clinical and immune responses to subsequent natural infection in children. *J. Infect. Dis.* 168:1024–1029.

315. Groothuis, J. R., S. J. King, D. A. Hogerman, P. R. Paradiso, and E. A. Simoes. 1998. Safety and immunogenicity of a purified F protein respiratory syncytial virus (PFP-2) vaccine in seropositive children with bronchopulmonary dysplasia. *J. Infect. Dis.* 177:467–469.

316. Piedra, P. A., S. Grace, A. Jewell, S. Spinelli, D. Bunting, D. A. Hogerman, F. Malinoski, and P. W. Hiatt. 1996. Purified fusion protein vaccine protects against lower respiratory tract illness during respiratory syncytial virus season in children with cystic fibrosis. *Pediatr. Infect. Dis. J.* 15:23–31.

317. Piedra, P. A., S. Grace, A. Jewell, S. Spinelli, D. A. Hogerman, F. Malinoski, and P. W. Hiatt. 1998. Sequential annual administration of purified fusion protein vaccine against respiratory syncytial virus in children with cystic fibrosis. *Pediatr. Infect. Dis. J.* 17:217–224.

318. Simoes, E. A., D. H. Tan, A. Ohlsson, V. Sales, and E. E. Wang. 2001. Respiratory syncytial virus vaccine: a systemic overview

with emphasis of respiratory syncytial virus subunit vaccines. *Vaccine* 20:954–960.

319. Karron, R. A., P. F. Wright, F. K. Newman, M. Makhene, J. Thompson, R. Samorodin, M. H. Wilson, E. L. Anderson, M. L. Clements, B. R. Murphy, et al. 1995. A live human parainfluenza type 3 virus vaccine is attenuated and immunogenic in healthy infants and children. *J. Infect. Dis.* 172:1445–1450.

320. Karron, R. A., M. Makhene, K. Gay, M. H. Wilson, M. L. Clements, and B. R. Murphy. 1996. Evaluation of a live attenuated bovine parainfluenza type 3 vaccine in two- to six-month-old infants. *Pediatr. Infect. Dis.* 15:650–654.

321. Karron, R. A., P. F. Wright, S. L. Hall, M. Makhene, J. Thompson, B. A. Burns, S. Tollefson, M. C. Steinhoff, M. H. Wilson, D. O. Harris, et al. 1995. A live attenuated bovine parainfluenza type 3 virus vaccine is safe, infectious, immunogenic and phenotypically stable in infants and children. *J. Infect. Dis.* 171:1107–1114.

322. Ewasyshyn, M., G. Cates, G. Jackson, N. Scollard, A. Symington, and M. Klein. 1997. Prospects for a parainfluenza virus vaccine. *Pediatr. Pulmonol. Suppl.* 16:280–1.

323. Murphy, B. R., and P. L. Collins. 1997. Current status of respiratory syncytial virus (RSV) and parainfluenza virus type 3 (PIV3) vaccine development: memorandum from a joint WHO/NIAID meeting. *Bull. World Health Org.* 75:307–313.

324. Durbin, A. P., L. S. Wyatt, J. Siew, B. Moss, and B. R. Murphy. 1998. The immunogenicity and efficacy of intranasally or parenterally administered replication-deficient vaccinia-parainfluenza virus type 3 recombinants in rhesus monkeys. *Vaccine* 16:1324–1330.

325. Nichols, W. G., L. Corey, T. Gooley, C. Davis, and M. Boeckh. 2001. Parainfluenza virus infections after hematopoietic stem cell transplantation: risk factors, response to antiviral therapy, and effect on transplant outcome. *Blood* 98:573–578.

326. Ellis, R. W. 2004. Technologies for making new vaccines. In: S. A. Plotkins and W. A. Orenstein (eds.). Vaccines 4th edition, Philadelphia: Elsevier, 2004, pp. 1177–1198.

327. Weltzin, R., and T. P. Monath. 1999. Intranasal antibody prophylaxis for protection against viral disease. *Clin. Microbiol. Rev.* 12:383–393.

328. Dickler, H. B., and E. W. Gelfand. 1996. Current perspectives on the use of intravenous immunoglobulin. *Adv. Intern. Med.* 41: 641–680.

329. Centers for Disease Control and Prevention. 1999. Renal insufficiency and failure associated with immune globulin intravenous therapy—United States, 1985–1998. *Morbid. Mortal Weekly Rep.* 48:518–521.

330. Bean, B. 1992. Antiviral therapy: current concepts and practices. *Clin. Microbiol. Rev.* 5:146–182.

331. Berkman, S. A., M. L. Lee, and R. P. Gale. 1990. Clinical uses of intravenous immunoglobulins. *Ann. Intern. Med.* 112:278–292.

332. Bass, E. B., N. R. Power, S. N. Goodman, R. I. Griffiths, T. S. Kickler, and J. R. Wingard. 1993. Efficacy of immune globulin in preventing complications of bone marrow transplantation: a meta-analysis. *Bone Marrow Transplant.* 12:273–282.

333. Blacklock, H. A., P. Griffiths, P. Stirk, and H. G. Prentice. 1985. Specific hyperimmune globulin for cytomegalovirus pneumonitis [letter]. *Lancet* 2:152–153.

334. Emanuel, D., I. Cunningham, K. Jules-Elysee, J. A. Brochstein, N. A. Kernan, J. Laver, D. Stover, D. A. White, A. Fels, B. Polsky, et al. 1988. Cytomegalovirus pneumonia after bone marrow transplantation successfully treated with the combination of ganciclovir and high-dose intravenous immune globulin. *Ann. Intern. Med.* 109:777–782.

335. Reed, E. C., R. A. Bowden, P. S. Dandliker, K. E. Lilleby, and J. D. Meyers. 1988. Treatment of cytomegalovirus pneumonia with ganciclovir and intravenous cytomegalovirus immunoglobulin in patients with bone marrow transplants. *Ann. Intern. Med.* 109:783–788.

336. Nicholls, A. J., C. B. Brown, N. Edward, B. Cuthbertson, P. L. Yap, and D. B. McClelland. 1983. Hyperimmune immunoglobulin for cytomegalovirus infections. *Lancet* 1:532–533.

337. Reed, E. C., R. A. Bowden, P. S. Dandliker, and J. D. Meyers. 1986. Efficacy of cytomegalovirus immune globulin in marrow transplant patients with cytomegalovirus pneumonia [abstract]. In: Program and Abstracts of the Twenty-Sixth Interscience Conference on Antimicrobial Agents and Chemotherapy, Washington DC, 1986, Abstract 731.

338. Graneto, D., C. Swift, D. R. Steinmuller, et al. 1988. Use of intravenous immunoglobulin (Ig) prophylaxis for primary cytomegalovirus (CMV) infection post living-related donor (LRD) renal transplantation [abstract]. Abstracts of the American Society of Transplant Physicians Annual Meeting, Chicago, 1988, Abstract 10.

339. Light, J. A., N. Khawand, W. Brems, A. Aquino, and A. Ali. 1988. Does IVIG prevent primary CMV disease in kidney transplant recipients? [abstract]. Abstracts of the American Society of Transplant Physicians Annual Meeting, Chicago, 1988, Abstract 11.

340. Bernstein, L. J., B. Z. Krieger, B. Novick, M. J. Sicklick, and A. Rubinstein. 1985. Bacterial infections in the acquired immunodeficiency syndrome of children. *Pediatr. Infect. Dis.* 4:472–475.

341. Calvelli, T. A., and A. Rubinstein. 1986. Intravenous gammaglobulin in infant acquired immunodeficiency syndrome. *Pediatr. Infect. Dis.* 5:S207–S210.

342. Gupta, A., B. E. Novick, and A. Rubinstein. 1986. Restoration of suppressor T-cell functions in children with AIDS following intravenous gamma globulin treatment. *Am. J. Dis. Child.* 140:143–146.

343. Oleski, J. M., E. M. Connor, R. Bohila, et al. 1987. Treatment of immunodeficiency virus antibody positive children with intravenous immunoglobulin. *Vox Sang* 52:162–175.

344. Spector, A., R. D. Gelber, N. McGrath, D. Wara, A. Barzilai, E. Abrams, Y. J. Bryson, W. M. Dankner, R. A. Livingston, and E. M. Connor. 1994. Controlled trial of intravenous immune globulin for the prevention of serious bacterial infections in children receiving zidovudine for advanced human immunodeficiency virus infection. *N. Engl. J. Med.* 331:1181–1187.

345. Hadler, S. C., J. J. Erben, D. Matthews, K. Starko, D. P. Francis, and J. E. Maynard. 1983. Effect of immunoglobulin on hepatitis A in day-care centers. *J. Am. Med. Assoc.* 249:48–53.

346. Krugman, S., R. Ward, J. P. Giles, and A. M. Jacobs. 1960. Infectious hepatitis: studies on the effect of gamma globulin and on the incidence of inapparent infection. *J. Am. Med. Assoc.* 174:883–890.

347. Woodson, R. D., and J. J. Clinton. 1976. Hepatitis prophylaxis abroad. *J. Am. Med. Assoc.* 209:1053–1059.

348. Lauchart, W., R. Muller, and R. Pichlmayr. 1987. Immunoprophylaxis of hepatitis B viral reinfection in recipients of human liver allografts. *Transplant. Proc.* 19:2387–2389.

349. Samuel, D., A. Bismuth, D. Mathieu, J. L. Arulnaden, M. Reynes, J. P. Benhamou, C. Brechot, and H. Bismuth. 1991. Passive immunoprophylaxis after liver transplantation in HBsAg-positive patients. *Lancet* 337:813–815.

350. Grellier, L., and G. M. Dusheiko. 1997. Hepatitis B virus and liver transplantation: concepts in antiviral prophylaxis. *J. Viral. Hepat.* 4(Suppl 1):111–116.

351. Centers for Disease Control and Prevention. 1996. Prevention of varicella: recommendations of the Advisory Committee on Immunization Practices (ACIP). *Morbid. Mortal Weekly Rep.* 45(No. RR-11):1–36.

352. Groothuis, J. R., E. A. Simoes, M. J. Levin, C. B. Hall, C. E. Long, W. J. Rodriguez, J. Arrobio, H. C. Meissner, D. R. Fulton, R. C. Welliver, et al., for the Respiratory Syncytial Virus Immune Globulin Study Group. 1993. Prophylactic administration of respiratory syncytial virus immune globulin to high-risk infants and young children. *N. Engl. J. Med.* 329:1524–1530.

353. For the PREVENT Study Group. 1997. Reduction of respiratory syncytial virus hospitalization among premature infants and infants with bronchopulmonary dysplasia using respiratory syncytial virus immune globulin prophylaxis. *Pediatrics* 99:93–99.

354. Burks, A. W., H. A. Sampson, and R. H. Buckley. 1986. Anaphylactic reactions after gamma globulin administration in patients with hypogammaglobulinemia: detection of IgE antibodies to IgA. *N. Engl. J. Med.* 314:560–563.

355. IGIV transmission of hepatitis C. 1994. *FDA. Med. Bull.* 24:3–4.

356. Hengster, P., M. D. Pescovitz, D. Hyatt, and R. Margreiter, for the Roche Study Group. 1999. Cytomegalovirus infections after treatment with daclizumab, an anti IL-2 receptor antibody, for prevention of renal allograft rejection. *Transplantation* 68:310–313.

357. Johnson, S., C. Oliver, G. A. Prince, V. G. Hemming, D. S. Pfarr, S. C. Wang, M. Dormitzer, J. O'Grady, S. Koenig, J. K. Tamura, R. Woods, G. Bansal, D. Couchenour, E. Tsao, W. C. Hall, and J. F. Young. 1997. Development of humanized monoclonal

antibody (MEDI-493) with potent in vitro and in vivo activity against respiratory syncytial virus. *J. Infect. Dis.* 176:1215–1224.

358. For the IMpact-RSV Study Group. 1998. Palivizumab, a humanized respiratory syncytial virus monoclonal antibody, reduces hospitalization from respiratory syncytial virus infection in high-risk infants. *Pediatrics* 102:531–537.

359. Subramanian, S. K., L. E. Weisman, T. Rhodes, R. Ariagno, P. J. Sanchez, J. Steichen, L. B. Givner, T. L. Jennings, F. H. Top, Jr., D. Carlin, and E. Connor. 1998. Safety, tolerance and pharmacokinetics of a humanized monoclonal antibody to respiratory syncytial virus in premature infants and infants with bronchopulmonary dysplasia. *Pediatr. Infect. Dis. J.* 17:110–115.

360. Prevention of respiratory syncytial virus infections: indications for the use of palivizumab and update on the use of RSV-IGIV. 1998. American Academy of Pediatrics Committee on Infectious Diseases and Committee of Fetus and Newborn. *Pediatrics* 102:1211–1216.

361. Lieu, T. A., S. L. Cochi, S. B. Black, M. E. Halloran, H. R. Shinefield, S. J. Holmes, M. Wharton, and A. E. Washington. 1994. Cost-effectiveness of a routine varicella vaccination program for US children. *J. Am. Med. Assoc.* 271:375–381.

362. Murphy, T. V., P. M. Gargiullo, M. S. Massoudi, D. B. Nelson, A. O. Jumaan, C. A. Okoro, L. R. Zanardi, S. Setia, E. Fair, C. W. LeBaron, M. Wharton, J. R. Livengood, and J. R. Livingood, for the Rotavirus Intussusception Investigation Team. 2001. Intussusception among infants given an oral rotavirus vaccine. *N. Engl. J. Med.* 344:564–572.

363. Dales, L., S. J. Hammer, and N. J. Smith. 2001. Time trends in autism and in MMR immunization coverage in California. *J. Am. Med. Assoc.* 285:1183–1185.

364. Kaye, J. A., M. del Mar Melero-Montes, and H. Jick. 2001. Mumps, measles, and rubella vaccine and the incidence of autism recorded by general practitioners: a time trend analysis. *Br. Med. J.* 322(7284):460–463.

365. Ascherio, A., S. M. Zhang, M. A. Hernan, M. J. Olek, P. M. Coplan, K. Brodovicz, and A. M. Walker. 2001. Hepatitis B vaccination and the risk of multiple sclerosis. *N. Engl. J. Med.* 344:372–373.

366. Confavreux, C., S. Suissa, P. Saddier, V. Bourdes, and S. Vukusic, for the Vaccines in Multiple Sclerosis Study Group. 2001. Vaccinations and the risk of relapse in multiple sclerosis. *N. Engl. J. Med.* 344:372–373.

367. Tacket, C. O., H. S. Mason, G. Losonsky, J. D. Clements, M. M. Levine, and C. J. Arntzen. 1998. Immunogenicity in humans of a recombinant bacterial antigen delivered in a transgenic potato. *Nat. Med.* 4:607–609.

368. Arakawa, T., and W. H. Langridge. 1998. Plants are not just passive creatures! *Nat. Med.* 4:550–551.

Index